Dr Chris Irons is a clinical psychologist, resear
co-director of Balanced Minds (www.balanced.
organisation providing compassion-focused psychological interventions
for individuals and organisations. He is the author of a number of books,
including *The Compassionate Mind Workbook*.

THE COMPASSIONATE MIND
APPROACH TO

Difficult Emotions

using **compassion focused therapy**

CHRIS IRONS

ROBINSON

ROBINSON

Published in Great Britain in 2019 by Robinson

1 3 5 7 9 10 8 6 4 2

A CIP catalogue record for this book
is available from the British Library.

ISBN: 978-1-84901-621-6

Typeset in Palatino by Initial Typesetting Services, Edinburgh
Printed and bound in Great Britain by Clays Ltd, Elcograf S.p.A

Papers used by Robinson are from well-managed forests and
other responsible sources

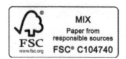

Robinson
An imprint of
Little, Brown Book Group
Carmelite House
50 Victoria Embankment
London EC4Y 0DZ

An Hachette UK Company
www.hachette.co.uk

www.littlebrown.co.uk

For my Dad, Paul Irons (MBE!).

*Thank you for being an inspiration to so many people,
and a role model for me in how to be a dedicated, caring
person in the world.*

Love you pops

Contents

Acknowledgements   xix

Foreword   xxi

Introduction   1

   Why are emotions important?   1

   What are emotional difficulties?   2

   Difficult emotions: A personal story   3

   How can compassion help with difficult emotions?   4

   How to use this book   6

   Practice   7

   Case examples used in the book   7

Section One
Learning about emotions   9

1 What are emotions?   11

Definition of emotion   11

Beyond definitions – emotions organise the body and mind   12

Tracking the 'story' of emotions   17

What's the difference between emotions and feelings?   19

What's the difference between emotions and moods?   20

Are there some emotions that are healthy or good, and some
that are unhealthy or bad?   21

Key reflections   22

2   **Why do we have emotions?**   23

   Emotions evolved to help us   24

   Emotions serve our motives   26

   What are the functions of our different emotions?   26

   The three system model of emotion   29

     Exercise: Anxiety vs anger   31

   Built for us, not by us   35

   Key reflections   36

Section Two
How and why we struggle with our emotions   37

3   **Evolution and our tricky brain**   39

   Our brain has inbuilt glitches   40

   Loops in the mind – when new and old collide   41

   Loops in the mind – not our fault   46

   Key reflections   47

4   **Emotions are shaped by life experiences**   48

   Difficult emotions – shaped for us, not by us   50

   How have your emotions been shaped?   50

   Caring, attachment and distress regulation   58

     Exercise: How have your relationships shaped your three systems?   61

   What can compassion, and CFT, do to help?   62

   Key reflections   64

5   **Emotion regulation problems**   65

What is emotion regulation?   65

What is emotion dysregulation?   66

Difficulties in regulating emotions – the emotion
    regulation model (ERM)   68

Section Three
What is compassion, and how might it help with
my difficult emotions?   83

6   **What is compassion, and how can it help with difficult**
    emotions?   85

What is compassion?   85

First psychology of compassion – engagement with distress   86

Second psychology of compassion – alleviation of distress   90

Bringing the two psychologies together   93

Compassion, shadow and difficult emotions   96

The benefits of cultivating a compassionate mind   97

The three flows of compassion   98

Key reflections   99

7   **How to develop a compassionate mind**   100

Starting the process – motivation   100

Exercise: Compassion-based motivation – why do I want
things to be different?   100

Is it possible to 'feed' our brains?   102

Getting the ball rolling – practice   103

Key reflections   105

8   Compassionate mind training – attention and mindfulness   106

Foundations of a compassionate mind: Attention,
  mindfulness and mind awareness   106

The power of attention   108

  Exercise: The nature of attention   108

A restless mind   109

  Exercise: Our restless mind   109

Strengthening attention: Mind awareness and stability
  through mindfulness   111

Ways to be mindful   113

Before you start – five steps of preparation   115

Core mindfulness practices   116

  Exercise: Mindfulness of sound   116

  Exercise: Mindful body scan   118

  Exercise: Mindfulness of breathing   120

Difficulties with mindfulness   122

Mindfulness in daily life   124

  Exercise: Mindful walking   124

  Exercise: Mindful eating   125

Key reflections   126

9   Compassionate mind training – building the soothing system   128

Body posture   128

  Exercise: Developing a grounded, stable body posture   129

Soothing rhythm breathing   130

  Exercise: Soothing rhythm breathing   133

Exercise: Learning to slow down – how to slow your breathing 135

Facial expression 137

Exercise: SRB with friendly facial expression 138

Voice tone and inner talk 138

*Exercise: Soothing rhythm breathing with inner speech and
caring inner voice tone* 139

Memory and imagery 140

Exercise: Soothing memory 141

Exercise: Soothing system imagery – creating a safe place 146

Key reflections 148

**10 Compassionate mind training – developing your
compassionate self** 149

Creating a compassionate mind 149

Core qualities of the compassionate self 150

Cultivating the compassionate self 153

Exercise: Compassionate memory 153

Developing your compassionate self – acting techniques 154

Exercise: Compassionate self 155

Embodying your compassionate self – bringing the
virtual into reality 159

Exercise: Bringing your compassionate self into daily life 159

Ideal compassionate other 161

Exercise: Creating your ideal compassionate other 164

Key reflections 167

11 Fears, blocks and resistances to compassion   168

Misunderstandings about compassion   169

The compassionate ladder   171

Key reflectioms   173

Section Four
Using your compassionate mind to manage your emotions –
compassion-focused emotion regulation   **175**

Example: Helpful emotion regulation   176

12 Compassion-focused emotion regulation skills (CERS) –
awareness of emotion triggers   181

1. Developing attention and awareness of triggers of
   difficult emotions   183

   Exercise: Learning from the past   184

   Exercise: Increasing awareness of external triggers   188

   Exercise: Noticing internal triggers to difficult emotions   190

2. Modifying triggers/emotionally stimulating situations   191

   Exercise: Using your compassionate mind to modify trigger
   situations   193

3. Wise selection of situations   196

   Exercise: Wise selection of situations   198

Key reflections   199

13 Compassion-focused emotion regulation skills (CERS) –
awareness of emotions   201

Emotion patterns   203

Awareness of emotion 205

Mindfulness of emotion 210

Exercise: Mindfulness of emotions – noticing their shape and pattern 211

Key reflections 213

14 Compassion-focused emotion regulation skills (CERS) – labelling emotions 214

Present moment labelling 217

Exercise: Present moment emotion labelling 217

Exercise: Emotion daily review 218

Range of emotional experience 219

How often do you experience different emotions? 222

Memory and emotion labelling 224

Exercise: Labelling emotional memories 224

Discriminating between emotions 225

Recognising mixed feelings 226

Exercise: Labelling mixed emotions 228

Key reflections 229

15 Compassion-focused emotion regulation skills (CERS) – understanding emotions 230

1. Validate 233

Exercise: Using the compassionate self to validate emotions 234

Receiving validation from someone else 237

*Exercise: Using memory and imagination to validate
your feelings* 238

Exercise: *Validation of emotion from the image of your
compassionate other*   239

2. Mentalising and understanding our emotions   240

   Exercise: *Mentalising from the compassionate self*   242

3. Listening to what our emotions are telling us – the
   wisdom of emotions   243

   Exercise: *Listening to the wisdom of emotions*   244

4. Recognition of, and working with, what maintains
   difficult emotions   247

Key reflections   250

16 **Compassion-focused emotion regulation skills (CERS) –
   coping with and using emotions**   251

16a: **Coping with emotions – tolerating and accepting**   255

Tolerating difficult emotions   255

Mindfulness   257

   Exercise: *Mindfulness of emotion – distress tolerance* 257

Stability of mind and body   259

   Exercise: *Distress tolerance – soothing breathing*   260

Compassionate intention   261

   Exercise: *Compassionate self – supporting distress tolerance*   262

Accepting difficult emotions   263

   Exercise: *Compassionate acceptance of difficult emotions*   265

Working with 'emotions about emotion'   267

Key reflections   268

16b: Modifying the intensity of emotions   270

Modifying the intensity of emotions   271

Decreasing the intensity of emotions   272

Increasing the intensity of emotions   277

   Exercise: Turning up the volume of emotional intensity   278

   Exercise: Using writing to increase emotional intensity   279

Developing your skills further – online material   280

Key reflections   281

**16c: Coping with emotions – expressing emotions
and assertiveness**   282

   Exercise: Exploring difficulties with emotional expression   284

   Exercise: Managing fears about expressing emotions   285

Three steps to emotion expression   286

Emotional expression – learning to be assertive   291

Key reflections   294

16d: Working with multiple emotional 'selves'   295

   Exercise: Multiple selves   298

Step 1: Listening to the angry part of you   298

Step 2: Listening to the anxious part of you   300

Step 3: Listening to the sad part of you   301

Step 4: How do the different parts relate to each other?
Emotions about emotions   306

Step 5: Bringing compassion to the party   307

   Exercise: Bringing compassion to the situation   308

Compassion for my angry self   309

    Exercise: Compassion for your angry self   309

Compassion for the anxious part of me   310

    Exercise: Compassion for your anxious self   310

Compassion for the sad part of me   311

    Exercise: Compassion for your sad self   312

Key reflections   313

16e: Managing shame and self-criticism   314

What is shame?   315

Why do we experience shame?   316

The shape of shame   317

What impact does shame have on our other emotions?   319

Shame can disconnect us   319

Compassion – an antidote for shame?   321

    Exercise: Bringing compassion to shame   324

Self-criticism – shame's best friend   327

Why do we become self-critical?   330

Self-criticism and feared emotions   332

Bringing your compassionate mind to help your self-critic   333

    Exercise: Using our compassionate self to work with self-criticism   339

Key reflections   343

Section Five
Deepening your emotion regulation skills   345

17 'Turning up for yourself' – the compassion PDA (Pre,
    During and After)   347

   Exercise: Your compassion PDA   350

   Key reflections   353

18 **Cultivating positive emotions**   354

   Pay attention to positive emotions   355

   Recalling positive emotions   357

   Exercise: Connecting with positive memories   357

   Exercise: Memory writing   358

   Gratitude and appreciation   358

   Exercise: Three good things   359

   Key reflections   360

19 **Compassionate letter writing**   361

   Before writing – engage your compassionate mind   361

   Exercise: Compassionate letter writing   362

   After writing – compassionate reading   366

   Key reflections   368

20 **Using compassionate thinking to manage your emotions**   369

   Understanding the way we think   370

   Taking perspective – not your fault   372

The relationship between threat emotions and
thinking patterns   373

Thought monitoring   374

Threat system thinking vs compassionate thinking   377

Developing compassionate, balanced thinking   378

Exercise: Thought-emotion form   379

Key reflections   389

Section Six
Compassionate futures – sustaining your compassionate mind   391

21 **Sustaining healthy emotion regulation**   393

Continue to work out!   393

Deepening emotion regulation skills – online chapters   394

Conclusion   395

References   397

Index   409

Acknowledgements

I've been supported in writing this book by so many wonderful friends and colleagues. I'm indebted to the input of Tobyn Bell, Syd Hiskey, Dennis Tirch, Roisin Joyce, Rachel Egan, Shelley Kerr, Jed Shamel, Chris Winson, Christine Dunkley, Sunil Lad, Brett Grellier and Sam Thompson.

Special thanks to Paul Gilbert for all your input – not just on this book, but throughout the twenty years I've been lucky enough to know and work with you! It's been quite a journey, and a real privilege to be part of how this wonderful approach to life has developed and grown.

I'd also like to extend my thanks to the many clients I've had the honour to work with, and who have shown great courage in sharing their emotional difficulties, and wisdom in teaching me how compassion can be a powerful way of alleviating distress.

A massive thanks to my wife, Korina. Without your ongoing support and encouragement, this book would have never seen the light of day. But even more than that, I've really appreciated discussing the ideas, structure and flow of this book with you, and you've helped to shape it in a wonderful way. Thank you!

And finally, to my son, Idris – you might only be a few months old, but you're teaching me so much about what love and compassion are about.

Foreword

Emotion gives texture and colour to our lives. Imagine what our lives would be like without emotions, if we were just run by logic. We would not experience joy, sexual desire, excitement, hope, fascination, humour, wonder and awe. These would be great losses. Some researchers believe it would be almost impossible for us to make decisions or have intuitions, while other researchers think that emotion is a basis of consciousness itself. On the other hand, we would also not experience intense anxiety, rage, vengeance and hopelessness. When you think about it, we spend a lot of our lives trying to create the feelings we like and avoid or get rid of the feelings we don't like. The problem is that our gene-built brains and socially choreographed minds did not build emotions into us just for the pleasure of experiencing emotion. Evolution built capacities for emotions that would direct actions that aided the struggle for survival and reproduction. Evolution did not build emotions to make us happy and many of them don't (although some do). Emotions are there to do a job. What emotion we may feel depends on how we need to act in certain contexts. Dr Irons offers masterly guidance in exploring the importance of understanding the evolutionary roots of our emotions. It is often said, that in biology and psychology, nothing makes sense without an evolutionary function analysis and Dr Irons does that expertly here. He also presents his unique model for understanding emotion.

Most, but not all, of the emotions that cause us trouble are linked to what we call 'threat processing'. These are the emotions we experience when there are dangers or obstacles and setbacks; when we fail rather than succeed; when we get rejected rather than accepted; when we become ill rather than stay healthy. The big four threat emotions or emotion states are: anxiety, anger, disgust and sadness. Although we might like to get rid of these emotions, because evolution has built them into us it's not possible to somehow take them out of our brain; we can't remove them like we might an appendix or cyst. Of course, this doesn't mean that people don't try to directly alter their brains so they don't have to feel certain emotions. Billions and billions are spent on drugs to control anxiety, depression or anger. And, of course, people also use drugs to help them feel good such as amphetamines, cocaine and heroin. And a substance that many use to change their emotional state is alcohol. The problem with all these methods are that they have a dark side linked to addiction, harmful behaviours, withdrawal and short-termism.

As Dr Irons describes, there are many reasons why we want to try to regulate some of our emotions. For example, we may find the unpleasant ones are too frequent and easily triggered in us, are too intense, seem to last for too long, or are difficult to recover from. We can also have beliefs about emotions that make them more difficult to deal with. For example, we may think that other people don't feel emotions as intensely as we do or that the emotions are intolerable and will overwhelm us. We might feel ashamed of our emotions or desires. We might not understand them so we don't know why we're feeling what we're feeling. We might experience many different emotions at the same time that seem to be in conflict with each other, causing us confusion. One emotion might block another, as, for example, when individuals feel rage to hide from grief or are comfortable with feeling sadness but not rage. All of these can orientate us towards trying to get rid of and avoid emotions rather than working with and through them.

However, if we are to take the journey of working with and through unpleasant or frightening emotions then clearly we need a way of doing that. As Dr Irons indicates, this is where compassion comes in. Compassion is a basic motivation to tune our attention to the things that are difficult or cause suffering and to try as best we can to be helpful and alleviate and prevent unnecessary suffering in the future. Compassion is not an emotion: it is a basic motive that will help us with our emotions. Part of the reason for this is because caring behaviour and compassion were designed by evolution to be soothing and down-regulate threat processing in appropriate circumstances. As Dr Irons explains, compassion helps us find the resources, the courage and the wisdom we need to be able to work with difficult emotions.

This leads to the core question of how we cultivate and utilise those compassionate circuits in our brain to help us with difficult emotions. This is where compassion focused therapy comes in because this is precisely what this therapy seeks to do: to stimulate the psychological and biological processes, associated with caring behaviour, that are wired in to threat processing and can help regulate it. Luckily, Dr Irons has been at the forefront of compassion focused therapy for over twenty years. He is an international compassion focused therapy trainer.

In this book, he brings his extensive experience and wisdom to help navigate us through the tricky territory of understanding our emotions and how compassion can be a wise guide. In the first section he takes us through the up-to-date research on what emotions are. Emotions are not static. Our emotions can depend on our background state: if we're already anxious then getting more anxious might be easy; if we're already in an irritable state, quite small things can upset us which perhaps they wouldn't if we were more relaxed – in a 'just returning from holiday' state, or having won a lot of money! So there may be no direct link between a situation and an emotion. How we express emotions may depend on the context. While we might be okay with expressing certain emotions to somebody we know, we might not be to somebody we don't know. Some emotions we might express to our close friends but not to our boss.

Dr Irons highlights the fact that emotions are partly built by our genes and therefore our potential and capacity to feel certain emotions is not our fault. We are all built by our genes to feel and want to do certain things; that's what makes us human and a representative of the species. It's called our common humanity. Without that, we would struggle to understand other people's emotions, and empathy would become strangely difficult. While, of course, there are important differences between the textures of emotions different people around the world may feel, it's important that we realise other human beings have the same feelings, wishes and needs that we do. They are not aliens and should not be treated as such. And today there are major debates on whether animals feel emotions and what that means for the (shocking) way we treat them.

Dr Irons also uses the insights from understanding the evolutionary roots of emotion to explore how and why we should not fuse our sense of self with what we feel. Because we have certain emotions, fantasies or thoughts, that doesn't make us a good or a bad person. Remember these potential feelings have been in existence for millions of years in millions of brains – you didn't build them or create them so don't claim them as 'yours' in a shameful way. Try, instead, to note them so you can stay with the compassionate living style of trying to be helpful, not harmful. As Dr Irons outlines in the book, we can take a step back and become a mindful observer of our emotions, a mindful observer of the shifting patterns of emotion of which our brains are capable. Then we are less caught up in them, less rushed along by them, and less fused into them. Then we can become more discerning, choosing whether to act on them or not, or even to act against them. For example, there are many times when we might wish to override anxiety. We might get anxious the day we take our driving test, but we override anxiety to take it anyway; or we go for that important job interview or we ask that particular person out for a date. We can also override anger. We choose not to act harmfully because that's important for us even though we may wish to.

Being mindful and aware of the nature of emotion and how it plays through us because of the way our brains are built is a step towards learning emotional tolerance. Probably one of the greatest strengths that will help us is developing emotional tolerance because then we need not be frightened of an emotion. Rather than feeling we 'must' get away from an emotion because it's so awful, emotional tolerance helps us no longer fear it, even if we don't like it.

In addition, within that tolerance we may learn new things about ourselves. For example, in tolerating anger we may begin to recognise unmet needs that we can seek out in other ways, or see that our anger is a mask for sadness and grieving. We can also learn that sometimes we can make our emotions worse by the way we think or ruminate. Although tolerance of emotion is important, it needs to be purposeful. Learning to tolerate emotions that are being generated by unhealthy ways of living or thinking is not purposeful and so it would be good to change them.

For example, I'm anxious about my weight but I'll just learn to tolerate the anxiety and not do anything about it. So compassion tolerance comes with compassionate wisdom for helpful action. This takes us into the territory of how to work with intense emotion, emotions that are too frequent or emotions that come on in the wrong context. For all these aspects of emotion, Dr Irons is a wonderful guide.

The book will also explore specific kinds of emotions, such as anger and anxiety, and how to create more positive emotions in your life. It is filled with up-to-date ways of mindfully tending to your emotions and generating compassionate ways of containing, holding and working with your emotions.

It is a great pleasure for me to recommend my esteemed colleague of many years who is one of the world's leading teachers of compassion focused therapy (for more, see www.compassionatemind.co.uk). This book comes to you textured by many years of clinical experience as well as working with general compassionate mind training groups.

Paul Gilbert

Introduction

First up, thanks for reading this book. I hope it will be a helpful guide for you. In the coming sections and chapters, we'll explore how and why we struggle with emotions, and introduce ideas and practices that might help you to find new ways of addressing common difficulties in life. But let's start with why this book is focused on emotion in the first place.

Why are emotions important?

Take a moment to think about the best moment in your life. Where you were, what you were doing, who you were with. Allow yourself a minute to connect with the memory as best as you can.

Now, if you're willing, bring to mind a time in life that was more difficult, a time that you're pleased is long in the past. If you can, allow yourself a minute or so to connect with that memory.

Now, with both of these memories in mind, consider how they're similar. Given their differences, what binds them together?

There has always been something inherently contradictory about emotions; we are both drawn to them, but at times, do our level best to avoid or stay away from them. We recognise that they are central to our life, bringing colour and texture to experiences, and that much in life would be drab and grey without them. But for many of us, given a choice, we would turn them off quicker than a light switch if it meant that we didn't have to *feel* – didn't have to feel the pain, discomfort, and heaviness that emotions like fear, sadness and shame can bring.

We can experience many joys in life: moments with close friends or family members, the birth of a child, falling in love, succeeding in a test or project that is important or meaningful for us. In contrast, we can face many struggles in life: poverty, loss of loved ones, failures and rejections, bullying, criticism or abuse, and a host of physical health problems, illnesses and diseases. What translates these events from being just 'experiences' to something that connects us with distress, suffering or happiness is often emotion – sadness, fear, anger, shame, joy or excitement that go *with* these experiences.

What are difficult emotions?

Sadly, rather than being confined to discrete situations and experiences, it is emotion that often causes us ongoing difficulties in life. In my work as a clinical psychologist, in one way or another, all of the clients I work with have some struggle with emotion. Sometimes this is someone battling with feelings of anxiety and panic, unable to speak up in meetings at work, go on dates, or attend parties with friends. Sometimes it's a person constantly on the edge of anger and rage, lashing out at loved ones and strangers alike, pushing people away and causing themselves and others pain. Sometimes it's someone weighed down by overwhelming sadness and grief, shut down to life following the death of a loved one or end of a relationship. Sometimes it's a person burdened with feelings of shame, caught up in painful memories of things that happened to them in the past, or crippled by feelings of inadequacy and inferiority. And for some people, it's the absence of emotion that is causing problems. For example, someone who is unable to experience anger, and therefore blocked to asserting and sticking up for themselves at work and with their partner. Or the person who is unable to express sadness or distress, and consequently struggles to allow others to get close to them and share meaningful relationships. Or finally, someone who is unable to experience excitement, contentment and happiness, and whose life is stripped of many of the pleasures and joys that can come with relationships, hobbies and learning.

So, this is a book that is for anyone who experiences difficulties with emotions – whether that's experiencing certain emotions too often or strongly, or if you're blocked to certain emotions that it could be helpful to experience more of. It's designed to help you understand more about what emotions are, why we experience them, and how they can cause us distress. We'll look at various models for working with emotions and learn how cultivating skills in mindfulness and compassion can help to bring a healthier emotional balance in your life.

Difficult emotions: A personal story

Although emotions often form the centre of what I encounter in other people's struggles, this book is partly a reflection of my own experience with emotional difficulties. Growing up, I was often described as a happy and laid-back person – and I guess in many ways, I was. What I struggled with was acknowledging, validating and expressing certain emotions – particularly those that were unpleasant, such as anger, anxiety and shame. My strategy – although I was not doing this consciously – was a 'keep them suppressed at all costs' approach. It wasn't that I couldn't get angry (ask my brother – we had some good arguments and fights growing up!) or anxious (I remember very clearly avoiding taking part in a football competition because I was scared of failing). Rather, I wasn't able to *acknowledge* that I was feeling how I was feeling, and if I did express these emotions, it was only at the level of an action or behaviour (for example, getting aggressive or avoiding something scary). Crucially, I found it very difficult to manage my emotions *effectively*. I found it difficult to tolerate and experience my anger in a way that could lead to expressing it in an assertive and helpful way. I also found it hard to tolerate my anxiety enough, and to seek help from others, so that I could have the courage and support to compete without getting overwhelmed with worries about failing. There are lots of reasons why I managed my emotions in these ways, many of which are linked to my history, relationships and experiences growing up in life. And to a certain extent, my strategy of suppressing unpleasant feelings was helpful at times; however, it also led to difficulties, and contributed to unhappy friendships and relationships, mismanagement of opportunities in life, and more generally, a sense that it was difficult to get my own needs met.

Over the years, I've worked hard to make progress in these areas. I spend less time suppressing and keeping feelings to myself (although I'm still quite good at this!) and am learning how to tolerate emotions like anger and shame, and try to bring compassion to my experiences in a helpful way. I still feel like I've got a distance to travel, but this is the beauty of developing your compassionate mind – getting to the destination would be great, but the main thing is that I'm heading in the right direction, I'm in the flow of the journey.

How did I do this? Well, like many things in life, there were multiple factors – friends, family, partners and mentors, as well as the ups and downs of experiences in life. But it turns out that many of the other things that helped outside of these people were linked to the ideas and skills of Compassion Focused Therapy (CFT). CFT was developed by Professor Paul Gilbert, initially to help people experiencing distress commonly associated with high levels of shame and self-criticism. I was lucky enough to start working with Paul on some of the ideas linked to CFT in 1999. So, it was through applying these ideas to clients that I saw how they also applied to me, and I started to make changes to the way I approached my own emotions.

How can compassion help with emotional difficulties?

In the last two decades or so, there has been an increasing interest in how training our minds in compassion can change the way we think, feel and behave. We're also learning through an increasing number of research studies that practising compassion can have a significant effect on our body, gene expression and immune response.

One of the difficulties with compassion can be the word itself. One of my clients used to say to me, partly with a smile on her face but also with a fair bit of anger, 'You're not going to talk about that f*cking C word again, are you?!' I never did find out if she was equating compassion with one of the most feared illnesses (cancer), or a word often seen as the most unpleasant of swear words in the English language! For some people, compassion can bring to mind weakness, fluffiness and just being 'nice'; for others, it evokes a sense of letting others (or themselves) off the hook, or indulgence.

But it turns out that compassion is none of these things. Compassion is the motivation that spurs a person on to risk their life as a firefighter or to dedicate their career to being a doctor or nurse. When a loved one, friend or even stranger is distressed and suffering, it's compassion that motivates us to pay attention to this and try to do something to help. So, the definition of compassion that we'll use in this book is: 'a sensitivity to the suffering of self and others, with a commitment to try to alleviate and prevent it' (Gilbert, 2014). This is a commonly used definition and suggests compassion requires certain qualities of mind. First up, we need to develop a desire to pay attention to and engage with things that are difficult, such as painful or overwhelming emotions, without turning away, avoiding, switching off, or turning towards the next chocolate bar or alcoholic drink. So, to help here, we need to develop the strength, courage and ability to tolerate our own distress and painful feelings, and those of others. Second, we need to cultivate understanding and wisdom to guide our desire to be caring and helpful; we also need to build a variety of skills that help us to work with our own difficulties and distress, so that we can find a new, more helpful way of working with this.

Throughout this book I'll help you to learn how to prepare your mind for, and in, compassion; and how by doing this, you can use your 'compassionate mind' to better manage difficult emotions. We will draw upon training exercises taken from Compassion Focused Therapy (CFT) that are known as compassionate mind training or 'CMT'. The key thing here is that you don't have to be in therapy, or feel that you need to be, to benefit from these. They've been developed from a variety of contemplative traditions and psychotherapeutic approaches, and are helpful for managing a range of life difficulties and emotional problems.

How to use this book

The book is divided into six sections. In the first section, we will explore what we mean by emotion, and why we experience them. In section two, we will explore the CFT model, and help you understand why you might be struggling with emotions in the way you are. The third section will outline what compassion is, what it involves, and how it can help with managing difficult emotions. We'll also explore a model of emotion regulation that will guide us later in the book. There are different ways of understanding what emotion regulation means, but for the purposes of this book, it refers to our ability to influence the type of emotions we have, when we have them, how we experience them, and how we express or use them.

Section four will focus on compassionate mind training and we will work through a series of exercises in mindfulness, breathing, imagery and compassion. Section five will return to the emotion regulation model introduced in section three, and in combination with the compassionate mind skills developed in section four, we will consider how these can help to bring balance to our emotions. The final section will focus on how we can sustain our compassionate mind going forward.

It's also worth noting that there are some extra, online materials that you might find helpful that supplement the chapters in this book. These go into more detail about specific emotions that you might struggle with, including anger, anxiety and sadness. You can access these at https://overcoming.co.uk/715/resources-to-download.

If you can, move through the book by section, taking your time to reflect on each chapter and, if it helps, making notes along the way. Although it is tempting to jump straight to the later sections that focus on working more specifically with difficult emotions, I would recommend holding off if you can until you've had a chance to work through the earlier sections first. It is through these initial chapters that you will learn how to develop the skills of your compassionate mind, and through doing so, be best placed to work with the ideas and exercises that come later in the book.

Practice

As you move through the book, particularly from section three onwards, you will be introduced to a variety of compassionate mind training exercises. These are evidence-based practices that are designed to help you learn to manage difficult emotions in a helpful way. You can find audio files for many of these at www.balancedminds.com to guide you with your practice.

Case examples used in the book

All case examples are amalgamations of real people that I've worked with in therapy or know personally. Any identifiable characteristics (e.g. name, gender, age, ethnicity) have been altered to protect anonymity.

SECTION ONE

Learning about emotions

In this first section, we're going to explore what emotions are, how they're defined, and what happens when we experience them (for example, to our attention, thinking or behaviour). We'll also look at why we experience emotions and learn about how they evolved to help us manage and tackle various challenges that we face as human beings.

1   What are emotions?

What is an emotion? Take a moment or two to think about it – to *really* think about it. How would you describe an emotion to someone who, for whatever reason, had no understanding about emotions? If an alien came down to earth and asked you what an emotion is, what would you tell them?

At first, this might seem a simple thing to explain. However, you might have noticed that, actually, it's harder than it initially appeared. Now, if you struggled to answer this, you are not the only one; it turns out that the same question has been causing philosophers, scientists, psychologists and therapists headaches for thousands of years! Given that we have landed people on the moon, discovered cures for deadly illnesses, and even mapped our genome, it's interesting that there is no consensus on what something so 'normal' and 'day-to-day' as emotions actually are. As a former client of mine said: 'Describing my feelings and emotions in any detailed way is like trying to use a nail to pin down water.'

The word 'emotion' was first used in the English language in the sixteenth century and replaced terms like 'passions' and 'affections' that had been used by the Greeks and other civilisations for millennia before. The origin of the word 'emotion' is actually from the French word *émouvoir*, which means 'to stir up', and before that, the Latin word *emovere*, which means to 'move out' or 'agitate'. So, in terms of the etymology of the word itself we can understand emotion as being linked to energy, movement and a type of physical tension.

Definition of emotion

There are almost a hundred different ways that psychologists have defined and conceptualised emotions. As one set of researchers in the area suggested: 'Everyone knows what an emotion is, until asked to give a definition' (Fehr & Russell, 1984, p. 464). Now clearly, we aren't going to try to outline all of these ways in this book. But this large number of definitions tells us something that you probably already know, and have intuitive wisdom about: *emotions are very complex*. And because they are complex and difficult to define, maybe it's no wonder that many of us find it difficult to understand, recognise, describe or manage them.

Let's take a look at a few definitions though. The online Oxford dictionary suggests that emotion is 'a strong feeling deriving from one's circumstances, mood, or relationships with others' (Oxford Dictionary, 2018). Hoffman (2016), a well-known psychologist in the emotion field, suggested that: 'an emotion is (1) a multidimensional experience that is (2) characterised by different levels of arousal and degrees of pleasure-displeasure; (3) associated with subjective experiences, somatic sensations and motivational tendencies; (4) coloured by contextual and cultural factors; and that (5) can be regulated to some degree through intra- and interpersonal processes'. While this is very thorough and captures how emotions are a complex combination of different components, it's probably true that for most of us, this isn't an easy or accessible definition of what an emotion is. In that sense, it's unlikely to be that helpful for our purposes of understanding and working with emotions. Given this, let's look at another way of understanding what emotions are.

Beyond definition – emotions organise the body and mind

It might be helpful to sketch out an example of how emotions, as defined above, can play out in real life. Imagine walking down a road, heading to a restaurant to meet a good friend. You're feeling excited about seeing this friend, and thinking about what you're going to eat and talk about. You are walking quickly, as it's been a long time since you've seen your friend, and you're eager to catch up. However, as you walk along the road, a car swerves to miss a young child who ran into the road, and is now heading straight for you. You suddenly shift from feeling excited, to fearful. This new emotion drags your mind to a new concern (your physical safety/preservation), focusing your attention on the car and motivating you to move quickly to one side. A moment later, once you're safe, you feel angry as you recognise that the driver was on his mobile phone, rather than watching the road. This angry feeling directs your attention to the driver (your current 'concern'), and you tell him, in no uncertain terms, what you think about him and his actions. Finally, you start to feel guilty, as you notice that the man has a young child in the car with him, who has started to cry because you're shouting so loudly. This directs your attention towards the child; you apologise and try to reassure them that everything is OK, using a softer voice tone.

As you can see from this example, our emotions can change as new situations and information emerge; yet they continue to act as a bridge between an event or trigger, and our concerns, behaviour and motives. You might have noticed that linked to each 'emotion' (here, excitement, fear, anger and guilt), are some common components. In other words, emotions involve a cluster of responses, including bodily feelings, facial expressions, a desire to act (behave) in a certain way, and a conscious way of describing the experience.

Another way of looking at this is to consider how emotions organise our mind (and body) in a particular way. Let's take a look at this with the aid of Figure 1 overleaf, and the example of a personal experience of anxiety I had a number of years ago. It was a dark winter's night, and I was walking back home after having a drink with a friend. It was late, and I wanted to get home as quickly as possible as it was really cold. I decided to take a shortcut through backstreets, rather than walk down the slightly longer, but better-lit main street. As I started to walk down a side street, I heard a noise and sensed someone walking behind me, seemingly getting closer to me.

Figure 1: Emotions organise the mind and body

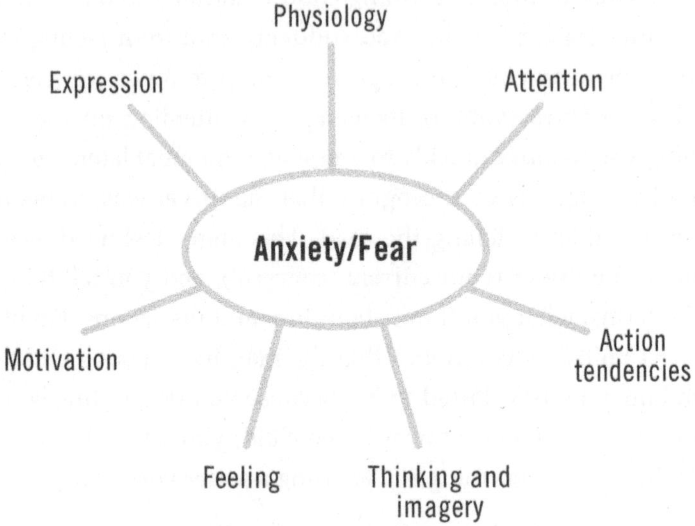

Physiology

Expression   Attention

Anxiety/Fear

Motivation   Action
                                                  tendencies

Feeling   Thinking and
                   imagery

Using this diagram, let's take a look at some of the different aspects of what happened to me in this situation:

Physiology	When we experience an emotion, there are a variety of physiological changes in our body that we may or may not be consciously aware of. These include changes in the brain (e.g. different areas of the brain become activated), and changes in the autonomic nervous system (e.g. change in heart rate, breathing, muscle tension). *My experience:* In this situation, I noticed that my hands started to sweat, my heart was racing, and my muscles were tense.
Action tendencies	With the experience of an emotion, there is often an action or urge in which the body becomes ready to engage in a response. This might include common evolved reactions such as fight, flight, freeze, submission, and so forth. *My experience:* I had the urge to flee the situation, to start running or cross the road to get away from the person following me.

Attention	Emotions guide attention, and depending on the type of emotion and the situation you're in, this could have a very different impact on the way attention is directed. For example, 'high arousal' anxiety and anger tend to narrow attention to the nature of the threat (Richards et al., 2014), whereas positive emotions like excitement and contentment may open and broaden attention (Fredrickson, 2013).
	My experience: My attention became narrow and fixed. I could hear the sound of footsteps behind me, I was aware that it was dark and that there was no one else was on the street in front of me. I was also aware of my heart beginning to beat faster.
Motivation	Emotions work in the service of motives (see Chapter 2), guiding us towards things that are important (e.g. acquiring things, safety, social relationships), and responding differently depending on whether we are successful or thwarted.
	My experience: I wanted to get away from the threat, to protect myself and be safe.
Thinking & imagery	A variety of studies have shown two important ways thinking is associated with emotion. One – the 'top-down' approach – has found the way we think about something can trigger an emotion. For example, if you consider what thoughts you might need to have to feel panicky, or to feel angry, you might start to notice that what you think (or what images you bring to mind) can have a big impact on your emotions. However, we also know that emotions influence the content of thoughts, and various research studies have found support for this 'bottom up' approach. For example, following the terrorist attacks on 11 September, 2001, researchers asked study participants to focus on what made them angry or sad about these attacks. Following this emotional priming, participants voiced more causal and blaming attributions about the attacks when asked to focus on feeling angry, than they did when feeling sad (Small et al., 2006).
	My experience: Various thoughts were flashing through my mind: 'It's a mugger, and they're catching up with me,' and 'They're going to attack.' I had an image that the person behind me was tall, strong and had a knife in his hand.

Expression	This involves the manifestation or overt display of the felt emotion verbally, through words, as well as non-verbally, through body posture, facial expression, eye gaze, voice tone and so forth. For example, the expression of anger (often involving physically expanding, gritting of the teeth, frowning, clenching of the fists, and raised voice tone) would be different to the expression of fear (often involving becoming physically smaller, averted eye gaze, loss of muscular control, and absence of, or softer speech).
	My experience: I was tense in my body, with my shoulders 'up' and hands balled into fists. My face was tight and probably showing fear. If I had spoken, my voice would have come laced with fear.
Feeling	Emotions turn up 'feeling' a certain way – a 'felt sense' that is *subjectively* experienced and often verbalised by describing what this is like. This 'putting words to' is sometimes dependent on the degree and clarity of the physiological component outlined above. This 'feeling' aspect of emotion can have different facets; for example, we can experience emotions that have a pleasant feel to them (sometimes known as 'positive' emotions such as joy or excitement), whereas others can feel unpleasant (sometimes known as 'negative' emotions, such as anger, anxiety or disgust). This does not mean that emotions are 'good' or 'bad' – just that they have pleasant or unpleasant feelings when we experience them. The feeling component can also vary in how long it is experienced for, as well as its intensity – for example, ranging from the lower-energy feeling of contentment to the higher-energy feel of excitement.
	My experience: I felt tense, on edge and panicky. I was definitely scared. It was a very unpleasant feeling.

So, you can see how this situation triggered fear in me, and how this fear 'showed up' in many different ways, all preparing my body to take action to keep safe. Emotion (fear) acted as a *relevance radar* to me –

tuning me into my safety and orientating me to find ways (actions) to make myself safe. In this sense, we can see that emotions are signals to us, helping us to focus on and respond to things that matter to us in the world – that we care about (in this example, my desire to avoid harm).

These components of emotions are not linear – so they don't necessarily arise in the order they're listed on the previous pages. In fact, in psychology and other related fields, there have been arguments for many, many decades, about which components of an emotion are *primary*, or come first. In other words, do we experience emotions because we appraise (think about) a situation in a certain way, or because we experience a change in our physiology and feelings, which then sets off changes in our behaviour and the way we think? Sometimes there can be a tendency to make the above process purely linear, with the implication that emotions always follow the same process. Rather than getting lost in a chicken-and-egg debate of what causes what, from the perspective of this book, we will take the approach that the seven components previously outlined are part of an integrated, coordinated system, or network. They emerge and are a patterned response to certain situations, and move us to manage or cope with emotions in ways that are consistent with our basic life motives – to avoid harm, to feel cared for, or to achieve things. We'll return to these points in Chapter 2.

Now, it turned out that when I came up to the traffic lights and had to stop and wait, the dangerous mugger did indeed catch up with me, but turned out to be an elderly lady taking her dog for a walk! Although realising this helped to calm my anxiety, my initial response was triggered not by what was actually happening (i.e. that there was no need to feel alarmed), but by my perception that I was in danger. We'll come back to look at how you can develop your own examples using Figure 11 in Chapter 13.

Tracking the 'story' of emotions

Alongside understanding how emotions orientate our mind and body, it's also helpful to hold in mind the process or 'story' of emotions: their beginning, middle and end. This includes:

1. **Triggers** – what starts or creates an emotion. This could be something external (e.g. a meeting, a conversation with a friend, a dark street late at night) or something internal (e.g. a thought, worry, memory or rumination).

2. **Frequency** – some emotions may show up in us as if they're frequent visitors or companions in our life. Others are like a distant aunt or uncle – we rarely get to meet them.

3. **Intensity** – emotions can show up at different volumes. Some are subtle, barely perceptible and operating like quiet music in the background of our lives. Others are like standing at the front row of a thrash metal music gig, loud, overpowering and overwhelming.

4. **Duration** – some emotions show up briefly, for a few moments, before being replaced by something else. Others tend to show up for longer – often because certain things keep them triggered inside us.

5. **Expression and action** – we may well experience an emotion, but that doesn't tell us much about whether we can express it to others or use it to guide our behaviour in an effective way. So, while some people can 'show' their emotion in a helpful way (both helpful to themselves, but as a signal communication to others), other people struggle to act upon or show their emotion, and instead keep it 'on the inside'.

6. **Settling** – as some emotions begin to pass, it can feel that this happens quickly and smoothly. We can feel ourselves settling from this experience relatively easily. In contrast, other emotions can have a longer half-life, and seem to go down like a bad meal.

7. **Regulate** – during the above process, some people feel that they are able to guide, manage and regulate their emotional experience, shaping each aspect in a way that is helpful given the context, situation or goal. Others feel like the emotion is entirely in charge, that they are at best an observer, along for the ride.

Although we'll come back to these ideas in Section Four, you might start to think about how each of the domains functions for you. So, if you took three emotions to begin with – anger, anxiety and excitement – you might consider the following questions:

1.   How easily are they triggered? What types of things tend to trigger them?

2.   How often (frequently) do you experience them (e.g. hourly, daily, weekly . . . less often?)

3.   When you encounter them, how intensely do they turn up? Low, medium, high? Do you feel you have much control over their 'volume' once triggered?

4.   When they start, how long do they tend to stay around for? Are you aware of things that might happen that reduce or prolong their duration?

5.   How able are you to act alongside or express each of these emotions, once you're experiencing them?

6.   How long does it take you to settle once an emotion arises? What helps each emotion to settle?

7.   How much do you feel able to guide the above steps, managing your emotions in a way that is helpful for you?

For some of us, there is a high degree of overlap between these domains, and different emotions like anger, anxiety and excitement. However, some of you might have noticed that these processes work in quite different ways for these emotions, and this may be the case if we extended this to other emotions (e.g. sadness, shame, guilt and so on). Key at this stage is that we're learning something about the shape and pattern of our emotions.

What's the difference between emotions and feelings?

The terms 'emotions' and 'feelings' are commonly used, sometimes to mean the same thing, other times to mean something slightly different.

Although not agreed by everyone, one way of discriminating them is to consider the different components of emotion that we described previously. Here, emotion affects all of the domains, from physiological through to behaviour and appraisal. Feelings, on the other hand, are the conscious, subjective awareness – the mental experience – of a physical state which we could describe in some way, and may or may not represent an emotion. When we say 'I feel crap', 'I feel awful' or 'I feel great', these are examples of a feeling, rather than an emotion (which we might think of as the entire experience). In comparison, while emotions make us feel something, they also make us want to do something (Frijda, 1986). You may notice this with phrases that are used to describe the action tendencies of an emotion: in anger, we can be 'hopping mad', 'lose our head' or want to 'blow our top', we can 'hang our head' in shame, and be 'flooded with tears' in sadness.

What's the difference between emotions and moods?

These are also terms that are often used interchangeably. In lay language, an 'emotional' person is often seen as someone who is quite reactive to a particular situation. For example, Paul was described by his friends as very 'emotional' – when positive situations occurred, he would often get very excited and happy and be the 'life and soul of the party', but when some slightly negative things happened, he would fly off in a rage. In comparison, a 'moody' person is seen to have a similar response (often negative, but not always) regardless of the situation itself. For example, Daniel was described by his friends as 'moody', a 'glass half empty' kind of guy as he tended to see the negatives, even in positive situations. Another way of thinking about the difference between emotions and moods is in terms of the duration of the experience. On the whole, emotions are seen as fleeting or passing experiences, whereas moods are seen as more persistent, and longer lasting, in nature.

Are there some emotions that are healthy or good, and some that are unhealthy or bad?

While classifying our emotions as 'good or bad', 'healthy or unhealthy' is common and understandable, it can be unhelpful. For example, although typically happiness and joy are seen as healthy and helpful emotions, can you conceive of when these might be unhelpful? A classic example would be if such 'positive' feelings persist (or stay 'online') when they are not warranted. Imagine that you are having a lovely meal with a good friend or loved one. You're particularly enjoying your main course, and the red wine is just divine! Suddenly there's a commotion, and you look up to see a man holding a knife, shouting that he wants your money, mobile phone and valuables. But rather than get anxious, you're still focused on the pleasure of your experience; after all, the wine and food are just so tasty! Although somewhat extreme, if our positive emotions stay online like this, this could be unhelpful or even dangerous. This can happen when people experience hypomania or mania, which are extended periods of elation and energy. Similarly, if our negative emotions stay online when they don't need to be, this can also cause problems. For example, in an intimate, sexual moment with a new partner, if high levels of anxiety kick in and persist, it is likely to get in the way of a potentially pleasurable and connecting experience.

So, we can begin to see here that while emotions have the potential to be helpful, it doesn't mean that they always are. In fact, there can be several reasons why we hit difficulties with our own (and others') emotions. We are going to spend more time together in the next chapter looking at just this – how we can get caught up in difficulties with our emotions. But, for now, the key thing is to return to the idea that it is the context in which our emotions occur, how quickly they are activated, how long they last, and our ability to manage them, that bears upon whether they are helpful or unhelpful.

Key reflections

- Emotions bring colour and energy to our life – without them, life would be stripped of meaning

- It's not easy to give a simple definition of emotions

- Emotions are multi-faceted – they emerge bringing changes to our physiology, attention, thinking, feelings, behaviour and motivation

- Emotions tend to have a 'story' – various processes such as triggers, intensity and duration

- Emotions are not the same as moods, and are neither good or bad

2   Why do we have emotions?

In the previous chapter, we explored what emotions are, how we might define them, and how they involve a patterning of different components. All this leads to an important question: why do we have emotions in the first place? Why, as a species, do we experience emotions like happiness, joy and excitement that can feel *so good*, but others that can cause us (and other people) so much pain, distress and suffering? How does having the ability to experience anxiety or anger contribute to our lives, other than bringing pain and distress?

Something I frequently hear from my patients is a version of: 'Life would be so much easier if I didn't have to feel anything.' While this is understandable, given how painful emotions and feelings can be, it can be a useful place to start thinking about why we experience emotions. Let's look at this with a thought experiment.

Thought experiment: Life without emotion

Let's imagine that we didn't have emotions or feelings; that we were like Mr Spock from *Star Trek*, or an android in a science-fiction film. What would life actually be like? Let's explore this through a number of scenarios:

- Imagine being indifferent to whether you were in a caring or abusive relationship.

- Imagine feeling unconcerned whether you completed a task, or succeeded in a job interview.

- What would it be like if you felt unmoved about whether a friend or loved one was healthy, or suffering from painful illness, or facing death?

> • What would it be like to feel nothing while seeing someone treat your child or loved one in a really unpleasant or unfair way?
>
> • Imagine not having any feelings about seeing a speeding car racing towards your daughter or son?

What ideas came to mind in that short experiment? Often when looked at like this, living life without emotions may not seem very attractive at all – in fact, living without emotions strips life of many of the things that we find *meaningful*. Without them, we would likely be apathetic and unresponsive; unmoved by life's pleasures, ills, and everything else in between. However, with them comes purpose; with them comes energy, need and hope. What this experiment may help us to see is that emotions serve an essential *function* in our life. Although it might not always feel like it, emotions are important as a type of signalling system, letting us know how we're getting on, whether our needs are being met, or whether there's something not working out quite right. They help to give us information between what's happening in the world around us, and the impact this is having on us. The tricky thing is that, because some emotions are painful, scary or overwhelming, we may try not to look at them. If this happens, we may find it difficult to listen to what they're telling us; we struggle to read their signals. So, although they can be challenging to experience and work with, as we'll come on to see throughout this book, the skill with working with emotions is learning how to experience them so we can listen to what they're telling us. When we are able to do this, we can then use emotions to respond to what's happening in our life in a way that's helpful for us.

Let's look at this idea further.

Emotions evolved to help us

One way to understand why we experience emotions is to look at the reasons they evolved in the first place. We can start this by comparing emotions – and particularly those that cause us distress – to physical pain. Let's take an example. Imagine you are looking forward to a nice hot bubble bath after a long, stressful day at work. You've put your favourite music on, and have a glass of wine by the side of the tub. You take your clothes off and slide your right foot into the water. Suddenly, you experience intense, excruciating pain, jump backwards shouting and swearing, hopping up and down on your other foot! Of course, you hadn't realised that the cold tap wasn't on correctly, and the bathwater is far too hot. So rather than experiencing the anticipated pleasure, you're now in pain, and maybe even feeling angry (at the 'water' for hurting you, or at yourself for not having paid better attention). While the feeling of pain is very unpleasant, and not something that you 'wanted', it also has an important function – it alerts your body to make a rapid response, to move away from the source of the pain. It protects your body from long-term damage – in this case, scalding. Take a moment to consider what would have happened if you didn't experience pain at that moment (which is actually the case for some people born with a rare and unfortunate genetic condition called congenital analgesia that prevents them from experiencing pain). Without pain, you wouldn't register that the water was too hot for your body, and likely to cause you a lot of damage.

We can see here then that pain evolved to signal to an organism – in this case, us – to stay away from things that could cause physical damage or death. From an evolutionary perspective, individuals who were more pain-sensitive may have had better survival chances. When this is coupled with the ability to learn and make associations of what is, and what isn't, painful, it can provide helpful information about what we need to be cautious about, or avoid.

So, what does this example have to tell us about why we experience emotions? Well, just like physical pain, emotions evolved to provide *adaptive advantages* to us. In the language of evolutionary theory, adaptive advantage describes how an animal is able to respond most effectively to its environment, which, as a result, increases its prospect of survival (e.g. by being able to run quickly, hide, or find food), and its likelihood to reproduce and, ultimately, pass on its genes successfully. So how do emotions help with this?

Emotions serve our motives

What this metaphor of pain helps us to understand is that emotions are bound up in and with our motives. Simply put, motives refer to the things that we want to do or achieve. The word itself comes from the Latin word *'motivus'*, which means 'to move' or 'moving'. Motives evolved in animals to move them towards certain biosocial goals, for example, survival and reproduction. We share basic motives with all other animals – for example, to avoid harm, and to approach resources (e.g. food, reproductive opportunities). But as mammals, we also have motives linked to caring and being cared for, group living, cooperation and competing for resources and social position/rank. So, some of our motives are non-social, such as harm avoidance (e.g. avoiding a falling rock or dangerous animal) or seeking food or shelter. Others are socially based (e.g. reproduction, attachment, social competition), and often involve more complex processing systems which need to track the flow from self to other, and then back from other to self (Gilbert, 2015).

If we didn't have motives (that is, we didn't have any drives, urges or wishes), then we wouldn't have emotions – we just wouldn't be bothered about anything. So, this helps us then to see that we often experience emotions in the pursuit of things that are important to us, or when our motives have been blocked or thwarted in some way. We will return to this later in the chapter.

What are the functions of our different emotions?

In Chapter 1 we outlined how emotions help navigate and bridge the gap between our environment and our concerns/goals. It may be helpful now to get a little more specific. What function does an emotion like anger have, or sadness? What about anxiety or joy? Let's explore this by looking at some of our common emotions.

Table 1: The evolved function of emotions

Anxiety	Signals potential danger and motivates to engage in a defensive response (e.g. to move, or run away).
Anger	Signals a potential threat to us or others. It may also indicate a block to our goals, or an injustice. It can energise and motivate us to stand up for ourselves and others, and to challenge, be assertive or fight.
Disgust	Signals something harmful or toxic (e.g. rotten food, faeces) and motivates us to stay away from it, or expel it (e.g. be sick) if consumed.
Sadness	Signals a loss of some type, and the need for reconnection or recovery of what was lost. This could be the loss of a loved one (e.g. through death) or temporary disconnection (e.g. the child being left for the first day at school). It can also emerge following a failure or setback (e.g. loss of money or a setback at work).
Happiness/joy	Signals that something is valued or important to us, and moves us towards pursuing goals with rewarding outcomes.
Shame	Signals that our behaviour or actions may lead to rejection or being outcast by others, and motivates us to engage in behaviours to ensure our belonging/that we won't be rejected (e.g. by paying attention to others' responses, or appeasing them).
Guilt	Signals that our behaviour or actions have brought harm to others (or ourselves). It connects us to a type of empathy and motivates us to repair the harm caused, or prevent it from happening in the future.
Contentment/ calm	Signals safeness in the absence of threat or danger, allowing the body to slow down, rest and repair.

So, by looking at the evolved function of these common emotions, we can see that they serve important functions. The list in Table 1 could have been much longer of course, as other emotions such as embarrassment, pride, envy, and jealousy also have important evolutionary functions. The key reflection here is that emotions help us (and of course, originally our ancestors) to navigate situations in life that promote and facilitate survival and/or gaining things (e.g. territory, food, sexual opportunities) and ultimately, opportunities to reproduce and pass on our genes. As we'll return to in Chapter 15, if we can learn to listen to our emotions, we may see that they can provide a type of wisdom about what is happening in our environment. If we're able to couple that with engaging in helpful ways of using emotion – in the way we tolerate them, express them and so on (see Chapters 16a, 16b and 16c) – we're more likely to navigate many of life's challenges skilfully.

One way that emotions help us is by boosting or amplifying our drives, motives or concerns – directing more energy and attention to them. They also help to give primacy of one motive or concern over another (Tomkins, 1970). For example, if you are messing around in the sea, and set a competition with a couple of friends to see who can swim to the buoy quickest, you might well experience a flush of energy, excitement and drive to win. But during the race, if you suddenly see a shark-fin approaching you, it's likely that the fear that you experience would reorientate your focus so that a new concern (self-preservation/safety) predominates over your previous concern (competitiveness, the excitement of winning the race). In other words, emotions help to give prominence to or prioritise one motivation over another – in this case, prioritising safety and survival over competition and winning. As we'll come to see throughout the book, while evolution has built into us a range of powerful emotions, this doesn't mean that we're in the driving seat of them; in fact, the reality is that often we can feel beholden to our emotions, a passenger in their car. We can feel they are too easily triggered or be quite overwhelmed when they turn up, or not know how to turn up or down their 'volume'.

Let's look at a model that helps to explore this link between emotion and motives.

The three system model of emotion

One way to look at this is by exploring the 'three system model' of emotion. This is a simplified model developed by Paul Gilbert (Gilbert, 2009; 2014; 2015) based on some quite complex research on the different types, evolution and neurophysiological basis of our motives and emotions (e.g. Panksepp, 1998; Dupue and Morrone-Strupinsky, 2005). At its heart, the model (Figure 2 overleaf) suggests that we can cluster emotions by what they evolved to help us do (their 'evolved function'):

- Emotions that serve the function of detecting threats and motivating defensive and protective responses or strategies (known as the *threat system*)

- Emotions that serve the function of detecting, energising, seeking and acquiring resources that are useful for survival and reproduction (known as the *drive system*)

- Emotions that serve the function of contentment, calming, slowing down and 'rest and digest' (known as the *soothing system*), and that also play a role in attachment and caring

Let's take a bit more time to explore each of these systems in turn.

The threat and self-protection system

This system – known as the threat system for short – evolved to alert and direct attention to things that are threatening in the world, and motivate a response (e.g. to protect oneself or others, and get to safety). It has a menu of responses. For example, in the presence of a threat, there is a quick-acting physiological response in the brain and body, outside of conscious awareness, that prepares the body to respond. The system has a variety of threat emotions – for example, anger, anxiety and disgust – that urge the body into action, and these can involve a range of behaviours, such as fight, flight, submission or freezing (among others). Our threat systems influence our *attention* (you are more likely to spot negative things), create 'better safe than sorry' forms of *thinking* (e.g. you see

Figure 2: Emotion regulation systems

Three Types of Affect Regulation System

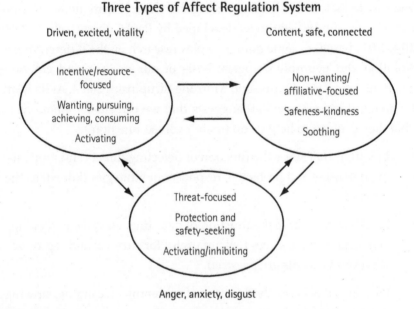

Anger, anxiety, disgust

From Gilbert, *The Compassionate Mind* (2009), reprinted with permission from Little, Brown Book Group

things in black and white ways, focus on the negative and not the positive) and *images* (e.g. you imagine worst-case scenarios).

We also know that the threat system is our most dominant emotion processing system and can powerfully impact what we pay attention to. For example, imagine that you are going shopping for a birthday present for your friend or family member. At the first nine shops you go in to, the shop assistants are very warm, friendly and helpful – they show you where to find what you are looking for and treat you in a kind way throughout. However, in the tenth and final shop, the shop assistant is very rude to you, they ignore your requests for assistance, speak down to you, and generally appear disrespectful and disinterested in you or in helping you. After these experiences, which do you talk about when you get home that night? Even though 90 per cent of your experiences were positive, you naturally pay attention to and re-rehearse threat-based experiences.

Conflicts in threat system emotions

Psychologists and scientists have developed many ideas about how parts of the threat system can get caught up in conflicts, and how these can create problems. This can happen on many levels, but we'll focus on the emotions of the threat system for now. So, if we take anger and anxiety, while it may seem at first that we just experience one of these at any given time, or about any given thing, it's not as simple as these emotions acting in discrete ways. Often, we can experience blends of emotions, in which we're both angry and anxious, or sad and angry, at the same time. We may also recognise that some of these emotions don't get on with each other very well. Let's do a quick exercise to look at this:

Exercise: Anxiety vs anger

Bring to mind a recent situation in which you had both anxious and angry feelings. It might be following a dispute with a colleague in a meeting, or a fallout or argument with a friend or loved one. Take 30 seconds or so bringing to mind the anxious part of you in this situation, what that felt like, what thoughts this part of you had about what was happening. Then take 30 seconds or so to do the same for your angry part. Now, focus on how the angry part of you feels about the anxious part of you and its reaction in the difficulty. What does it feel for the anxious part? Is it happy that the anxious part is there? Does it like the anxious part? Now shift the other way around. What does your anxious part think and feel about your angry reactions to this difficult situation? Does your anxious part like the angry part? Is it happy for anger to have space to do its thing?

Often in this exercise people recognise that these two threat emotions don't get on very well. We'll explore this in more detail in Chapter 16d, but you might have noticed that your angry part was quite contemptuous of the reactions of the anxious part. In turn, the anxious part is often quite worried and fearful about what angry part thinks or wants to do (e.g. lashing out) in a situation. In fact, depending on which threat emotion is stronger for you, this can mean that you even struggle to let in other threat emotions. None of this is our fault – this system is set up to be quite basic in many ways, and as we'll work on later in the book, compassion is about how we can learn to regulate and balance our emotions in a helpful way.

As we'll find out in Chapter 5, and throughout Sections Four and Five, problems with threat emotions – including how they are triggered, how intense they are, how long they last, and their impact on various aspects of life and relationships – are often the reason people seek psychological help, and may well be why you've picked up this book.

The drive-excitement system

This system – often known as the drive system for short – evolved to motivate animals to pay attention to things that are helpful for them (e.g. food, shelter, sexual opportunities) and motivate and energise them into pursuing these. When activated, this system can leave us experiencing positive emotions and feelings such as excitement, joy and elation, which may make it more likely that we engage in similar behaviours in the future. In our brains and bodies, this system is associated with chemicals that are associated with motivation, activation and pleasure.

Here are a few examples of when the drive system might be activated. Remember how you felt when you passed a test or got a good grade in an exam. Or imagine that you've just found out that you've won ten million pounds on the lottery. It's probably your drive system, with a sense of excitement and energy, that grabs you here. It's also likely to be the system that gets activated when your favourite team wins, or when you've been working hard to achieve something with which you're ultimately successful. But it's also this system that's involved in relationships – so imagine that you're seeing some of your best friends tonight, whom you haven't seen for ages; that anticipatory excitement of seeing people we like, and then the joy and pleasure we have upon spending time with them, are all linked to this system too. So, it's these types of experiences that might help you resonate with this system. However, problems can arise with this system if our drives and goals are blocked, or we are striving to achieve these to prevent ourselves from feeling inferior or being rejected – situations that bring the threat system online alongside the drive system.

The contentment, soothing and affiliative-focused system

This system – often known as the soothing system for short – is similar to the drive system in the sense that it is related to positive emotions. However, this isn't a system that gets activated in the pursuit of resources or achievements. While it's essential for animals to be able to respond to threats and be driven to pursue and achieve things, it's also important for them to conserve energy, slow down, and experience periods of calmness and peacefulness that may facilitate rest and recuperation. For this reason, this system is sometimes referred to as the 'rest and digest' system, and is linked to various physiological responses (e.g. the parasympathetic nervous system) associated with calming and slowing the body down.

Over time, it is hypothesised that this system adapted in mammals to be linked to the experience of attachment, caring, bonding and interpersonal connection. In this sense, it may well be that the soothing system is also associated with a 'tend and befriend', caring motivation. This is likely to have initially involved caring for offspring, but there is anthropological evidence clearly showing extended caring (that is, not just to offspring when they are young, and potentially, not just to direct genetic relatives) in many mammals, including ourselves (Spinkins, 2017). From what we understand, this care-based reproductive strategy may be (in part at least) underpinned by neuropeptides like oxytocin and vasopressin, which have also been implicated in mammalian caregiving and receiving, and with bonding and trust (e.g. Carter, 2017).

As we'll come back to explore in Chapter 9, and important for working with difficult emotions, the soothing system has an important role to play in regulating the other two systems. Because the soothing system is linked to the parasympathetic nervous system, which has a powerful role in regulating the sympathetic nervous system (which underpins in part the threat system, as well as the drive system), harnessing this system can be an important focus of the compassionate mind approach. However, rather than being experienced as helpful and grounding, some people don't find activation of this system a source of soothing and contentment. Instead, they find slowing down, resting and receiving care triggers a threat-system response. This may be because they have been taught that resting and relaxing is 'lazy' and bad, and that we should instead focus on being busy and working hard (think of the saying 'the devil makes work for idle hands'). For other people, the environment they live in (or even grew up in) may be quite threat-based, and therefore they have not learned, or do not have the opportunity, to experience the soothing system. And sadly, for some people, there has been an absence of feeling cared for and loved which can mean that the soothing system is associated with difficult, threat system emotions such as anxiety, anger and loss.

Self-reflection: Applying the three system model to yourself

Given what we've been discussing, at this point it might be helpful to think about how these three systems are working *in your life*. To do this, it can be useful to consider the following steps and questions:

1. To start, draw the three systems out on a piece of paper, but with the size of each circle representing how much of that system you experience in life (or how much time you spend in it). How big would each system be?

2. Secondly, for each system in turn (threat, drive and soothing), consider the following questions:

- How often do you experience this system?

- What type of things tend to trigger this system?

- Which emotion(s) do you experience or recognise from this system?

3. Finally, reviewing what you've just done, consider the following questions:

- Is one system triggered more frequently or powerfully than others?

- Is one system – or maybe more than one – not experienced very often?

- Which system may need cultivating so that there's more balance between them?

You may want to do the above exercise on life on the whole, life at a particular time (e.g. in the last week/month), or a specific part of life – for example, what the three systems are like when you are at work, or with friends, or with your family at home. Remember, it's not that one system is bad or good, but that we can sometimes get out of shape or balance with our emotion systems, and when this happens (especially if over a longer period) this can cause us and others distress. We'll return to this model frequently throughout the book, and see how compassion, and compassionate mind training, may help to bring more balance to these systems.

Built for us, not by us

It's important that we hold the insights discussed in this chapter in a broad frame. While our emotions may cause us problems, and be quite painful to experience at the time, they serve important functions linked to survival. In this sense, a theme we'll return to throughout the book is that if you struggle with difficult emotions, *this is not your fault*. You didn't decide to have emotions or choose how they function in you. Rather, you – like me and the other seven billion people on this earth (not to mention countless millions of animals) – have emotions because they were built into our genes over millions of years of evolutionary processes. You, just like me, had no influence over this process. So, it's useful sometimes to hold this insight in mind, as it can help us step back from judgements that we have about ourselves and our emotions, judgements that often add extra weight to something that we're already finding heavy. We'll return to this theme in Sections Four and Five.

Key reflections

- Emotions evolved to serve certain functions, such as avoiding harm, survival, reproduction and caring

- Emotions can be clustered by those that function to help manage threats, those that help us to pursue and achieve things, and those that help us slow down and engage in caring relationships

- We may experience different patterns of activation within these systems

- Sometimes these systems get out of balance, and this may be at the heart of psychological difficulties

SECTION TWO

How and why we struggle with our emotions

3 Evolution and our tricky brain

In Chapter 2, we learned that emotions evolved to serve important functions, and that without them, many things in life would lose meaning. However, we also learned that like many evolved processes, emotions can operate in a way that becomes unhelpful and even harmful to our self and others. There are many examples in nature of how a helpful evolutionary adaptation can also lead to problematic by-products or unintended consequences. Let's look at an example that might help to outline this.

Giraffes born with the gene for a longer neck are likely to have had an advantage over those who weren't, as a long neck helped them to reach leaves in trees that shorter giraffes couldn't. This advantage meant that they were more likely to consume food, and therefore more likely to stay alive, and possibly reproduce and pass on their genes. However, while having a longer neck helps gain access to food, having too long a neck (and legs) also creates problems. If you YouTube a video of giraffes drinking water, you'll see quickly that an essential task like this doesn't come easy for them. Moreover, when they drink they become very vulnerable to attack – they have to angle their front legs and neck to reach down to get the water, which can limit quick responses to danger. So, like other adaptations, evolution can bring solutions to one problem, but can inadvertently leave problems in other areas. Just as our immune system evolved to help fight off infections and pathogens, sometimes it misfires or attacks something that it doesn't need to (e.g. as in certain autoimmune disorders such as rheumatoid arthritis or lupus). It turns out that our emotions may be similar, in that they have essential adaptive functions, but can cause us pain and suffering in a variety of ways. How does this relate to problems with our emotions though?

Our brain has inbuilt glitches

To understand this further, it can be useful to spend some time considering how our brains work, and in particular, how they evolved in a way that can contribute to some of the emotional struggles we experience. We can explore this in the following way:

Old brain competencies

Our brains are the products of hundreds of millions of years of evolution. Some parts – particularly those linked to the brain stem and an area sometimes referred to as the limbic system – are very ancient, and in fact, are structurally similar to those of other animals (e.g. reptiles and mammals) that we have a shared evolutionary heritage with. These old parts of our brain give rise to certain old brain competencies – for example, *behaviours* (e.g. fight-flight system), *motives* (e.g. avoiding harm, seeking food, sexual opportunities, status) and *emotions* (e.g. anger, anxiety, sadness and disgust). Now, it's important to recognise that this is a simplification – the brain is highly complex and interconnected so that one 'area' doesn't specifically control any given ability – but you get the picture.

We have a more recently evolved 'new brain'

Approximately two million years or so ago, our ancestors began to evolve along a line (the genus 'homo') that led to a rapid expansion of cognitive abilities. They began to develop increasingly complex and sophisticated abilities to think, plan and imagine. It was this process that led ultimately to our human intelligence and gave rise to the ability to:

- Imagine things – we can create sensory information inside our minds that may or may not be real

- Be self-aware and self-monitor – we can think about and form judgements about our feelings, and form a sense of an 'I' and self (e.g. I'm a good person; I'm stupid; I'm ugly)

- Plan – we can consider something that is going to happen in the future, play through our minds different conclusions/outcomes, and start to take action/prepare based upon that

- Ruminate – we can cast our minds into the past, playing through memories and reflecting upon our actions, decisions and their consequences

These new brain abilities have allowed us to do amazing things – to write great works of poetry and fiction, to paint, sculpt, and make music, and gain a scientific understanding of the world and universe. We have developed cures for illnesses, learned about our genome, and sent men and women into space. While these new brain abilities are astonishing, under certain conditions, they can also create significant problems for our mental and physical health (Sapolsky, 2004). Let's look at how this works.

Loops in the mind – when new and old collide

Because our new brain abilities for thinking, imagining, ruminating, anticipating and self-monitoring have neuronal connections both to and from the old brain (with its capacity for emotions and basic motives), we can quite quickly get caught up in old brain–new brain loops. These loops can cause us a lot of distress. In terms of our emotions, this means that we can stay 'online' with a feeling, when the initial situation that triggered it is long gone, and the emotion is no longer functional or helpful to us. We can also stay connected with a motive (e.g. harm-avoidance) in a way that other animals could never experience. Let's look at an example of how this plays out:

Imagine a zebra happily chewing away at the grass in the African savannah, when it sees a lion approaching. Understandably, the zebra gets quite anxious and runs away (so, old brain emotions and defensive/protective behaviours kick in, linked to the motive of harm-avoidance). Luckily, this zebra happens to be very fast and manages to get away from the lion. So now the zebra is safe, what do you think it will go back to doing relatively quickly after the threat of the lion has disappeared? Maybe go back to eating the grass again? Now, imagine that you're sitting in the sun outside a café, enjoying some lunch and your favourite drink. Just as you're tucking in and enjoying things, you notice a lion running down the pavement towards the café! Like the zebra, the sight of the lion approaching also stirs up the same old brain responses in you – harm-avoidance, anxiety and flight – and just like the zebra, you manage to get out of the way of the lion by running into the café and locking the door. So now that you're safe and sound inside the café, do you – like the zebra – calm down relatively quickly, and go back to eating your lunch and sipping on your drink? Well, probably not – although if the café has a bottle of vodka, you might turn to that!

So why don't we calm down and go back to eating, as the zebra does? Well, it turns out that because of our new brain abilities (which you don't choose to have of course), we're able to do something that zebras can't – we can keep the threat going even though it has passed. For example, we might start thinking: 'What if it had caught me, and started ripping my limbs off!', or 'What if it's still out there ... how am I going to get back to work on time!' or even, 'I've heard they hang out with other lions – I wonder whether the other ones are.' In each of these scenarios, our capacity to think and imagine (which in this situation is being shaped by old brain anxiety) is directed towards 'worst-case scenarios' and 'what ifs', and these can operate to keep the threat going, re-stimulating the old brain emotion of anxiety. So, for humans, our new brain abilities can work in such a way that a previous external threat is now internalised – brought inside our minds – and this can keep the threat going. In terms of our emotions, it means that we can continue to be caught up with anxious feelings, even though the threat has long past.

While it's fair to say most of us don't have to deal with the threat of lions on a day-to-day basis, we do have to navigate a variety of other situations that are threatening to us – for example, building and maintaining relationships; handling rejection and failure; trying to compete with other people. These – and many other situations – can all lead to the emergence of thinking-feeling loops. You might have experienced this when lying in bed at night, feeling anxious and worrying about a talk or meeting you need to go to the next day. Or lying on a beautiful beach on the first day of your holiday, but finding yourself caught up with anger, ruminating about how your boss spoke to you in a disrespectful and demeaning way in a meeting a few days earlier.

Figure 3: Old and new brain competencies

New Brain Competencies

Imagination, Planning, Rumination, Worry,
Self-awareness

Old Brain Competencies

Motives (e.g. for caring, competition, harm-avoidance)
Emotions (e.g. anger, anxiety, sadness, joy)
Behaviours (e.g. fight, flight and submission)

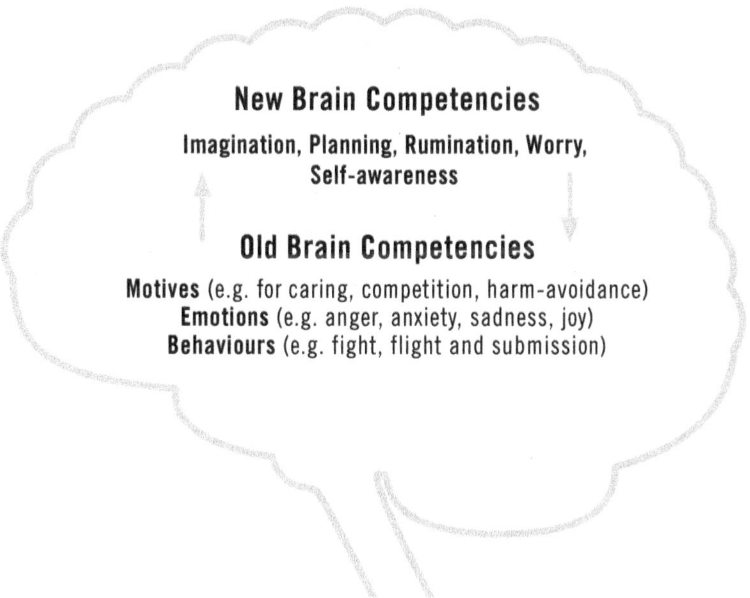

While the capacity to consider events that haven't happened yet, or those that have passed, might have brought adaptive advantages to our species (e.g. by allowing us to learn from mistakes, or prepare for upcoming difficulties), it can mean that some of us get stuck with particular emotions like anger, anxiety and shame. It's unlikely that these emotions were initially evolved to work in this way, and various problems can occur when this plays out in our life. Let's take a look at an example of how this can lead to or maintain difficult emotions:

Example 1: Hassan was lying in bed, feeling tired and ready to fall asleep. Suddenly, a memory came to mind from earlier in the day, when he was telling a story to some colleagues who he'd gone for some food with after work. An image came into his new brain of his colleague's faces looking bored when he was telling the story, which, lying in bed at 11pm now, gave him a flush of anxiety in his old brain. This, in turn, led to various new brain thoughts, such as: 'People don't like me, they think I'm boring,' and 'They won't invite me to come next time.' Rather than getting a restful night's sleep, for the next couple of hours, Hassan was trapped in a variety of loops in the mind, all of which heated up unpleasant emotions like anxiety and shame.

Figure 4: Some of Hassan's loops drawn out

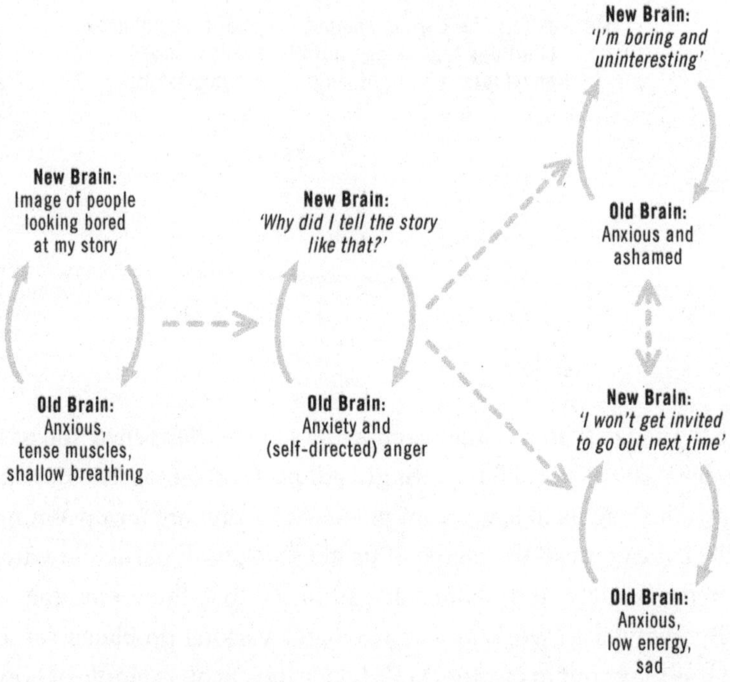

New Brain:
'I'm boring and
uninteresting'

New Brain:
Image of people
looking bored
at my story

New Brain:
'Why did I tell the story
like that?'

Old Brain:
Anxious and
ashamed

Old Brain:
Anxious,
tense muscles,
shallow breathing

Old Brain:
Anxiety and
(self-directed) anger

New Brain:
'I won't get invited
to go out next time'

Old Brain:
Anxious,
low energy,
sad

Example 2: Kate was checking Facebook when she saw a picture of a group of close friends out for a meal together. Next to the picture it read: 'Such an amazing night; great food, and best mates back together again.' As Kate saw the post, she had a flush of feeling left out, uncared for and sad: 'How come I wasn't invited?', and 'Why did I get left out again?' After a while, this shifted to a different, anger-based loop: 'Typical – they're so thoughtless about these things, what sort of friends are they anyway, proper friends wouldn't do this.' Kate was caught in this loop for a while, so much so she put a response to the picture of Facebook saying: 'Thanks for the invite, I don't like that restaurant anyway.' After an hour of no one responding to her post, she then shifted from anger into a different type of loop: 'What's wrong with me? Why don't people include me in these things?' and 'I'm such an idiot, why did I post that message, I've just made it worse now.' Understandably, this left her feeling low in mood, anxious and ashamed. Figure 5 shows Kate's loops drawn out.

Figure 5: Some of Kate's loops drawn out

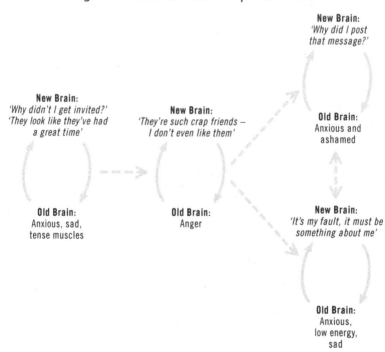

New Brain:
'Why did I post that message?'

New Brain:
'Why didn't I get invited?'
'They look like they've had a great time'

New Brain:
'They're such crap friends – I don't even like them'

Old Brain:
Anxious and ashamed

Old Brain:
Anxious, sad, tense muscles

Old Brain:
Anger

New Brain:
'It's my fault, it must be something about me'

Old Brain:
Anxious, low energy, sad

Self-reflection: Given what we have been discussing about the 'loops' that can form in our minds, it can be helpful to consider the common loops that you experience. What loops do you get caught in that are linked to unpleasant or painful emotions? Maybe you get caught in thinking about and judging your own emotions (e.g. blaming yourself for feeling like you do, or feeling that you shouldn't be experiencing the emotion you are)? Or maybe you worry about being too anxious or angry in a particular situation? Or maybe you recognise that you often get caught up in rumination and self-criticism about previous things you've done or said, and that this stirs up anxiety, shame or (self-directed) anger.

If it helps, draw out your own old brain–new brain loops on a piece of paper, a bit like Hassan and Kate did.

Loops in the mind – not our fault

An important aspect of the compassionate mind approach is to recognise that these 'loops' between your new brain and old brain are not your fault. In fact, it's no one's fault that this happens; we didn't choose to have brains that could get caught up in this way. Moreover, I'm guessing that at no time have you woken in the morning and thought: 'I know what I'll do today, I'm going to start focusing in my new brain on all the things that are wrong with me in life, and that will then start to stimulate my old brain emotions of sadness and demotivate me. And then because the old brain can influence the way I think, I'll start to focus on how hopeless everything is…!' Like me, rather than wanting and planning to engage in these types of loops, we often just find that our minds start to operate in this way. We can see then that quite a lot of what goes on in our mind is not of our choosing – it's a little like it has a mind of its own! But seriously, the realisation here is that our minds are vulnerable to this type of thinking-feeling loop, that this can often operate in the background of conscious awareness, and can drive quite a lot of further distress and difficulties for us.

Loops in the mind – what can we do?

Just because it's not our fault that we get caught in mind loops, it doesn't mean that it's compassionate just to allow them to continue without trying to do something helpful with them. In fact, self-compassion involves learning how to take responsibility for things we struggle with in life. So, in Chapter 8 we're going to explore how working with attention training and mindfulness may help you to notice these thinking-feeling loops, and learn what we can do to step out of them. First, we need to think a little more about other factors that tend to shape how our emotions work.

Key reflections

- Our minds and bodies emerged as part of the flow of life, designed by evolution for survival and to reproduce

- We have relatively 'new' abilities for thinking, imagination, planning and self-monitoring

- We naturally get caught up in loops in the mind, and this can drive problematic experiences with our emotions and feelings

- Much of this has been designed for us, and not by us – it's not our fault, but we have a responsibility to work with it to alleviate emotional struggles

4 Emotions are shaped by life experiences

There are lots of different ways to think about or describe ourselves. For example, some people see themselves as a particular type of person – confident, happy, anxious, angry. For others, there's not a clear description, and instead, just a sense that 'I'm just "me"'. An important insight within the compassionate mind approach is that whatever sense of 'identity' we may or may not have, much of this will not have been through our choice. The way we see ourselves – and often the way we see others – is likely to have been shaped by many things that we had little control over. Crucially, the way our emotions work, and any struggles we have with them, are also likely to have been shaped by things we've had little control over. Let's have a look at this in more detail.

Although you probably don't know anything about my background, imagine for a moment that rather than being brought up by my parents and family, I was instead abducted as a three-day-old child by a couple who were part of a violent drug gang. Imagine that as a child, I saw my parents do some pretty terrible things; I witnessed them being violent to others, hurting each other and sadly, that they both were physically abusive to me. Imagine that I didn't receive any encouragement to pursue things that I might enjoy in life, and didn't receive any warmth, love or affection. If this had been my upbringing, do you think I'd be exactly the same version of me that is typing these words now? Well, it's improbable, as the version of me that's typing at the moment was shaped and influenced by all the things that I've been through: my parents, my family, my friends and my experiences in life. If I'd had different experiences and relationships in life (even with the same genes), *I would be a different person.* You might also begin to imagine not only what type of person I might be, but also how my emotions might operate. Maybe I'd be someone quick to anger, and once angry, could say and do some quite unpleasant things to others? Or maybe you could imagine that I could be quite an anxious person, and have learned to stay out of people's way, keep my head down and behave in very passive ways in life. In each case, you might see that these emotional repertoires and strategies make sense – they serve to try to protect me and keep me safe.

Consider another scenario, this time using yourself as the example. Rather than being brought up in your house, with your parents, caregivers or family, imagine instead that you were raised by your next-door neighbours, in their home. Spend a moment thinking about this, as best as you can do with what you know about them. Now, try to consider that, if this was the case, how might you be different as a person today? Think about how your personality, your beliefs, politics or religion, and even the things that you enjoy doing as a person, might be different.

Of course, we can never know for sure how you would be if you were raised by your neighbours, but what we can know is that you would be a different person to the one that is reading this book today. And in terms of the difficult emotions you struggle with, can you imagine that this might be different if you'd had a very different set of life experiences? The version of you reading this book today is dependent upon the experiences you've had in life, but so many of these experiences are those that you had little control over (such as what type of house you were raised in). Change those experiences, and you'd be a different person – there would be a *different version* of you in the world, with a different experience of your emotions. You can extend this exercise if you like. Rather than imagining being raised by your next-door neighbour, instead imagine being raised in a different part of the town you live in, or a very different part of the country (e.g. in the countryside if you were born in the city, and vice versa; or being raised in a wealthy area if you were raised in a poor one and so on). You may even want to imagine being raised in a completely different country to the one you were. In each of these, you're using your imagination to lead to certain insights about yourself – that this version is just one of many that could have been.

Difficult emotions – shaped for us, not by us

What these examples move us towards is an understanding that much of our sense of self – the way we think about ourselves, the way we behave, the type of emotions we may or may not struggle with – *is shaped for us, not by us*. There could be thousands of different versions of us in the world today if we'd been through different events and experiences in life. So, the difficulties you might have with your emotions – or more broadly, your sense of self – is just one version of you that emerged in the world. If you'd had a different set of experiences in the past, there would be a different 'you' reading this, who might have a very different type of relationship with their emotions.

How have your emotions been shaped?

These examples can also help us to understand how our emotion systems have been shaped. Let's take a moment to return back to the idea of the three system model of emotion that we outlined in Chapter 2. If you remember, we discussed how this model describes three basic emotion-motive systems – threat, drive and soothing. While these systems are evolutionary shaped and biologically rooted, they are also open to learning and shaping processes linked to the experiences and environments that we have grown up in. Let's spend a bit of time exploring how each system might be sensitised in more detail.

Threat system emotions

While the threat system (and the emotions that come with it, like anger and anxiety) evolved to protect us, it can also create many problems for us. In fact, many relationship problems, mental health problems and conflicts in the world are linked to difficulties with this system. This is because the threat system was designed for quick, rapid and 'rough and ready' responses, rather than for fine-grained thinking and decision-making. Here's an example. Imagine having a lovely walk in a wood or forest. As you step over a log, you notice an object on the path that looks like a snake. Automatically, you quickly jump backwards. Now it turns out that on second look, this was an unnecessary response – it's only an old piece of rope, so nothing to bother about. However, your mind cannot afford to take the chance *not to respond like this*. Rather than reacting quickly and jumping backwards, if you instead reacted with 'That's strange, I've walked on this path hundreds of time, and never seen a snake' or 'I wonder if this is a poisonous snake or a different type . . .', it's likely the time taken to work out the answer could leave you in big trouble if there was a snake, especially a poisonous one. This threat-based, 'better safe than sorry' approach is designed by evolution to keep us safe. It's likely that species that were able to respond in this self-protective way to dangerous situations were more likely to survive and pass their genes on. But we end up paying the price for this 'better safe than sorry' thinking. In modern-day contexts, where survival threats might be less pervasive, our minds continue to operate in the same way with thoughts that might be illogical, unrealistic and ultimately unhelpful. It's this sensitivity to overestimating danger and threats that can lead to major problems with anxiety. It's useful though to recognise that our brains are designed to make these mistakes – it's not our fault, but it can get us into problems in our lives and with our emotions if we don't become aware of this and learn to work with it.

But it's not just that our threat systems are designed to be non-rational, 'better safe than sorry'-based – they are also highly sensitive to learning and shaping through experiences we encounter in life. So, while we all have threat systems, the *type* of threat systems we develop is greatly dependent on the kind of experiences we have in life. It might be that for some of us, our threat systems become more sensitive and reactive because the environment we live in (e.g. an area affected by war or sectarian violence) *is* very dangerous. There are also specific processes that shape this. For example, one process is called body learning, or in psychology speak, classical conditioning. Some of you might have experienced this without realising. For instance, if you've had a fish curry that made you quite sick afterwards, or drank a few too many glasses of cider, or whisky and coke (just saying, of course . . . not that this ever happened to me!) and were very sick afterwards, what happens to your body the next time you smell fish, cider or whisky and coke? That automatic flush of nausea is your body remembering – it's likely not to be conscious, but rather an automatic, 'learned' association that 'fish/cider/whisky and coke = pain'.

This classically conditioned process can play out in our relationships, and texture our threat system and its emotions in powerful ways. Charles Ferster – an American psychologist – suggested that if a young child is punished for showing anger to their parent, they may become anxious about being punished. Over time and repetitions of this interaction, anxiety will become associated with anger, to the extent that angry feelings will no longer be consciously processed anymore. In effect, as the child begins to move into angry feelings, they 'flip' to anxiety instead, almost as if this emotion is turning up to protect them (from punishment). Compassion here would be to recognise that it's not the child's fault that this is happening, and in some ways, it's quite helpful to have systems in our body and brain that help us adapt to our environments in this way. However, if later in life they encounter problems in using angry feelings to assert or to stick up for themselves or others, or more generally, feel anxious about getting angry, we would want to help that person learn how to tolerate these fears, understand why they have them, and support themselves to practise and expose themselves to angry feelings again. We'll come back to this idea in Section Four.

So, our threat system and its emotions can get textured by other people. For example, if one of your parents is very emotionally or physically abusive, or you are bullied for years at school, your threat system is learning: people aren't safe, they hurt you, they cause you pain. Under these circumstances, it may be that different aspects of your threat system might be sensitised. For example, it's likely you'll be more attentive to people, including small changes in their voice tone, facial expression or body posture that might signal that they are going to be a threat to you. It might be that your thinking will be influenced in particular ways, such as expecting people to hold bad intentions towards you or holding specific beliefs such as 'people can't be trusted, they always end up hurting me'. Emotionally, it might be that you are primed and quick to respond with anxiety in certain situations, or for others, react with anger and aggressiveness when it appears someone may be threatening to you.

We can also learn certain beliefs about threat emotions; for example, we can get raised in a family in which we're taught that 'big boys don't cry', or that showing fear or anger is shameful. Over time, we may internalise and 'believe' these ideas ourselves. If this happens, we essentially shift to having a threat system reaction to threat system emotions, and this tends to lead to various problems in managing emotions in a helpful way.

Our culture will also affect how the threat system and its emotions operate. For example, researchers have found differences in cardiovascular responses to anger in people from different cultures studying at the same university in Singapore. While Caucasian participants (with European or North American parents, and raised in these countries) showed stronger cardiovascular responses to suppressing rather than expressing anger, Chinese participants (who had Chinese parents and were raised in Asia) showed the opposite physiological profile – stronger cardiovascular responses to expressing anger, rather than suppressing it (Zhou & Bishop, 2012). It's thought this effect is linked to how these different cultures view these emotions, and how much they prioritise the individual or group harmony as most important.

Drive system emotions

If you recall from Chapter 2, the drive system evolved to energise us to achieve things that are important for our survival and reproduction. And when we achieve these, we get a buzz of pleasurable feelings such as joy and excitement. It's because of this 'buzz' (a type of 'positive reinforcement') that we're more likely to want to go out and repeat the process again. While this is essential for our success and survival, if you think about major achievements and excitement you've experienced in life, how long did that last? Often these experiences are quite short-lasting, but because they feel so pleasurable, we are motivated to have them again.

The above is fine when in balance, but just like the threat system, our drive system and its emotions are also influenced by our experiences in life. For many people growing up and living in Western cultures, it's likely the drive system may have been stimulated a lot. This is because Western cultures tend to put a lot of emphasis on the importance of competition, succeeding, winning and pleasure. We're taught that being happy is a good thing, something that we should pursue, and that getting and achieving things (e.g. qualifications, friends, nice clothes, cars) are essential for our self-esteem. The drive system and its emotions can also be shaped by your experiences with your parents, peers, school or workplace. Crucially, our capacity to experience the emotions linked to this system – for example, anticipation, excitement, joy – can be affected by what we learn about whether these emotions are valued or shunned. Let's look at a couple of examples here:

> Asha was brought up by parents who not only worked hard but who took a lot of pleasure from working, trying hard and success. As a child, she recalled her parents encouraging her and her sisters to try out different activities and saw them take great pleasure at exploring new foods, cultures and life experiences more broadly. They took time as a family to look forward to events coming up (for example, the excitement at seeing family members at an upcoming wedding), and to talk about things they enjoyed from events in the past. Positive emotions like these (and emotions generally) were encouraged, and Asha recalled how it felt very natural for her to feel them.

> Steve was in the same class at school as Asha but had a very different experience of drive emotions. He was naturally intelligent, but upon getting good grades or results, would have his pleasure and excitement extinguished by his parents: 'Don't get too big for your boots – it was only an exam,' and 'Don't get carried away with yourself, what happened with the 10 per cent you got wrong?'

At home, things often felt quite constricted, and there was lit-
tle opportunity to laugh, play or look forward to anything. At
Christmas, he recalled his mother telling him that if he didn't stop
talking excitedly about opening presents Santa wouldn't come.
Steve grew up to feel drive emotions were somehow shameful or
indulgent, and that if he allowed himself to get too excited or joy-
ful, something terrible would happen instead.

As you might have noticed, the background experiences of Asha and Steve had a very different impact on their ability to experience and enjoy certain types of positive emotion linked to the drive system. For Steve, drive emotions were associated with the threat system. In comparison, Asha had been brought up to feel safe and at ease with these types of feelings, and in fact, had been encouraged that these were feelings that were healthy to experience and seek out.

Now, it's not to imply that there is anything wrong with competitive cultures, or certain styles of upbringing per se. Rather, it's considering how these can place greater emphasis on aspects of the drive system in comparison to other cultures (e.g. that are less competitive, and more focused on cooperation, content and well-being), and how too much stimulation of the drive system and its emotions can land us in trouble. For example, the buzz of winning a bet, passing an exam, or buying something nice can become quite addictive, so much so that we get caught up in needing to repeat the process again and again, leading to addiction problems. We can get caught up in imagining and daydreaming about future successes and excitement in an anticipatory way, and find that we're not living in the present moment in a helpful way (e.g. 'I can't wait until "x" happens, things will be better then'). For some of us, the striving process of the drive system is bypassed, and the emotions are achieved in a more immediate way (e.g. through pornography or drug taking).

Compassionate mind training involves learning to recognise how our drive systems and their emotions can get caught up in an overly competitive, self-focused, materialistic and achievement orientation. While not our fault, this can be an ongoing fuel to the fire of our threat systems, which are primed to monitor signals of inferiority, failure, defeat and rejection. Compassion involves creating the inner capacity to tolerate the excesses that the drive system can bring, and allow for a healthy, more balanced connection with its emotions. It also means being able to appreciate and savour these positive feelings, rather than immediately searching for the next dose of excitement or distraction. Social media and the internet have created problems for our drive and threat systems in this regard, so we really need compassion to help us work with how our brains are easily overstimulated, and as a consequence, we can struggle with a hangover of difficult emotions.

Soothing affiliative system emotions

In contrast to the drive system and its emotions, the soothing system and its emotions of contentment, peacefulness and calmness are often undervalued and unappreciated in Western societies. As we learned in Chapter 2, this system is more about 'being and non-wanting', rather than striving and achieving. In Western countries, we even have sayings that give an idea about the lack of value this system has, for example: 'the devil makes work for idle hands'. In fact, this idiom also highlights that 'not doing' can be viewed in threat-system-based, negative terms as being associated with being lazy or bad in some way. However, from an evolutionary point of view, it is essential for animals to be able to experience periods of rest, recuperation and slowing down.

In comparison to the threat and drive system, this slowing and resting aspect of the soothing system is underpinned by the parasympathetic nervous system (Gilbert, 2015; Porges, 2007). When people are able to take time out of their busy lives to allow this system to come online, it naturally helps to provide balance to the sympathetic nervous system. Some people grow up in families and societies that actively encourage exactly this, whereas this may be absent for many others. For example, researchers have found that people from Hong Kong valued low-arousal positive emotions more highly than European Americans (Tsai et al., 2006).

However, over evolutionary time and particularly with the emergence of mammals 200 million years ago, this 'rest and digest' system adapted to be linked to forming attachments to other people, and to caring for offspring and vulnerable family members (Gilbert, 2015). It's likely that this was related to the evolution of the neuropeptide oxytocin. Oxytocin has been found to have an important role in moderating the physiology of the threat system (Heinrichs et al., 2003; Uvnäs Moberg, 2013). It is associated with affection, touch and bonding, and has been hypothesised to be important in the emergence of the human nervous system and social behaviour (Carter, 2017). It is because of this evolutionary function that the soothing system and its emotions are so clearly linked to our relational experiences with others. The development of this system is sensitive to signals of care, affection and kindness from other people. For most of us, this takes the form of relationships with our parents or caregivers, but it can also extend to other influential people who are part of our development (e.g. grandparents, aunts/uncles, neighbours and friends). Because this system is experience-dependent (that is, it is linked to needing inputs in the form of care, affection and so forth), its development is contingent upon receiving those inputs from others. Consider another couple of examples below:

> Fahima was the youngest of four children. She was raised by loving parents and lived near to her maternal grandparents and many other relatives. Growing up, she experienced lots of nurturance, affection and care from her immediate and extended family, and described feeling that she was raised by a 'village' of people who had her best interests at heart. When distressed, Fahima felt confident that someone would be available and sensitive to her difficulties, and that more broadly, her family was supportive and encouraging.

> In contrast, Olivia was raised by her father in a small town that they had moved to after her mother had died following a heart attack. They did not know anyone in the new town, and had moved there for a 'new start'. Her father worked hard to raise

her but was so busy that any 'care' he gave her was more about providing food, clothes and heating for the house. He worked very long hours, so much so that from a young age Olivia would leave and return home after school without seeing her father, and would spend long hours on her own. When her father was in the house, he was so tired that he was unable to respond to any difficulties she was having. He did not show any interest in spending time with her or showing any affection or love, but instead, would spend time watching the TV and drinking beer.

You might appreciate that given these experiences, Fahima and Olivia might have entirely different experiences of the soothing system as adults. As you might be able to guess, Fahima described feeling comfortable turning towards and trusting others, but also had an 'internal' sense of safeness and when needed, could soothe her own distress without turning to others. Sadly, Olivia found both of these very difficult. She described feeling anxious about turning to others for support and care, and if someone did express affection or care to her, this would often leave her feeling tense, scared and wary. If distressed, she did not feel able to manage her own distress, but instead tried to suppress her feelings, and often turned to wine or work to numb her feelings.

Caring, attachment and distress regulation

In the middle of the twentieth century, a British psychologist called John Bowlby started to develop ideas that went on to revolutionise the psychology and psychotherapy field, and more generally, our understanding of the nature of caregiving, care-receiving and attachments between parents and children. Bowlby (1988) suggested that evolution created an innate attachment system in the brains of mammals (and therefore humans), in which infants were orientated to seek closeness and contact with caregivers (parents), and likewise, parents were also motivated to be sensitive to the needs, distress and well-being of their offspring.

Bowlby suggested that the attachment system led the parent to provide three important functions to the infant:

- *Proximity seeking*: Here, the child actively seeks out their parent or caregiver, having a desire to know where they are and seek closeness

- *Secure base:* Here the parents' presence and encouragement provide the foundations for the child to move away (physically) from the parent and explore the world around them. You might have noticed infants and young children doing this in a new environment, checking out new sights, sounds and objects to be discovered, while checking that their parent is still available if needed. If the parent left for any reason, the child would likely stop exploring, and become distressed

- *Safe haven:* If the child's threat system is activated and they become distressed, they can move back towards their parent who is available but also sensitive to their distress, offering physical contact, affection, or a reassuring facial expression or voice tone. Essentially, in the language we've been using in this book, the caring actions of the parent stimulates the soothing system in the child's brain and body, helping to gradually turn off the firing of the threat system and consequentially, the child's distress

It is, of course, these types of interactions – an infant's emotional distress being met with signals of care and affection – that form our first examples of our emotions being regulated and managed effectively. Bowlby suggested that over hundreds and thousands of these interactions, the child begins to lay down memories and models in their mind (called working models) that represent a sense of how other people are likely to respond when they're distressed (e.g. caring/loving vs absent or unresponsive). Essentially, the child begins to recognise (non-consciously at first) that when they get distressed, someone will be there to help them. In other words, a representation forms that when I meet my threat system, someone will help to stimulate my soothing system and things will be OK. But it's more than just soothing and regulating threat system-based distress. If you remember, the secure base aspect of the attachment system also links to the parent providing the conditions (e.g. availability, consistency but also encouragement) for the infant to go out and explore the world (drive system), even if they are anxious (threat system). So, you can begin to see that the three systems work in constant interaction.

Of course, all the above is shaped differently if our parents or caregivers are unavailable when needed, respond inconsistently when turned to for support (e.g. are affectionate one time, or not at all the next) or become a generator of threat themselves (e.g. they shout at us, show anger or fear or physically punish us as children for showing distress). In these conditions, the infant's brain becomes confused; there is a biological urge to seek out the parent via the attachment system, but this figure then creates distress, rather than soothing. Under these conditions Bowlby suggested a number of things can happen:

- The child can become more sensitive to the availability, responses and feelings of the parent, needing to monitor and 'check' this frequently, and can be emotionally distressed easily if they perceive an absence of the attachment figure

- The child shuts down to the importance of seeking care from the parent, and over time, becomes more reliant on themselves for support and begins to inhibit signs of distress

These responses are referred to as insecure attachment styles and represent the child's best attempts at trying to manage stressful situations in which there is too much threat system activation and/or not enough soothing system experiences.

In recent decades, research into attachment theory has expanded significantly, and much interest now focuses on how attachment theory has a lot to teach us about how adults manage their distress. Think about it for a moment; when upset or anxious, many adults also turn to others (friends, family members, colleagues) to act as their safe haven and as a way of receiving care, support and reassurance. However, this isn't the case for everyone, and research suggests that insecure attachment styles may persist from childhood (Fraley, 2002) and are associated with maladaptive ways of managing or regulating emotions and distress as adults (Pascuzzo et al., 2015).

How have your emotion systems been shaped by experiences in life?

So, given what we've been exploring, it might be helpful now to think about how your experiences have affected the patterning or your connection to each of the three systems. Take some time to complete the following exercise:

Exercise: How have your relationships shaped your three systems?

Although the three systems are all innate systems that we're born with, we've explored in this chapter how they're all susceptible to shaping through experience. Given this, take some time to think about the following questions:

Threat system

What experiences in life have shaped your threat system and its emotions? What relationships (e.g. parents, friends, partners, work colleagues) come to mind that were associated with your threat system? How did these experiences of relationships impact your threat system? What did you learn about threat emotions (e.g. anger, anxiety) when you were growing up? Were these permitted and validated, or seen as bad, weak or unacceptable for some reason?

Drive system

What experiences in life have shaped your drive system and its emotions? What relationships (e.g. parents, friends, partners, work colleagues) come to mind that were associated with your drive system? How did these experiences of relationships impact your drive system? What did you learn about the acceptability of drive system emotions (e.g. joy, excitement)?

Soothing system

What experiences in life have shaped your soothing system and its emotions? What relationships (e.g. parents, friends, partners, work colleagues) come to mind that were associated with your soothing system? How did these experiences of relationships impact your soothing system? What did you learn about the acceptability of the soothing system emotions (e.g. contentment, calmness)?

If it helps, draw out three circles to represent the three systems on a blank piece of paper, and write down different experiences 'inside' the system that you feel they might be linked to.

For some people, spending time on this can be very illuminating. They are able to see how life experiences have shaped a particular system (e.g. threat), and maybe even a specific part of that system (e.g. anxiety rather than anger). It can also be helpful to see that although pleasurable, there may be understandable reasons why experiencing the emotions linked to the drive system or soothing system may be quite tricky for you.

What can compassion, and CFT, do to help?

In CFT we are interested in how to bring *balance* to these different systems. So, the aim is not to get rid of any of them, but rather, see if we can:

- Understand why they work in the way they do

- Understand how they impact on each other

- Consider ways to reduce those that may be overactive and causing us difficulties (e.g. the threat system)

- Seek to build the soothing affiliative system

- See how developing compassion may bring the systems into greater balance

Of particular interest to us is how developing access to the soothing system (underpinned by the parasympathetic nervous system) may help to manage our difficult emotions. Research has found that the soothing system – both on the level of its underpinning physiology, the feelings associated with it (soothing, calming, safeness) and the experiences that trigger it (e.g. affection and kindness from others) – has powerful regulating effects upon the threat system. Unfortunately, this isn't easy. For some people, slowing down and resting is associated with agitation, and for others, they would quite like time for this but find themselves constantly distracted and stimulated by life – by TV, social media, advertisements, emails, work and so forth. These can rev up the threat and drive system emotions, and actually cut us off from a sense of connectedness and care of each other. Consider a child who is anxious or distressed about something. It is the care, affection and soothing of another (usually their parent) that helps the threat system to calm down. But even as adults, we often turn to someone who makes us feel cared for if we get distressed, upset or anxious. We know that our brains and bodies are highly sensitive to the care and presence of others, and in fact, research has found that we are less threatened by physical pain if we're holding the hand of someone else (Coan et al., 2006). Unfortunately, for some people who have had threatening and complicated relationships with people in life, it's not easy to experience others as calming, soothing agents. In fact, for some of us, other people *trigger* threat emotions – anger, anxiety, shame. So, Sections Three, Four and Five of this book will focus on how we can develop skills that can build the soothing system, and more broadly, a more caring way of relating to ourselves and our emotions.

Key reflections

- This version of 'you' reading this book is just one of many versions that you could have been, and might be in the future

- Although biologically based, the way our emotions and emotion regulation systems function is influenced by our experiences in life, much of which we did not choose

- At times, our emotion system can get out of balance, and be overly dominated by threat and drive system

- Compassion can help to balance our emotions

5 Emotion regulation problems

An umbrella term for some of the types of difficulties outlined in Chapters 3 and 4 is *emotion regulation problems*. Emotion regulation may not be a term that you've heard before, but it turns out that it plays a central role in many of the challenges and struggles we face in life.

What is emotion regulation?

Although emotions are often triggered automatically, that doesn't mean that we're impotent bystanders during the process. Psychologists coined the term 'emotion regulation' relatively recently to refer to our ability (or relative inability) to notice, monitor, understand and modify our emotional responses to meet our goals or follow our motives. James Gross (2015), a psychologist who has spent much of his career studying emotion regulation, suggests it is a process in which people can influence:

• The type of emotions they have

• When they have an emotion

• How they experience an emotion

• How they express or use an emotion

It's likely that you have intuitive knowledge about emotion regulation. For example, have you ever felt very anxious, maybe before giving a speech or going to an interview, and managed to hold these feelings in, and look assured and calm on the outside? Have you ever felt sad and tearful, but stopped yourself crying because you were in a situation (e.g. a meeting) where it wasn't appropriate to express your feelings in this way? Or have you ever felt angry, but stopped yourself swearing or shouting at someone who had treated you disrespectfully?

Each of these situations involves an aspect of emotion regulation – doing something to impact or influence the emotion we're experiencing. In this sense, emotion regulation can include any action taken to influence or change emotions – including those that might be helpful and adaptive, and those actions that prove unhelpful or maladaptive. There is growing evidence that for a variety of reasons, some of us may struggle to manage emotions in an effective way and in fact, do things that actually cause ourselves (and others) more distress and suffering. This is known as emotion regulation problems, or alternatively, emotion dysregulation.

What is emotion dysregulation?

Emotion dysregulation refers to the unhelpful handling of aspects of our emotional experience. Let's take a look at an example: Tom has had a stressful day at work and then got stuck in a long traffic jam on the way home. He finally arrives home at 8pm, tired and stressed. His wife Anaya has been cooking Tom's favourite meal (chicken curry) all afternoon, and as Tom walks in the door, tells him that she is upset as he's taken so long to get home that the curry has dried out. At this moment, given the stressful day he has had, Tom's emotional regulation skills are compromised. Rather than calmly apologising and showing his empathy for how her hard efforts to cook have been thwarted, and explaining what made him late (the traffic jam) and his tough day, he instead shouts: 'Typical, I can't even have a minute to take my coat off before you start at me! I don't even like your bloody curries anyway.' As you can imagine, this leads to a big argument, and Tom storms out of the house and heads to the pub.

How can we understand this example in terms of emotion dysregulation? Well, we can see that Tom:

- Struggled to recognise that his experiences in the day were impacting upon his emotions

- Seemed to lack an awareness into what emotion (e.g. anger) was present

- Seemed to lack an awareness that his anger was influencing his thinking and actions (e.g. shouting)

- Was unable to understand how his wife might be feeling, and try to adjust his response in a caring and supportive way

- Was unable to find a way to manage (regulate) his anger so that he could recognise feelings of stress and unhappiness from the day he had just experienced, rather than shouting at his wife and criticising her food

We all struggle to regulate our emotions from time to time, so this is not a weakness or something to beat yourself up about. In fact, I struggle to regulate my emotions on a regular basis! Here's a recent example. Yesterday, before writing this part of the chapter, I was unable to regulate my emotions after being woken late in the night by noisy neighbours. Rather than going out and speaking to them assertively, I ended up lying in bed, awake, struggling with a mixture of anger and fear, for over an hour. Finally, my anger captured me, and I ended up going out and shouting at them and generally causing a bigger fuss than was necessary. Afterwards, when I was back in bed, I found it difficult to step back from my angry feelings, and continued to ruminate about why the neighbours had done what they had done. I had various thoughts ('Don't they know I have to get up early tomorrow and write my book?') and judgements about what I should have done ('Why didn't I tell them that I'd call their landlord . . . that would have made them listen'). My heart rate remained high, my muscles tense, and my threat system very active; it took another 2 hours or so to fall back to sleep.

The point here is not that we struggle to regulate our emotions, but whether we can notice when this is happening or has happened, try to do something about it at the time (if we can), or if not, learn from it and try to bring a different, more helpful way of dealing with things in the future. There have been many psychological theories about emotion regulation, along with tens of thousands of research papers. Below we're going to explore a model of emotion regulation that we'll continue to use throughout this book.

Difficulties in regulating emotions – the emotion regulation model (ERM)

In the face of intense emotion, many of us can struggle to cope. There are many ways this can play out. At times, like Tom and the example of my noisy neighbours, we may get caught up or lost in our emotions, so much so that the emotion 'runs the show' (e.g. our behaviour, actions, thoughts). At other times, we may try to stop ourselves from feeling, maybe by trying to force the feeling down or control it, or by suppressing thoughts and memories related to difficult emotions. Some of us may try to distract ourselves (e.g. by watching TV), or by 'doing' something rather than staying with the feeling (e.g. cleaning, shopping, working), or by numbing our feelings – for example through drinking, or taking drugs. On other occasions, we may try to protect ourselves from problems occurring in the future (for instance, by worrying about things that might happen and trying to come up with solutions), or solve past mistakes (by churning over and ruminating about why certain things happened, or why we acted in the way we did). Compounding this struggle in coping with difficult emotions, is often a tendency to blame others for this dysregulation, and/or beat ourselves up for not coping, or getting too emotional.

Research studies have highlighted a number of emotion regulation strategies (e.g. rumination, avoidance and suppression) which, while fine when used sparingly, can lead to increased distress, unhappiness and interpersonal problems when used in a more generalised way of managing emotions. They also seem to be linked to a variety of mental health problems, including depression, anxiety disorders (e.g. social anxiety), borderline personality disorder, eating disorders and psychosis (e.g. Aldao, 2010).

There are many different models of problematic emotion regulation. In this book, and the Compassionate Mind approach, we pull some of these ideas together in a simple model which outlines five aspects of the emotion regulation process that we can struggle with. This is not meant to cover all aspects of emotion regulation, just some of the main ones that have an important bearing on the experience we have with emotion:

1.   Awareness of triggers

2.   Awareness of emotions

3.   Labelling of emotion

4.   Understanding emotion

5.   Coping with and using emotion

This model is displayed visually in Figure 6. We will explore this by taking each step in order, but it's not to say that emotion regulation always needs to, or even could follow this linear, step-by-step sequence. The arrows pointing in both directions highlight that this is not a linear or sequential way of conceptualising the difficulties we have with managing our emotions, but rather an interactive process. We'll use the example of Kirsty (see box overleaf) to help illustrate the types of difficulties that would reflect each step of the model.

Figure 6: Emotion regulation model (ERM)

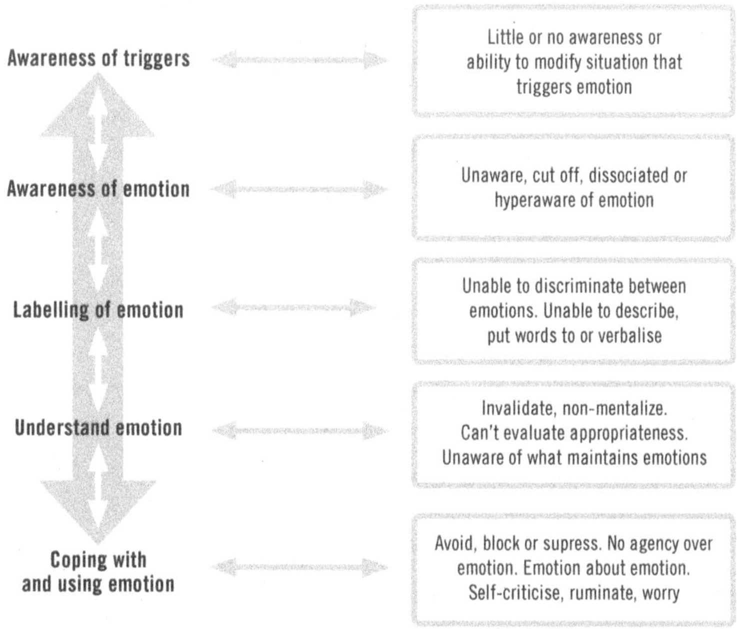

Awareness of triggers	Little or no awareness or ability to modify situation that triggers emotion
Awareness of emotion	Unaware, cut off, dissociated or hyperaware of emotion
Labelling of emotion	Unable to discriminate between emotions. Unable to describe, put words to or verbalise
Understand emotion	Invalidate, non-mentalize. Can't evaluate appropriateness. Unaware of what maintains emotions
Coping with and using emotion	Avoid, block or supress. No agency over emotion. Emotion about emotion. Self-criticise, ruminate, worry

Example: Emotion dysregulation

Kirsty, a twenty-five-year-old woman from London, worked in a junior position in a management consultancy firm. She had been involved in a difficult project with a team of colleagues, including her boss, a very charismatic and confident presenter. They were working towards pitching for a potentially lucrative contract, and her boss was due to lead on the presentation. Two days before it was due, Kirsty's boss told her that she would have to make the pitch instead, as he had decided he was going to go on a last-minute golfing holiday. Kirsty always experienced anxiety when public speaking, and had never given a presentation at work before. She began feeling on edge, unable to concentrate and had difficulty sleeping at night. When asked about how she was, she told her friends and colleagues that things were 'fine', but that she was feeling 'a bit run down'.

1. Awareness of emotional triggers

When we are aware of what is currently happening in our environment, or what might be emerging in the hours or days ahead, we may be able to start navigating these situations in a way that helps manage emotions that might naturally occur as a consequence. So just like checking the weather report might help to prepare us to choose whether shorts, T-shirt and flip flops or a big coat, boots and an umbrella are the most appropriate clothing, so too can we take this approach to the circumstances that may lead to our emotions. However, a problem that some people face in managing their emotions starts with a lack of awareness that a situation is about to arise, or is currently happening, that might trigger or has triggered, an emotional response. This can take the form of a type of 'situational blindness', in which a lack of awareness of emotional triggers may mean that we lack the ability to take early steps to do something helpful about this. There is an aspect of self-awareness that comes at this stage, linked to an understanding of ourselves and our personality. For example, you might be OK giving an impromptu talk, if that's something you're used to doing, whereas I might recognise that for me, given my personality or lack of experience in this area, this would be a potent trigger for difficult emotions. But it's not just an awareness of triggers. Step 1 also involves difficulties in modifying situations that have the potential to be emotionally difficult, so that they either don't cause (unecessary) distressing emotions or that the impact of the situation is lessened in some way. Let's look at Kirsty's example here:

> Kirsty struggled to appreciate how the situation she found herself in was a potential trigger for her threat system. She struggled to link how having to give an impromptu presentation was likely to activate stress and anxiety, or hold in mind that giving presentations was something she'd always found hard in the past. Because she did not recognise that this was a potentially difficult situation, she did not hand over another project that she was working on to a colleague who asked if that would be helpful. Moreover, she didn't consider talking about how to approach the speech with more experienced people in her team.

2. Awareness of emotions as they arise

If you have your eyes closed and you're handed a coffee mug, it's likely that you'll know what it is by noticing core aspects of the object (its shape, handle, feel of the material it's made of). But of course, if you've never seen or held a cup before, you wouldn't know what it is – you'd have to learn the different features of it so that in the future you can make that association. It can be a little similar with the shape or characteristics of emotions.

Developing skills in mindfulness, and becoming more aware of how your emotions show up in your body and mind, can improve your ability to deal with them in a helpful way. However, having difficulties in paying attention to, noticing and recognising emotions when they show up can compromise the emotion regulation process. This may involve a lack of awareness of how they show up or arrive with a particular 'pattern' in our bodies. It might also reflect an inability to notice the impulses or urges that come with emotions, or how they shape our minds in particular ways (e.g. that we are paying attention to certain things more than we usually would, or that we are caught up with ruminating or worrying). Other people can struggle at this step in the opposite way, becoming hypersensitive to or fused (overly connected) with different aspects of emotion as they arise. For example, someone might become preoccupied with a physical sensation that they associate with a health problem or panic, and be unable to shift their mind away from this. Let's have a look at Kirsty's difficulty at this step:

> *Kirsty found it difficult to notice her emotions (particularly anxiety) as they arose in her. She didn't notice that her muscles were more tense than usual, or that her breathing was quicker and shallower. She also failed to notice how anxiety had started to shape her new brain into repetitive worrying and imagining 'worst-case scenarios' about the presentation.*

3. Labelling emotions

Researchers have found that when people are able to name or label the feeling they are having – even under unpleasant circumstances like approaching a spider – it can help to reduce stress (Kircanski et al., 2012). In contrast, struggling to discriminate between emotions, and difficulties in being able to describe or verbalise our emotions and feelings, has been found to compromise emotion regulation. Sometimes this type of difficulty has been described as *alexithymia*. Alexithymia is a Greek word which means 'without words for emotions', and describes people who have difficulties in identifying, describing, understanding and expressing their emotions. Research has found that around 5 per cent of women, and approximately 9 per cent of men, may struggle with these difficulties (Kokkonen et al., 2001). People with alexithymia often describe feeling an emotion in general terms – such as feeling 'uncomfortable', 'horrible' or 'bad' – but can struggle to put more descriptive emotional labels to their feeling (for example, they may struggle to label this as 'I feel anxious' or 'I'm angry at the moment'). They might also refer to a physical expression of their experience, for example, 'my stomach is tense' or 'I feel tight', but not be able to describe this in emotion words (e.g. 'I'm feeling anxious'). There have been a number of studies that have found that the more people struggle with either of these dimensions, the more they're likely to experience various emotional and mental health difficulties, including anxiety and depression. Let's return to Kirsty to see how she struggled at this step:

> Rupa, a good colleague, noticed that Kirsty seemed to be out of sorts, and asked her if she was feeling OK. Kirsty responded with confusion: 'I don't understand – what do you mean? I'm just normal.' When Rupa suggested that it would be understandable to be anxious or stressed out given the upcoming presentation, Kirsty replied: 'I don't feel great, but I think I'm probably just coming down with something.' Kirsty was unable to label what she was feeling (e.g. anxiety, tension), or discriminate the difference between feeling anxious and physically unwell (i.e. having a cold).

4. Understanding emotions

Just like a doctor or car mechanic diagnosing a problem with a patient or a car, when we understand what is causing a problem, this can lead to helpful steps for doing something about it. To a certain extent, a similar process applies to our own (or other people's) emotions. However, some people can find this very difficult, and struggle to understand why they're feeling as they are, or tend to think about their emotions (or the situation that led to them) in a way that exacerbates their distress and makes it harder to manage feelings in a wise, helpful way. For example, some people tend to invalidate their emotions, believing that they shouldn't be feeling as they are, or that nothing has happened that would warrant the feeling they have.

Some of the difficulties that arise at this step are sometimes referred to as problems with *mentalization* or *mentalizing*. These words may sound odd but describe an ability that overlaps with terms like empathy, psychological mindedness, and mindfulness. Mentalizing has sometimes been described as the ability to see ourselves from the 'outside', and other people from the 'inside'. It has been defined as a 'form of imaginative mental activity' through which people can imagine and interpret their own or other people's behaviour in terms of intentional mental states (e.g. needs, desires, feelings, beliefs, goals, purposes and reasons; Fonagy et al., 2007; p. 288). When we struggle to mentalize, we find it difficult to understand our own minds, including how our emotions, motives and behaviour are linked, and how these are shaped by different (internal and external) factors. Research has found that problems in mentalizing are associated with increased emotion regulation problems, as well as a variety of mental health problems. Let's look at how Kirsty struggled at this step:

> On the morning of the presentation, Kirsty began to realise something wasn't right with how she was feeling, and took herself to the kitchen to make a cup of coffee. She started to think: 'What the hell is wrong with me? This is stupid, there's no reason to be like this, now, just be happy and get on with things.' She continued to invalidate her unpleasant feeling, and was unable to understand what had led her to be struggling like she was, nor why the feeling wouldn't go away.

5. Coping with and using emotions

While a doctor may understand what is causing a physical health problem, some may be more skilful or competent in how they go about treating the issue than others. There are many ways that we can try to cope with our emotions, and researchers have found that some of these can be quite helpful. For example, if we can tolerate and accept our emotions – even when they are unpleasant – this has been found to reduce how distressing it is to experience them. At other times, listening to what our emotions are telling us about a situation can be used to help to problem-solve or express our feelings in a way that is helpful. However, we may also engage in strategies to deal with our emotions that can make it harder for us to manage them in a wise, helpful way. There are various styles of coping that can lead to problems:

Avoidance, blocking and suppression: for many people, emotions can feel overwhelming and scary. In fact, we can even fear our emotions, so much so that this can interfere with (or block) our capacity to pay attention to, verbalise, express, or manage them in a helpful way. There are different reasons why people can be fearful of their emotions:

- I'll be overwhelmed – for some people, there can be a sense that if they allow themselves to feel or experience an emotion, it would be so powerful or long-lasting that it would overwhelm their capacity to cope.

- I won't be able to control myself – certain emotions (e.g. anger) can generate a fear that we will do something bad or harmful if we allow ourselves to feel them (for example, become violent or hurt someone).

- Other people won't like me – we can fear that if we show a particular emotion or feeling, other people will react negatively (e.g. with anger, or even violence, ridicule, or rejection). There may also be a fear – that may have been shaped through lived experience and/ or through what we've been told about emotions by others – that our emotions might overwhelm or burden others in a way that will change the way they respond to us.

We may seek to block or suppress our emotions in many ways. For example, some people may turn to excessive eating, alcohol, or drug use to quell unpleasant feelings, whereas others may spend money, gamble or use pornography as an escape. Although these strategies are not *always* detrimental, research has found that they tend to cause further distress or even an increase in negative feelings.

Emotion about emotion

As far as we know, no other animal can have emotions about their emotions, or feelings about their feelings. We don't think your pet dog feels anxious about whether they'll get angry with a strange dog they meet on their walk in the park today. We don't think your pet cat gets angry for how they anxiously ran away from the bigger next-door neighbour cat. However, the problem is that we *can* and *do* have these secondary emotional reactions about an initial emotional response. In fact, many of the difficulties we have with managing distressing emotions relate to secondary emotions – emotions about other emotions, or that emerge after the initial emotion. Although we don't choose to have this ability, unfortunately this means we can have a threat emotion (e.g. anger or anxiety) about another threat system emotion (e.g. anger or anxiety). For example, if you'd learned – maybe from your parents, school or broader culture – that anger was a 'bad' or dangerous emotion, you might learn to be quite fearful of your own anger. Unfortunately, while understandable, this is a bit like trying to put out a fire with fire, and tends only to bring more heat. It's possible to have a wide range of emotions about other emotions, but common ones that emerge for many of my clients are *anxiety* (fear), *anger* and *shame*. As one of my patients quipped, this 'unholy trinity' tends to have an exacerbating effect on initial emotions and feelings that were already difficult to manage. But some of us may also have a threat emotion (e.g. anger, fear, disgust, shame) about a drive (e.g. excitement, joy) or soothing system (e.g. calm, content) emotion.

There are different ways of thinking about and measuring whether we're fearful of our emotions, and whether we feel we need to avoid them. One way to do this is to consider the following questions (adapted from a research study by Paul Gilbert and colleagues; Gilbert et al., 2014).

	Not at all like me			Extremely like me	
	1	2	3	4	5
Sadness					
I am frightened of my feelings of sadness					
I am angry about my feelings of sadness					
I am ashamed of my feelings of sadness					
I go out of my way to avoid feeling sad					
Anxiety					
I am frightened of my feelings of anxiety					
I am angry about my feelings of anxiety					
I am ashamed of my feelings of anxiety					
I go out of my way to avoid feeling anxious					
Anger					
I am frightened of my feelings of anger					
I am angry about my feelings of anger					
I am ashamed of my feelings of anger					
I go out of my way to avoid feeling angry					
Shame					
I am frightened of my feelings of shame					
I am angry about my feelings of shame					
I am ashamed of my feelings of shame					
I go out of my way to avoid feeling shame					
Happiness					
I am frightened of my feelings of happiness					
I am angry about my feelings of happiness					
I am ashamed of my feelings of happiness					
I go out of my way to avoid feeling happy					

It might be helpful to take a look through your responses to the questions on the previous page. Which emotion do you most commonly have about other emotions? Which emotion do you feel most fearful of? Which emotion do you feel most angry about? Which emotion do you feel most ashamed about? Which emotion do you try to avoid the most? We'll return to how to help with this in Chapters 16d and Chapter 16e.

Often, if we are fearful, angry or ashamed of certain emotions, we tend to have to put a lot of effort into not feeling these, by *suppressing or avoiding* them in some way. We can do this through different routes:

• Psychologically – for example, by trying hard to battle or push feelings from our minds or by distracting ourselves

• Physically – for example, by staying away from certain situations or people that trigger strong feelings in us

• Physiologically – for example, by drinking, taking drugs, shopping or even hurting ourselves (sometimes known as self-harm)

On one level this makes complete sense – we are trying our best to find ways not to experience something that brings discomfort, pain and suffering. However, it turns out that this avoidance, suppression of, or rigid control over emotions can bring its own difficulties, compounding the initial problem. We will return to these ideas later in the book, in Chapter 16a.

Lack of control of emotion/ability to use emotions: Here, people may find it difficult to modify the intensity or duration of their emotions. Sometimes this is referred to as difficulty in downregulating emotion (when an emotion is experienced strongly), or to upregulate an emotion (when it is blocked or not experienced in a situation in which it might be useful to experience it).

Alongside the inability to modify or have some control over emotions, we may also struggle to know how best to use them in a helpful way. So, in a situation in which anger could facilitate an assertive 'sticking up for ourselves' or protecting someone else who is vulnerable (for example, a situation where your child or partner is being mistreated), we can struggle to use or express our anger in a way that could be helpful. Instead, we might end up feeling frozen or unable to help. Sometimes, if we struggle to use or effectively express our feelings, we can get stuck or trapped with them. An example here might be feeling anxious and caught up in worry, but not knowing how to express this to someone else in a way that might help us to feel supported, to work through ways of dealing with the situation that is causing the anxiety, and so forth.

Self-criticism and rumination: Finally, we can bring new brain abilities (Chapter 3) to our emotions. Commonly this involves self-criticism, worry or rumination. Blaming ourselves and ruminating about why we're struggling with our difficult feelings tends not only to keep the emotion activated inside us, but may also trigger feelings about our feelings – for example, angry about why we're feeling anxious. We know from various research studies that when this happens, it's likely to be more difficult to cope effectively with our feelings and emotions (e.g. Priel & Shahar, 2000).

Let's look at how Kirsty tried to cope with her anxiety:

> *Feeling overwhelmed and tetchy, Kirsty tried to distract herself by checking her emails, an online newspaper, and Facebook. None of these helped her feel better, and she also turned down Rupa's second attempt to talk about what was going on for her. The night before the presentation she drank a bottle of wine by herself (she would only usually have a glass at most). As time passed, she began to become increasingly critical with herself: 'You're so weak and pathetic – no wonder you haven't been promoted for ages.'*

Self-reflection – do you have difficulties with emotion regulation?

Given what we've just been exploring, take a look at the different steps of the ERM model again, and see whether any of the difficulties with these steps sound familiar in any way. It can be useful to identify an emotion that you know you find difficult, or think about a situation that happened recently in which you struggled and had a strong emotional reaction to (for example, a job interview, an argument or a setback or failure of some type). With this in mind, go through each step of the model and see what you learn about your own emotion regulation problems. Sometimes people find it helps to start by focusing on a situation that they felt they handled relatively well, noting whether there were difficulties with any of the steps as they hold this in mind. Following this, it's then helpful to use the model to work through a situation that didn't go so well, in which you experienced difficulties with your emotions. If it helps, make some notes on Worksheet 1 (p. 81).

Remember, it might be that there are variations here across emotions. For example, some people find that one emotion (say anxiety) is relatively easy to be in the presence of, and that they don't really struggle with any of the emotion regulation steps described in this chapter. However, when considering another emotion (e.g. anger or sadness), things become much trickier, and the difficulties with emotion regulation are more familiar. Try to hold this in mind as you reflect on this model.

We're going to return to how we might engage in more helpful types of emotion regulation across each of the five steps discussed in this chapter in Section Four, and in particular, will look to see how someone else (Simone) managed to navigate a similar stressful situation to the one Kirsty was struggling to deal with here. Key at this stage – as has been the focus in this chapter – is the exploration and understanding of aspects of emotion and emotion regulation that you might struggle with at times.

WORKSHEET 1: WHAT PROBLEMS DO I HAVE WITH EMOTION REGULATION?

STEP	DESCRIPTION	DO I HAVE ANY DIFFICULTIES AT THIS STEP? (If so, make notes about what these are)
Awareness of triggers	Little or no awareness or ability to modify situation that triggers emotion	
Awareness of emotion	Unaware, cut off, dissociated or hyperaware of emotion	
Labelling of emotion	Unable to discriminate between emotions. Unable to describe, put words to or verbalise	
Understand emotion	Invalidate, non-mentalize. Can't evaluate appropriateness. Unaware of what maintains emotions	
Coping with and using emotion	Avoid, block or supress. No agency over emotion. Emotion about emotion. Self-criticise, ruminate, worry	

SECTION THREE

What is compassion, and how might it help with my difficult emotions?

Now that we've discussed some of the common difficulties we can have with emotions, and looked particularly at certain types of emotion regulation problems, it's useful to consider how compassion – and developing a compassionate mind – might help with this.

6 What is compassion, and how can it help with difficult emotions?

Given our understanding of the struggles we can have with regulating our emotions in helpful ways, it's important to consider how compassion – and developing a compassionate mind – may help with this. To start with, let's spend some time thinking about what we mean by compassion.

What is compassion?

We began to explore the concept of compassion in the Introduction to this book. Let's take a bit more time on this now. When you hear the word compassion, what comes to mind? What other words pop into your head?

Often people say things like caring, warmth and kindness. However, some mention other words such as pity, weakness or indulgence. As you might be able to guess, given that this is a book on how compassion can help you with your difficulties, I'm not going to suggest that it's anything to do with this second set of words! Actually, often when we are compassionate, we bring many qualities that are *opposite* to pity, weakness and indulgence. We'll come back to this later in the chapter.

There are numerous definitions of compassion, but the one we use in the Compassionate Mind approach is:

A sensitivity to the suffering of self and others,
with a commitment to try to alleviate and prevent it.

Let's spend a little while thinking about this definition, and how we might use it to guide some of our ideas throughout the rest of the book. In CFT we suggest that this definition holds two separate but interrelated psychologies – known as the two psychologies of compassion.

First psychology of compassion – engagement with distress

The first psychology reflects the first line of the definition above, that compassion involves noticing, tolerating, turning towards and engaging with distress (rather than, for example, turning away or blocking our pain and suffering).

There are six core attributes or competencies that contribute to the first psychology of compassion. We'll explore them using the example of Anita:

> *Anita came to therapy as she was struggling at work and in her marriage, and because she was feeling depressed. As we explored these difficulties, it became clear that she found it hard to articulate various aspects of her emotional experience. She described having come from a family who never talked about emotions, and recalled being told by her mother, 'Don't show your emotions, it makes you weak and vulnerable.'*

Care for well-being (motivation)

Developing a compassionate mind starts with a basic motivation to be caring and interested in well-being – whether that is someone else's, or our own. So, with a compassionate mind comes an intention and desire to be caring, to try to be helpful and find ways to alleviate distress. Unfortunately, when we struggle with emotional difficulties, our threat system can block or shut down this motivation.

> *Anita recognised that she rarely took care of herself, and instead, would often work extremely long hours and get very little sleep at night. To care for her well-being would mean acknowledging that*

there was something wrong, which in turn would bring vulner-
ability, anxiety and shame. Coming to therapy had taken a lot of
effort and courage on her part, but was an initial step in caring for
and being interested in her own well-being.

Sensitivity to distress

When we are motivated to be caring, it's helpful if we can direct this intention in a sensitive way. This means being able to pay attention to our (or
someone else's) distress in an open, moment-by-moment way. Developing
sensitivity allows us to be open to and notice our own (and others') feelings, emotions, thoughts and behaviours. While some people can be
motivated to care for their distress, they can struggle to notice things that
trigger emotions and feelings, and may not be aware when a distressing
emotion is present (e.g. sadness, shame, anxiety). So, developing distress
sensitivity can help with various stages of the emotion regulation model
(Chapter 5), and help to guide our compassionate, caring motivation.

Anita described how she would often go through her day without
noticing basic things about herself, such as hunger, tiredness or
stress levels. At work, in particular, she could go the whole day
without a coffee or lunch break, and struggled to recognise how
certain situations (e.g. difficult meetings) led to her feeling an
increase in anxiety and stress. Over time in therapy, Anita prac-
tised attention training and mindfulness exercises. These helped
her to become more sensitive and aware of how feelings and emo-
tions turned up in her body (e.g. sensations, urges to behave/act),
how these shaped her mind (e.g. what she paid attention to, how
she thought), and the type of situations that would commonly
trigger these responses.

Sympathy

If we are blocked or disconnected from our own or other people's
distress, it can be difficult to be compassionate. Sympathy involves

being emotionally moved by our own or other people's distress, discomfort or emotions. In the CMT approach, sympathy is a relatively automatic and immediate emotional reaction we have – it's the flush of feeling you get when you see someone else you care for hurt themselves, or hearing news that a friend has been rushed to hospital. This automatic emotional response can be tricky though, as sometimes it can leave people feeling overwhelmed by their own or someone else's pain, and as a consequence, they can try to block out or suppress their sympathetic responses. However, when we allow ourselves to connect with and be emotionally moved by our own or others distress, this can bring an immediate impulse of wanting to do something about the distress.

> Anita initially described herself as 'cold' and 'frozen'. She couldn't remember the last time she had been moved by someone else's difficulties, and, at first, found it difficult to understand what it would be like to be moved by her own struggles. Over time, she began to 'feel' her struggles – to allow herself not only to notice, but also to experience the feelings and be moved by and feel sad about the stress and anxiety of work, and the pain and loss of her marriage breakdown.

Distress tolerance

If we are sensitive to and emotionally moved by our own or others' difficulties, this might stimulate our threat system and leave us feeling distressed. And if this distress becomes too intense, or is activated over a long period, our capacity for compassion may be blocked. To help mitigate this, we need to make sure that our compassion comes with, or is underpinned by, the ability to tolerate and hold distress so that it doesn't overwhelm us. This may involve developing strength, acceptance of difficult or painful feelings, and a recognition that we can ride these feelings as they come and go.

> Anita described herself as a strong woman, but when we explored the concept of distress tolerance she recognised that her idea of

strength was more linked to non-feeling and 'coping', rather than being able to tolerate being with distress. In therapy, we discussed how true strength was sometimes related to remaining in contact with distress, so as to do something about it. We practised ways to help her tolerate painful and difficult feelings, and as therapy progressed, Anita became more able to tolerate and remain grounded in the presence of difficult emotions.

Empathy

There can be a number of different aspects of empathy. One involves being emotionally in tune with someone – a type of 'feeling with' in which we get a sense of the feelings and emotions that they are experiencing. Another involves a type of perspective-taking that gives rise to understanding the reasons why someone is suffering – to look at what sits behind someone's emotional distress, and consider what might have led them to feel the way they do. Given these factors, empathy guided by a compassionate motivation can help us to begin to understand what it is we need to tune in to, and how we might go about helping someone – for example, through the things we might say to them, or through our behaviour or actions. It can help us to appreciate that another person's mind is not necessarily the same as ours; that what causes you fear and distress, may not cause me fear and distress. Like the other qualities of compassion, empathy can also be directed towards our own suffering, in which we learn to take perspective and develop an understanding stance to what our struggle is like, and what may have led us to feel as we do.

Although Anita felt she empathised well with other people's difficulties, she thought the idea of self-empathy was odd; she struggled to see how her distress and emotional reactions at work and home were understandable, and in fact, regarded them as a sign of weakness. Over time, we worked on how she could validate and see that, given what was happening in her job, and the breakdown of her marriage, it was understandable that she was feeling low, sad and on edge.

Non-judgement

Finally, non-judgement means that we recognise that we have tricky brains and emotions that can be difficult to understand and manage. However, rather than getting caught up in criticism, hostility and blame, non-judgement involves trying to step back from these. Instead, we try to bring a type of acceptance and understanding to our experiences. This acceptance is by no means an indifference, or passive resignation to our difficulties. Instead, guided by our compassionate mind, we hold on to our desire to do something to overcome our difficult emotions, and alleviate our suffering.

> To begin with, Anita was very critical of herself for her emotional struggles, and for coming to therapy in the first place (rather than being 'strong' and carrying on). Over time, she learned through various skills training practices (see Chapters 8, 9 and 10) how to step back from self-directed hostility, and rather than battling herself for struggling in the way she was, accepting the distress that she was experiencing, and focusing on what she could do to bring helpful changes to her life.

Second psychology of compassion – alleviation of distress

The second psychology of compassion involves a desire to acquire the skills, wisdom and dedication to do something about our own and other people's distress – to alleviate it, uproot the factors that caused it, and prevent it from returning. If you slipped on a patch of ice in front of your house one winter morning, it would probably be helpful to have a doctor at the local hospital who was caring, empathetic and non-judgemental. However, you'd probably also want them to have spent many years at medical school developing their knowledge, experience, confidence and skills for how best to treat your broken leg. So, in this sense, a caring motivation on its own is not enough to alleviate suffering; wisdom and specific skills are required as well. In this section, we'll be focusing on some of the skills necessary to alleviate suffering. These skills involve the domains of attention, imagery, thinking, behaviour, sensory focusing and feelings. Let's briefly look at these below:

Compassionate attention: As we explored in Chapter 2, our threat systems can often hijack our attention and keep us locked into focusing on things in a way that can perpetuate our distress, and the difficult emotions associated with it. From an evolutionary perspective, this, of course, makes sense, as our ancestors who could pay attention in a focused, narrow way to potential threats were more likely to survive than those who struggled to do this. So, compassionate attention involves learning how to focus on things that are helpful, finding ways to helpfully bridge out of difficult emotions or loops in the mind that may be fuelling our emotional difficulties. Some of these skills are referred to as mindfulness, which has been described as 'paying attention, in the present moment, without judgement'. We will return to mindfulness in Chapter 8.

Compassionate imagery: In Chapter 3 we explored how our new brain capacity to imagine and fantasise can have a powerful impact on stimulating old brain emotions (remember the example of what would happen if we escaped from a lion). While our imagination can stimulate difficult emotions like anxiety and anger, it can also be used in a way that is helpful and conducive to alleviating our suffering. As we will come on to see in this section, developing and using various compassionate images can have a powerful effect on our feelings, by way of regulating our threat system, and difficult emotions.

Compassionate reasoning and thinking: When our threat systems become activated, this can create a particular type of thinking (e.g. ruminating, self-criticism or worry) that can make emotion regulation difficult, and in fact may directly contribute to emotional difficulties. Learning to bring a more balanced and compassionate approach to the way we are thinking about our own and other people's difficulties can help to contain our threat system, and regulate our feelings. Compassionate reasoning and thinking involve training our minds so that we can deliberately engage in more helpful, caring and compassionate ways of thinking about ourselves, other people, and situations we find ourselves in. We'll explore this in more detail in Chapters 15, 16 and 20.

Compassionate behaviour: The way we behave and act in the world can have important benefits to our emotions, and our capacity to regulate them in a helpful way. Compassionate behaviour involves acting in ways that are helpful to self and others, motivated by a genuine interest in one's well-being and best interests. While this can involve 'being nice' and 'kind' at times, sometimes this type of response can be motivated by a wish to make people like us, or from a fear of being rejected in some way. For example, compassion is not saying 'yes' every time your child asks for sweets or a pizza; rather, it would be how to tolerate saying 'no' while knowing this might upset or make them angry with you, because *your wisdom* helps you to understand that it's not healthy for them to eat junk food regularly. Given that compassion often entails having to connect with difficult and distressing emotions or situations (as discussed in the engagement with distress section), compassionate behaviours often require a great deal of strength, courage and assertiveness to face fears, and do things that are likely to be helpful, despite the difficulties. Moreover, compassionate behaviour to deal with current distress might be different from what is required to manage difficulties in the long term. We will explore how to engage in compassionate behaviour in Chapter 16c, and in the online material which is accessible at https://overcoming.co.uk/715/resources-to-download.

Compassionate sensory focusing: Using our different senses – for example, smell, touch and hearing – may be a powerful way of stimulating our physiology. If, for example, we can use our sensory experiences to bring our soothing system online, this may facilitate healthy emotion regulation. For example, learning how to breathe in ways that help the body slow down, or adopting certain body postures that may help us to feel more grounded, balanced and strong.

Compassionate feelings: In recent years, researchers have found that spending time developing and experiencing certain types of positive emotion and feelings (e.g. warmth, safeness, gratitude, joy) can have a powerful impact on our ability to tolerate and reduce our distress, regulate our emotions and enhance our well-being. In CMT we spend time generating and practising certain positive emotions linked to compassion, including warmth, kindness, friendliness and contentment.

Bringing the two psychologies together

We can see how the two psychologies come together in Figure 7 (overleaf). The inner circle represents the qualities of the first psychology of compassion, while the outer circle reflects the skills training of the second psychology. This figure and the different components of compassion can seem a little overwhelming at first. A helpful analogy here may be recalling what it is like to learn to drive a car. You have to remember to juggle a number of things: which pedal to press to speed up, which to push to brake, how to change gears, indicate and look in the mirrors, all while doing your best not to hit anything or anyone! At first, all this can feel like a lot to remember and execute, but with practice, these tasks and skills come together in an integrated, and less effortful way. This is similar to developing the attributes and skills of compassion. It can feel tricky to start with, but as you practise, things begin to fall into place. For the time being it's worth holding onto two key aspects that lay at the heart of compassion: learning how to be sensitive and engage with our own and other people's suffering and difficulties, and developing skills and wisdom to work out what might be the most useful way to help, to ease this suffering.

Just like learning to drive, learning a new sport or learning how to play a musical instrument, developing your compassionate mind rests on understanding what the required qualities and skills are, and developing these through repetition, practice and commitment. Practising specific skills and behaviours over time activates a pattern of responses in the brain and body. The more we practise these, the more likely these patterns firm up and strengthen. For some of us, it may be that, unintentionally,

Figure 7: The compassion circles – the key attributes (1st psychology – inner circle) and skills of compassion (2nd psychology – outer circle)

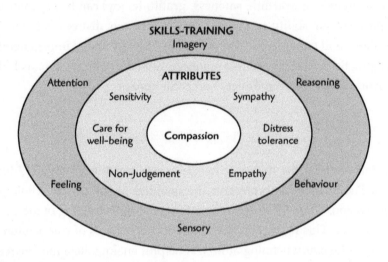

From Gilbert, *The Compassionate Mind* (2009), reprinted with permission from Little, Brown Book Group.

we've been practising, activating and hardening patterns of anger or anxiety for many years; and therefore, it's no surprise that we struggle to manage our emotions at times. The 'compassion pattern' may be less rehearsed, and therefore less elaborated. Developing this pattern (our compassionate mind) through focused practice and commitment can help us to regulate our emotions and difficulties better. In fact, colleagues of mine have found that after practising some of these exercises for two weeks, we can experience reductions in self-criticism, shame and stress, and increases in self-compassion (Matos et al., 2017). We will return to how we do this in the next chapters.

Many faces of compassion

When we look at the two psychologies of compassion, it becomes clear that rather than feeling weak or pitiful, compassion actually gives rise to a motivation to find ways to approach and work with distress. It is important to hold in mind that there are *different faces of compassion* depending on the situation. Let's look at some examples:

> *Imagine that your child (or a child you care for) falls over, cuts their knee and starts crying. What would be a compassion thing to do in this situation? Well, for most people this might be to give them a hug or use a warm and kind voice tone to reassure them and help them calm down. This is one face of compassion.*

> *Imagine now that the same child has a metal fork in their hand, and is trying to insert it into a plug socket. What would your compassionate response be here? A similar, reassuring, gentle voice tone and a hug? Probably not. It's likely that in this second scenario you would have a loud, authoritative voice tone, and you might even pull the child back from the potential danger. So, this is a very different 'face' of compassion to the first example.*

Compassion can come in very different forms and can look very different depending on the situation, the relationship between the giver and recipient, and the type of distress/suffering (or threat) requiring attention. However, compassion always rests in the ability to be sensitive to distress, and the motivation to prevent or alleviate this. Both the above examples have this in common. It's important to see that from this approach, compassion is a motive, not an emotion. That's not to say that compassion doesn't come with emotions, but rather, it can't be reduced to a single emotion. Although difficult, it's possible to be compassionate to people that you don't have positive feelings for, and some compassionate acts (e.g. fundraising for starving children) are triggered by threat emotions like anger at the awful conditions people are living in.

It might also be helpful to think about people you know in your life who are compassionate, or well-known people in the world who are/ were seen as compassionate – for example, Nelson Mandela, Mahatma Gandhi, Desmond Tutu or the Dalai Lama. While these people are often described as warm, kind and caring, they're never seen as weak, pitiful or indulgent. In fact, their compassion is deeply intertwined with the bravery to stand up to world injustices, the confidence to confront difficult issues in a respectful and dignified manner, and an enormous capacity to fight actively for people who were suffering and had little power of their own. This is not to say that these are perfect, superhuman people, who never experience fears, doubts or frustrations, or never act in ways that are unpleasant; however, when engaged in compassionate actions, these people exhibit strength, commitment, and a willingness to engage with pain and suffering.

Compassion, shadow and difficult emotions

Sometimes when people think about compassion, they can get caught in a trap of focusing on feeling good – that compassion is about being positive and happy, or alternatively, *in not feeling bad* (for example, not experiencing painful emotions such as anger, anxiety and sadness). Instead, compassion involves the recognition that we all get angry at times because we are born with the capacity to experience this emotion. We all experience sadness because we've evolved to want to connect, and as a consequence, find separation distressing and painful. So rather than getting away from – or not experiencing – emotions that can feel unpleasant, compassion instead involves accepting that we will experience them at times, and working out how we can notice them when they turn up, tolerate and understand them, and respond in a way that is helpful and conducive to our (and others') well-being.

In compassionate mind training, we learn how we can be with the reality of being able to experience emotions and feelings, and to hold a sense of common humanity of what it's like to be an animal with a body and brain that we did not choose, but can leave us *feeling*. Yes, feeling emotions that can bring us (and others) pain and distress. And yes, when this happens, it can feel that these emotions are overwhelming, destructive and unending. But with a sense of compassionate wisdom, we can also recognise that emotions have important functions in our life; and that there are things we can do to help us manage them in healthy, effective ways. So, compassion involves developing a variety of emotion regulation skills to cope with our anger, our sadness, our fear, our shame. Compassion involves turning towards those things in our lives that are in the shadow, things that cause us distress, pain and suffering, that we would prefer to stay away from. It also involves finding ways to bring these things into the light, to turn towards and embrace them, and learn how to navigate either living life alongside them, or finding healthy ways to alleviate them.

The benefits of cultivating a compassionate mind

There are many studies now looking at the *science of compassion*. Although I won't explore these in detail here, they have shown that developing compassion is associated with:

- Reductions in mental health symptoms, such as depression, anxiety and PTSD (see Graser & Stangier, 2018)

- Increases in motivation to be caring of others (e.g. Condon et al., 2013)

- Increase in heart rate variability, a measure of parasympathetic influence on the nervous system (Matos et al., 2017)

With regards to emotion regulation, compassion has been associated with reductions in levels of 'negative' emotions such as anger, anxiety and shame (Neff & Vonk, 2009; Johnson & O'Brien, 2013), and with increases in 'positive' emotions, such as happiness, joy and more generally, well-being (e.g. Baer et al., 2012; Trompetter et al., 2016). The ability to be compassionate to ourselves (self-compassion) has also been associated with lower levels of self-criticism, rumination and worry, reductions in emotion dysregulation (Jazaieri et al., 2014), and, crucially, with improved emotion regulation skills (e.g. Finlay-Jones et al., 2015; Scoglio et al., 2016, and Diedrich et al., 2016).

The three flows of compassion

When first asked about compassion, most people think about it as something they would feel for, or towards, someone else. While it's true that this is an important flow of compassion, it turns out that in the compassionate mind approach, having compassion towards someone else is only one of three potential flows. Let's take a look at these below:

1. Compassion for others

Compassion for others involves being aware of and sensitive to suffering in other people, being able to engage with it and tolerate their distress, and having the motivation and commitment to try to alleviate their distress and suffering. Scientific studies have found that various brain systems are activated when we respond to the distress of others compassionately.

2. Compassion from others

We can also be recipients of compassion, being directed to us from someone else. For many, receiving compassion can produce a reassuring or calming effect, and can help us feel connected. If we were lucky, some of our earliest experiences are likely to have involved this flow of compassion – someone else (usually our parents) noticing our distress (e.g. hunger, too hot/cold) and taking steps to alleviate this in some way. Research studies have shown that experiencing care and kindness from others can have powerful physiological effects upon our brains and bodies, and have a significant impact on regulating our threat system.

3. Compassion for oneself (self-compassion)

The third flow of compassion involves directing compassion to ourselves, commonly known as self-compassion. In self-compassion, we try to become sensitive to and witness the nature of our own pain, engage with it, and then commit to alleviating it, through active intention and motivation. Interestingly, while science has time and time again shown us the powerful and positive impact of self-compassion on various areas of our lives (including managing difficult emotions), many of us have never had much (if any) guidance or teaching on how to be compassionate to ourselves.

Key reflections

- There are two 'psychologies' of compassion – one that involves being sensitive to and engaging in distress, and a second that involves various skills that help to alleviate it

- Compassion has many faces, and is not just about being 'nice' – it is central to helping us turn towards and bring light to things that we find difficult and scary

- Training our minds in and for compassion can have significant effects upon our physiology and emotions

- Compassion has three flows – compassion for others, being open to the compassion from others, and self-compassion

7 How to develop a compassionate mind

Before we start the process of compassionate mind skills training, it's useful to consider why this is important, and what motivation we're recruiting as we go on this journey.

Starting the process – motivation

As you might have recognised from what we've covered so far, motivation sits at the heart of compassion. Compassion is a motive which helps to organise the other faculties of our minds, such as attention, thinking, behaviour and so forth, enabling us to engage with and try to alleviate difficulties in life. It is therefore important to clarify what your compassionate motivation is. Let's explore this together.

Exercise: Compassion-based motivation – why do I want things to be different?

Sit in an upright and comfortable position, and take a moment to allow your breathing to slow a little, in a way that feels soothing to your body. When you feel ready, see if you can connect to your motivation and intention to grow your compassionate mind:

- Why is it important for you to develop your compassionate mind?

- What would you like your compassionate mind to help you change in your life?

- How would you like to manage your emotional difficulties in the future?

- How would you handle the things that cause you distress if you were guided by your compassionate mind?

- What might challenge you in developing your skills in compassion? How will you manage these challenges?

- How would you treat yourself – and your difficult emotions – differently if you had a more compassionate mind?

Compassionate motivation – the two wolves story

For millennia, poetry, fables, stories and art have emotionally moved and motivated their audiences. One short story in particular that gets to the heart of compassionate motivation is that of the 'two wolves'. The story goes like this:

One evening a grandfather was teaching his young grandson about the internal battle that each person faces. 'There are two wolves struggling inside each of us,' the old man said. 'One wolf is vengeful, angry, resentful, self-pitying and scared . . . the other wolf is compassionate, faithful, hopeful, and caring.' The grandson sat thinking, then asked: 'Which wolf wins, Grandfather?' His grandfather replied, 'The one you feed.'

Compassionate motivation – which garden do you want?

We can further think about motivation through an analogy that scientist and Buddhist monk Matthieu Ricard sometimes uses. In some ways, our minds are like gardens. Left to themselves, like gardens, they grow in all sorts of ways, depending on the type of soil, amount of rain and sunlight they get, and types of plants, weeds or grass already present. They also change depending on how they are maintained – how they are looked after, nourished, what has been planted and so forth. It might be that you're perfectly happy with your garden growing as it does – with grass, shrubs, flowers, weeds, and anything else that happens to find its way into it! But if you want your garden to look different – to look a certain way – you need to cultivate it, by putting effort and energy in to shape it. Similarly, left to their own devices, our minds also 'grow' naturally depending on our genes, experiences, relationships, and environment. However, the end product may not always be as we'd like it; our minds may get swamped by the wilderness of overwhelming emotions and distress – rage, shame, panic – *unless* we spend time and effort cultivating, nourishing and shaping them in specific ways. Developing a compassionate mind involves intentionally cultivating our minds – developing a 'pattern' or mind state that shapes different aspects of our minds: attention, thinking, behaviour, imagery, and emotions – that in turn can help us to manage painful emotions in life.

Is it possible to 'feed' our brains?

In recent years, scientists have learned much more about how our brains work. One particularly interesting finding has been that our brains are actually far more malleable than we previously thought. What this means is that the connections between the cells in our brain (called neurons) have an amazing ability to organise and reorganise themselves into different patterns based on our experiences. Just like our bodies can change shape and strengthen depending on which machines we use at the gym, so too can our brains change if we exercise them using various compassionate mind training exercises. As the saying goes: 'neurons that fire together, wire together' (Hebb, 1949), so it's important to consider which version or pattern of 'mind' you've been practising. Maybe an angry and critical pattern? Or an anxious or emotionally suppressing one? Maybe it's been a pattern linked to shame and self-hatred. And here's the rub: for many of us, it's these patterns that have had the most air space to develop – the most opportunity to develop and grow strong. While this isn't our fault, these patterns may be distorting the way we view ourselves, how we interact with other people, and how we live our life. Moreover, they are likely to be continuously stimulating and fuelling our threat system, or creating an imbalance in our emotions. So, in the coming chapters, we're going to learn how to feed the brain with compassion – to practise new sets of patterns that naturally help to regulate our emotions in a different way.

Although it is still unclear just how much time we need to practise these new patterns, what is clear is the importance of creating motivation and commitment to do so. This makes intuitive sense. If you want to learn a new language, play an instrument, or pick up a new skill, what do you have to do? Practise, of course! This is paramount. Let's see how we can do this through an example.

Getting the ball rolling – practice

In the following chapters, I'll introduce you to some core compassionate mind training practices in a step-by-step way. Given this, it's useful to consider how we might go about practising our compassionate minds.

How to practise

A bit like exercise, it's helpful to do a little bit of practice regularly. Of course, each person finds their own way with this, but to start with, try to find 5 to 10 minutes each day to practise some of the exercises in the following chapters.

Speaking of exercise, if you've ever been to a gym, it's likely you found there were many different machines to try out. A treadmill to run on, an exercise bike or rowing machine, and lots of different weight machines, many of which seem quite confusing to know how to use correctly! Each of these machines helps to train parts of our body to get fitter or stronger in some way. Similarly, there are many ways that we can help to train your compassionate mind. In the coming chapters, I'll introduce a number of different exercises and skills practices. Just like gym equipment, you may find some of the exercises easier, or more pleasurable, than others. Although it's natural to focus on just doing those, it's wise to spend enough time on each one so that you give them a chance to know if they are helpful, rather than giving up too quickly.

It's also useful to remember what it's like trying to develop a new habit (whether it's learning a language, or a new skill, or getting into exercise to lose weight or get fit); to start with, you might stumble on challenges, or not readily notice positive changes. You might even think, 'What's the point . . . this isn't going to work.' While this is an understandable reaction, if we can tap into our wisdom and understanding about how change happens, this can help us when we're starting our practice. So, try not to become defeated if it's hard to do regular practice – it's always better to do a little practice than none at all.

Compassion starts with intention. It may be that you don't notice a shift in your feelings to begin with, but over time, with clear intention and continued practice, just like with fitness training, positive changes will become more apparent.

Where to practise

This can vary. It might be helpful to begin by practising in a quiet and comfortable environment, where you are unlikely to be disturbed (a bit like how we learn to swim in the shallow end of the pool). However, over time it might feel possible to practise in different environments – on the bus, train or even when walking.

When to practise

This can also vary, but again, it may be helpful to start off by blocking out a part of the day when you can fully commit yourself to your practice, when you are alert enough (to avoid falling asleep during the exercise), and not likely to be rushed, or disturbed by other daily demands.

It might also help to let others close to you know that you're embarking on this journey of developing new skills, so that they can support you in any way possible. This could be by reminding you to practice, respecting and granting your need for time and space to practise, and being sensitive to the likely changes you'll experience throughout the journey.

Keeping the ball rolling – dealing with blocks and setbacks

One of the common problems when developing compassionate mind skills is how to keep the practice going, particularly if and when we hit setbacks. As with life, setbacks are inevitable when embarking on these types of mind training practices. It's important to remember this, rather than seeing them as signs that you're not 'doing it right'. As you progress with your practice, keep an eye out for your threat system (for example, through experiences of self-criticism, fear, or frustration), and remember to try to bring some compassion to the fact that you're struggling with the practice at that moment. We'll have various tips and suggestions for how to manage specific difficulties and setbacks as we go along.

Key reflections

- Our minds are full of patterns – some of these may have had more practice than others

- Motivation sits at the heart of compassion

- Like many things in life, it takes practice and effort to develop a compassionate 'pattern' of mind

8 Compassionate mind training – attention and mindfulness

If you've ever gone out looking to rent or buy somewhere to live, it's likely you've had certain criteria in mind – the size of the place, the number of rooms, the style of its design and so on. While these are all important, what is less obvious (and perhaps less exciting!) but essential, is that the place you're looking at has been constructed well. Unless the property is supported by a solid foundation, it's likely that it'll develop problems over the years, that no fancy kitchen or funky bathroom will make up for. So, an important early step in working with emotional difficulties is to develop a strong, solid foundation from which to engage these.

Foundations of a compassionate mind: Attention, mindfulness and mind awareness

What does attention mean? *The Oxford Dictionary of English* (Oxford University Press, 2018) suggests a number of definitions of attention. In terms of how we will be using this term, three, in particular, stand out:

- The mental ability to take notice, or consider someone or something

- Regarding someone or something as interesting, or important

- Taking special care of someone or something

This suggests that attention relates to a mental ability to notice something consciously in a particular way. From a CFT perspective, this is an important quality that can lead to greater understanding of why we struggle with our emotions, and how we can bring compassion to managing them. Let's explore this further:

1. *Attention can get hijacked:* As we explored in Chapters 2 and 3, emotions and feelings often drag at our attention, bringing greater focus to whatever it is we are feeling. Just as when you stub your toe, and your attention is suddenly pulled to the pain in your foot, attention can also be captured or seized by strong emotions or feelings. If you've ever fallen in love, you'll know how frequently and powerfully your attention and thinking returns to focus on this person – so much so, it can feel as if 'you' no longer have any control of your mind. Similarly, if you're very anxious about something (for example, a presentation or speech you've got to give), you might have noticed your attention returning to and focusing on this, even when you're doing something completely unrelated to it.

2. *Attention can bring greater mind awareness:* As we learned in Chapter 3, through no fault of our own, our mind (and therefore our attention and our thoughts) often gets caught up in the gravitational pull of 'old brain–new brain' loops that can keep painful emotions or feelings going. Paying attention to these loops as they emerge in our minds, and then redirecting our attention to the present moment (often referred to as mindfulness) has been found to have a powerful impact on how we experience our emotions and distress. So, attention plays an important role in a type of *mind-mindedness* or *mind awareness*, which enables us to notice the workings of our mind, and find helpful ways of responding to them.

3. *Attention 'plays the body':* While attention can be captured by strong emotions, conversely, if we guide our attention in a particular way, it can also trigger specific emotions, feelings and physiological changes in our body. For example, if you spend some time focusing your attention on the happiest time of your life, it's quite likely you'll start to experience positive feelings, similar to those you had at the time of the experience. If I ask you to pay attention to someone you find very sexually attractive, you may notice a different type of change in your body! In other words, by consciously directing our attention, we can 'play' different physiological and emotional

tunes in our body. This intentional directing of attention is a central component of emotion regulation in CFT.

The power of attention

We can explore the power of attention – and in particular, how it can be consciously directed and 'play our body' – through the following short exercise.

Exercise: The nature of attention

When we discuss the concept of attention, it can be helpful to consider how it is similar to a spotlight in a dark room. Just like a spotlight, attention can be moved around, and 'shone' in different directions. And just like a spotlight, whatever you pay attention to 'lights up' in your mind and body. We will explore this in a few short steps.

To start with, place all of your attention on your right foot. Spend 15 seconds or so really paying attention to whatever sensations you can notice in this part of your body. After 15 seconds, move your attention to your left foot, and try to notice whatever sensations are present in this part of your body. OK, now move your focus to your right hand. Pay attention to whatever sensations are present in this area of your body. Again, after 15 seconds or so, shift your focus to your left hand, and notice whatever is present there. Finally, move your attention to your face. Try to notice whatever sensations are present there.

What did you notice during this exercise? Although people have different experiences with this exercise, there are some common themes that often emerge:

- We can consciously direct attention – it is 'moveable'

- It isn't easy to hold attention in one place – the mind tends to wander away or be distracted by thoughts, or external events (e.g. sounds)

- Paying attention in a particular area of the body is likely to trigger or enhance specific physical sensations in that part of the body. Attention can 'play the body', just like a spotlight 'lights up' whatever it shines on in a darkened room

- Like the camera on your phone, attention has a 'zoom lens'-like quality to it, enlarging and giving greater detail to what it focuses on. It can open, expand or narrow our consciousness. As we have discussed earlier in the chapter, it then depends what grabs the focus of attention – this could be something neutral (e.g. an article in a free newspaper), pleasant (e.g. a happy memory) or for some of us, unpleasant emotions and feelings like rage, shame and fear.

A restless mind

The nature of our minds is far more like a choppy, churning sea than a calm, tranquil lake. The Buddha is said to have referred to the mind as being full of drunken monkeys, as it's always moving, jumping around, restless, unsettled and chattering (often about nonsense!). It can be useful to recognise this for yourself through a short exercise:

Exercise: Our restless mind

Find a comfortable place to sit on a cushion or a chair, in a room where you will not be disturbed. Gently bring your awareness to the present moment by engaging your basic senses. Take some time to notice the sounds that you can hear around you. Notice the sensations in your body as you are sitting, and how the air feels on your skin. Notice what you can see in the room around you, the different objects, the colours and the light. Draw your attention to any smells around you, and any particular taste in your mouth. Continue doing this for the next minute or so.

Now, as you're doing this, notice what happens to your attention. Does it easily remain focused on sounds, bodily feelings or what you can see? Or do you notice that it naturally begins to wander, almost as if it has a mind of its own?

Continue to this focus on your senses for another minute or two, noticing as you do what happens to attention.

How long were you able to keep your attention in the present moment, focused on your senses? Was this easy, or did you notice that it began to wander as if it has a mind of its own? If you're anything like me – or the many people I've guided through this exercise – it's likely that you didn't find it easy to remain focused on your present, sensory experiences for very long. You probably noticed your mind wandering, to random thoughts relating to the future, your to-do list, or things that happened earlier in the day, or some time ago. In other words, it's likely that your mind was not always in the present moment. This is not because of some problem with your mind, but because *our minds are naturally restless*. As we discussed in Chapter 3, our minds often get caught up in loops between old brain feelings and motivations, and new brain thoughts and images. It's useful to hold in mind that this is not our fault; we did not choose to have a brain that is naturally so restless and unruly, and in fact, there are likely to be good evolutionary reasons why having a mind that wanders like this was helpful to spotting danger and threats. What is clear is that we were not the author of how our minds work; we did not choose to have a brain which, without effortful guidance, can take over, often wreaking havoc in our minds.

As we become more aware of the naturally restless nature of our minds, we also need to consider the type of context we live in. For many people, modern life involves constant stimulation and a sense of always needing to be on the go. Work, travel, family, friends, technology – all of these make it difficult to find time and space to slow down, to just *be*. Not only does this pour more fuel on the 'fire' of our naturally restless minds, but we also have little opportunity to notice, observe and learn about what our minds are actually like. Given this, it can be important to learn how to become more aware of your mind, what your attention is focused on, and develop skills in being able to calm and settle your mind as a helpful way of working with difficult emotions. One way of doing this is through practising something called mindfulness.

Strengthening attention: Mind awareness and stability through mindfulness

In the past decade or two, an emerging theme in the research and therapy literature is that like other skills, attention can be practised, trained and strengthened. Research now suggests that when we train our attention, this can lead to greater awareness of our emotions, and some of the factors that make it difficult for us to regulate them in a helpful way (see Chapter 5).

What is mindfulness?

There are lots of definitions of mindfulness, although the most common one in the West is that it involves:

> An awareness that emerges through paying attention on purpose, in the present moment, and non-judgmentally, to the unfolding of experience moment by moment.
>
> *(Kabat-Zinn, 2003, p. 145).*

The actual word mindfulness is derived from an ancient Indian Pali word that means *awareness, attention and remembering*. This, along with Kabat-Zinn's definition, suggests that mindfulness involves a particular intention (remembering) to pay attention in a specific way (e.g. in the present moment) without judging ourselves, our experience, or others.

Personally, I've always found the description that mindfulness involves 'knowing what you're experiencing, as you're experiencing it' a particularly helpful explanation.

When we practise mindfulness, this can lead to a greater mind mindedness; that is, we become wiser about the *nature of our minds*, how they function, and the loops they tend to get in to. This wisdom also enables us to appreciate the natural design of our minds; that they have been *designed for us, not by us*, through evolutionary processes, and contain a variety of motives, emotions, desires and thoughts that can be very complex (recall Chapter 2 and 3).

Through a variety of practices (for example, learning to root one's attention to an anchor, such as the breath or body), mindfulness helps us to become more aware of what is present in our minds and bodies (e.g. difficult emotions and feelings), and what might have triggered these experiences or what might be maintaining them. This, in turn, can help us to become less reactive in the face of often powerful, or distressing, feelings.

How does mindfulness help to manage emotions that can be painful and distressing?

Sometimes my clients ask how focusing attention, and practising mindfulness, is worth spending time on, particularly when they've got lots of other things to prioritise in life. Over the past twenty years, there has been an explosion in research looking at the potential benefits of mindfulness. We don't have space here to outline or review the literature in detail, but on the whole, there appear to be some consistent and significant findings. These suggest that, over time, consistent mindfulness practise can lead to:

- A reduction in stress, anxiety and depression symptoms

- A reduction in worry and rumination

- Improved emotion regulation skills

- Increased levels of self-compassion

- Management of pain and addiction difficulties

(see Goldberg et al., 2017; Kuyken et al., 2010; Opialla et al., 2015)

So, although mindfulness isn't a miracle cure or panacea to life's difficulties, there is good evidence that practising and developing such skills may be a helpful step in managing difficult emotions.

Ways to be mindful

There are various types of mindfulness practice, but broadly, these fall under two related but separate categories:

1. *Focused attention:* During focused-attention mindfulness practice, we learn to focus our attention in a very specific and focused way. These types of exercises usually involve anchoring attention to the breath, body, sounds or images, and then to notice when our mind is distracted from its initial focus. Typically, we can get distracted by discomfort or pain in the body, sounds around us (e.g. a ticking clock), random thoughts about something (e.g. about what we need to do later that day, about a friend or family member, or about work). Sometimes the distraction is because of an intense or unpleasant emotion (e.g. anger, sadness), or particular 'loops in the mind' (see Chapter 3) particularly linked to worry, rumination or self-criticism. Key to this type of mindfulness practice is to notice when we become distracted, and the reaction that we have to this distraction (e.g. frustration, self-criticism for 'not doing it right'). Then, rather than getting caught up with this, to have the intention to bring awareness kindly and gently back to the initial focus of attention

(e.g. the breath or a sound). I have tried to depict this 'process' of mindfulness in Figure 8.

Figure 8: The cycle of mindfulness

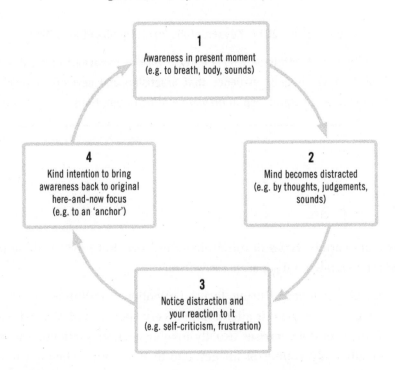

2.   *Open awareness:* During open-awareness mindfulness practice, we learn to hold our attention and awareness in an open manner, so that whatever emerges in it – an emotion, a thought, a memory – can exist in our minds without us having to push it away, fight it off, ignore it, or get (overly) captured by it. Like the clouds moving through the sky, over time we can learn to remain open to these experiences, observe, recognise and appreciate them, without trying to interfere with them, or change them in any way.

In this chapter, we'll focus on developing skills in focused-attention practices.

Before you start – five steps of preparation

Just as it's wise to warm up before exercising, it's important that before we start our mindfulness practice, we spend a few moments preparing our minds for what is to follow and creating conditions that are most conducive to the practice. The preparatory steps that we will use are:

Step 1 – if possible, find a place that is quiet and in which you are unlikely to be disturbed

Step 2 – find a comfortable place to sit (this could be a chair or a cushion on the floor)

Step 3 – try to sit with an upright yet comfortable posture, in which your spine is lengthened slightly (imagine a piece of string tied to the top of your head, that is gently being pulled upwards), with your head at an alert position. Try to allow your shoulders to open, and place your feet on the floor (roughly shoulder-width apart), with your hands resting on the chair or your lap

Step 4 – if you feel comfortable, close your eyes, otherwise pick a point to focus on in front of you

Step 5 – hold in mind for 30 seconds your wise, compassionate intention for the practice you're about to take. For example, hold in mind the intention to engage in the practice from a grounded, non-threat or drive system position, and that regardless of whether the practice goes 'well' or not, it is the intention to spend time cultivating the compassionate mind that is most important

These are, of course, just guidelines – adapt them to fit what you need and find helpful, and allow for any physical limitations such as pain or breathing problems you may have. It's important that while remaining upright, you are not holding your posture in a way that is creating strain or discomfort in any body parts. As you are finding this posture, you may realise that you are tightening particular areas of your body (for example, your brow, or jaw, or shoulders). If so, see if you can loosen around this as best as you can. As you are embarking on these practices, and until you are more familiar with them, it may be easier to listen to audio guides. Later, with increased practice and familiarity, you can silently guide yourself.

Core mindfulness practices

We will start with practising a number of focused-attention mindfulness exercises – if you can, try these in order, and if possible, once a day over the coming weeks, to get as much benefit from them as you can. Audio files of these exercises are available under the 'resources' section at www.balancedminds.com if you find that more helpful to use as a guide.

Mindfulness: External focus

In this initial exercise, we'll start with directing attention outside of the body, as sometimes this can be a slightly easier place to start.

Exercise: Mindfulness of sound

To begin this practice, remind yourself of the 'five steps of preparation' outlined on the previous page – quiet place, comfortable seat, upright posture, closing your eyes/resting your gaze in front of you, and compassionate intention for the practice. Give yourself enough time to settle into your posture and prepare your body and mind.

When you feel ready, draw your attention to the sounds that you can hear around you. Try not to force or reach out to the sounds – but instead, become aware of the sounds as they arise and disappear around you. Spend 30 seconds or so noticing this.

As you notice the sounds around you, try to become aware of when your mind moves away from these, when it gets distracted by thoughts (about the sounds or random and unrelated) or physical sensations (for example, discomfort in your back or leg). When you notice that your mind has drifted from sound, remember that this is just what minds do . . . remember the idea of your attention acting like a spotlight.

Then, gently and kindly, bring your awareness back to noticing the sounds around you. Again, spend 30 seconds just focusing on the sounds around you.

As you are paying attention to the sounds around you, you might slowly start to notice different qualities of these sounds. For example, you might pay attention to:

- The direction they are coming from

- How loud they are

- What pitch or tone they have

- Whether they are constant or intermittent

Spend 60 seconds or so just noticing this. Again, notice when your mind becomes distracted and, gently and kindly, bring your mind back to noticing the sounds around you.

Now, for 60 seconds or so, see if you can focus your attention more purposefully on just one sound that you can hear around you. Really try to focus on this, using it as an anchor for your attention, noticing with curiosity the nature and characteristics of this, and returning to this sound if your mind wanders.

After a while, gently pull back from focusing on this sound as you would bring the zoom of a camera to a wider focus. Now, see if you can broaden your attention to notice all of the sounds around you so that no sound is paid more attention than another. Repeat this process – focusing on just one sound for a period, and then pulling the focus back to become aware of all sounds.

It can be helpful after doing a practice – particularly to begin with – to make a few notes about what the experience was like; what you noticed, what you found difficult, how the practice left you feeling, what you have learned about the nature of your mind from doing it. Try to maintain your compassionate intention here about practice, recalling why you're doing this (e.g. to help to create the conditions in which you can manage difficult emotions differently), and to recognise if you're getting caught up in a threat-based drive goal. For example: 'I should be able to do this right' or 'I should have been able to keep my focus throughout the practice'. Remember that you *will* get distracted during mindfulness practice. This happens to everyone, and as outlined in Figure 8 (p. 114), mind distraction is an essential aspect of mindfulness – if your mind didn't get distracted, then we couldn't engage in all of the four steps of mindfulness.

Mindfulness: Internal anchor

One way of thinking about mindfulness is in terms of providing an *anchor for the mind*. Just like anchors serve as a point of stability for boats, helping to keep them steady in the face of winds and water currents, present-moment, non-judgemental awareness to our body and breath can offer an anchor to our minds, grounding and stabilising them. This is because our body and breath are always present for us and can, therefore, bring a here-and-now experience to our minds. Let's give this a go.

Exercise: Mindful body scan

Start with the five steps of your preparation (p. 115), finding a comfortable place to sit in an upright, grounded position. In this exercise, we are going to direct the spotlight of attention to the body, and in a step-by-step way, 'scan' different parts of it. As you do this, try to keep an open awareness to how the sensations in different parts of the body feel (pleasant, unpleasant, neutral) – try to step back from the temptation to cling onto, push against, or move away from these if they arise, holding instead to purely noticing the sensations themselves.

To begin, as best as you can, focus upon the 'outline' of your body – maybe you can just get a quick sense of the points of your body that connect with the chair you're sitting on, and how your skin feels where it contacts your clothing. Spend a few moments trying to get an outline of your posture, the space that your body takes, and the weight of your body as it pushes down into the chair. Spend 30 seconds or so just becoming familiar with this.

We are now going to pay mindful attention to different parts of your body in a progressive manner. To start with, pay attention to the sensation in the area around your feet and ankles. Spend 30–60 seconds just noticing whatever sensations are present in this part of your body. If you feel your attention being pulled away – to thoughts, feelings, sounds or sensations in other parts of your body – just become aware of this and, without judging or being critical of this, gently bring your attention back to the sensations present in your feet and ankles.

Now slowly move your attention to the area around your shins, calves and knees. Try to pay attention to the different sensations that are present in this area of your body. Spend 30–60 seconds noticing whatever sensations are present there. Now shift your attention to the area around your upper legs and bottom, paying attention to the sensations you can notice in this part of your body. Spend 30–60 seconds doing this.

Now gently shift your attention further up your body, to the area around your stomach and lower back. Notice any sensations that are present here, again for 30–60 seconds. When you're ready, slowly move your attention to your chest and upper back area, gently holding awareness to the sensations that are present here for 30 seconds or so. Notice if and when your attention is distracted from this focus, and try gently to move awareness back to your upper body.

Now, allow your attention to move down into your arms and hands, allowing awareness of the different sensations that arise in this part of your body.

Finally, slowly shift your attention to the area around your neck, face and head. For 30 seconds or so just try to be aware of whatever sensations are present.

Once you've completed this, remain seated, in your grounded posture, breathing gently. Take a moment to bring your attention back to the present moment and the environment you are in by opening your eyes (if they've been closed) and having a good look around you. Give your body a gentle stretch if that feels helpful.

Again, it can be helpful to make a few notes after this practice. What did you notice about your attention? Were there particular times when your mind drifted, or made passing judgements about your experience? Were there parts of your body that were easier or harder to focus on? As you practise this exercise further, see what it's like to shorten or extend the time you spend on each area of the body. Sometimes people find it helpful to start at their feet and move up to their head, before moving back down the body, and finishing the exercise back at the point of their feet.

Alongside the body, the breath is a constant partner in our life. Let's look at how we can use this as an anchor point for mindfulness practice.

Exercise: Mindfulness of breathing

Start this exercise with the five-step preparation (p. 115). When you are ready, gently direct your attention towards your breath. Begin to notice the sensation of breathing in and out, becoming aware of the sensations that are present as you do this. If it helps, try finding a point of focus to concentrate on. For example:

- Some people find it helpful to focus on the area around the tip of their nose, noticing as the cool air flows in on the in-breath, and the warm air moves outwards with the out-breath

- Some people find it helpful to pick a point in the centre of the chest, noticing the sensations as the chest expands on the in-breath, and contracts on the out-breath

- Some find it helpful to follow the flow of the breath, from the point of entry at the nose, through the nostrils, down the throat and into the lungs on the inhale, and then the flow out of the lungs, up through the throat, and finally out of the nose on the exhale

Don't worry about having to change the frequency, pace or depth of your breathing. For now, see if you can simply pay attention to the breath, however it is, and wherever it's felt in your body.

Continue to notice the sensation of the in- and out-breath, following the flow of the breath in a curious, open way. As you do this, there will be times when your attention might be taken away from your breath. This may be because thoughts pop into your mind (for example, 'This is boring' or 'I think I'm doing this wrong', or other random thoughts), you become distracted by sounds or other external events, or you become aware of pain or discomfort in your body.

When you notice your attention drifting in this way, try to acknowledge this has happened, and gently, without judgement, draw your attention back to your breathing. If the mind drifts again, notice, acknowledge this as normal, and with care and kindness return to your breath as best as you can.

Continue this process for another 5 minutes if you can, gently noticing the sensations and passage of the breath, and when the attention moves away from the breath. Treat your breath as the anchor for your attention, something that you can bring your mind back to again and again if your mind wanders away. It doesn't matter whether your attention drifts just once, a hundred or a thousand times during this exercise. The key thing is not whether your mind wanders (because it will), but rather, noticing when this happens, and gently, intentionally bringing your attention back to the breath again.

Once you've completed this, remain seated, in your grounded posture, breathing gently. Take a moment to bring your attention back to the present moment and the environment you are in by opening your eyes (if they've been closed) and having a good look around you. Give your body a gentle stretch if that feels helpful.

We will focus on using mindfulness explicitly to manage difficult emotions throughout Section Four. For now, it might be helpful to notice your emotional experiences and reactions in engaging in these exercises. Common emotional responses are:

- 'This is so annoying, I should be better at this' (frustration, anger)

- 'I don't like this, focusing on my breathing feels uncomfortable and makes me feel I can't breathe properly' (anxiety)

- 'This is going really well – I'm getting it right already' (excitement or pride)

While all of these are completely understandable reactions to practising mindfulness, they also provide opportunities to notice these as distractions from the focus on the anchor (the breath or body), and invitations to bring our awareness back to the initial focus (see Figure 8, p. 114). This process is important, as it helps to build confidence and capacity to notice and step back from our reactions (thoughts, emotions).

Difficulties with mindfulness

Struggles with mindfulness practice are common – in fact, everyone who has ever tried mindfulness has encountered difficulties in one way or another, so you're in good company if you have some too! Here are some tips and hints that might help as you continue with your practice in the coming days and weeks.

Top tips – attention and mindfulness

1. While it might sound easy and straightforward, try to remember that mindfulness practice can be tricky, particularly if we get caught in high expectations or a belief that we should 'do it right'

2. Your attention will get distracted and drift away when you are practising mindfulness – this is absolutely normal and happens to everyone who practises these exercises. Because our minds are not used to staying still, and in fact are naturally restless, it's useful to hold this insight in mind in a 'this is just how minds work' kind-of-way

3. Whether your attention drifts away just once, ten times or a hundred times during practice, this doesn't matter. The key thing is to try to be aware of when your attention drifts away, and as best as you can, kindly and gently try to bring your attention back to the initial focus (e.g. your breath)

4. Like learning any other skill in life, it takes effort to practise and develop the ability to be mindful. However, remember that this isn't a 'forcing' or a critical 'Come on, you should be better at this, you idiot', as that is going to activate your threat system. When practising mindfulness, it's an opportunity to notice these patterns and bring a compassionate approach to yourself – stepping back from judging and bringing a kind and caring approach to the challenge

5. Mindfulness isn't about trying to clear your mind, or trying not to think – your mind will always get distracted, and the thoughts will keep on coming! It can be helpful just to know that this will happen, and that it happens to all of us

6.   Remember that just like getting fit, it will take a while for you to notice changes and the benefits of your practice

7.   My first mindfulness teacher used to say that there is no such thing as a 'bad' practice. As long as the intention to 'notice and return' is present, that *is* a mindful practice. That's why, I think, it's called 'practice' because we're always working at it. This has always helped me to engage with the practice and tolerate frustration when it feels like 'it's not working'

Mindfulness in daily life

We can practise mindfulness in many ways throughout our daily life. This means engaging our intention to bring our full attention to *this* moment – observing our experience, moment by moment, just as it is, in the here and now. Body movement can help us do this.

Exercise: Mindful walking

To try mindful walking, the first thing you need to do is just that – walk! If you can, find a place where you have enough space to take at least ten steps before having to turn around. As you begin to walk around, notice the physical sensations that are present in your body. Gently become aware of what it feels like, physically, to be walking around the space that you're in. See if you can slow down your walking, and pay as much attention as you can to what this feels like in your body. Now draw your attention to the sensations at the soles of your feet, where your heels touch the floor, the centre part of your feet, and your toes, and notice one of your heels lifting as the other foot is still in contact with the floor. Go through the same process of being aware of contact – heel, centre and toes – and notice how the weight of your body shifts from the back of the foot to the front, and from one foot to the other. Notice any thoughts that come into your head and when your mind becomes distracted. When this happens, gently bring your attention and awareness back to the physical movement of walking. As you continue this process, see if you can become aware of the subtle sensations in your feet, ankles, legs and body.

You can bring this mindful, curious stance to any activity in your day; for example, you can engage your senses (sight, hearing, smell, touch, taste), and notice physical sensations on your body as you're having a shower, brushing your teeth in the morning, washing the dishes, or as you're taking your clothes off before bed. A common way of practising mindfulness is when eating. To do this, you need to do a little preparation and get some food ready for the exercise. It doesn't matter what food you have, although it may be easier to start with something you can hold with your fingers, such as a grape or raisin.

Exercise: Mindful eating

Spend a few moments looking at the food in front of you. Pick up the food, and notice its texture. Turn it around in your fingers, noticing its shape, contours and colour. Really pay attention to this as much as you can, as if this is the first time you've held this object in your hands. Squeeze it gently, and notice its size and weight. Slowly and mindfully, noticing the sensations in your arm, move the food up to your nose. Take your time to take in the smell of this food. Now gently put the food in your mouth, on your tongue, and take a moment to hold it in your mouth and savour its texture as you are moving it around your mouth, refraining from biting into it. In a moment, take a gentle bite into this food, and notice its taste as you're slowly chewing it. When you have finished chewing, notice how it feels to swallow the food. Complete this practice by paying attention to the taste and sensations in your mouth in the absence of the food.

As we discussed earlier, starting to practise any new skill can be tough. With this in mind, it may be helpful to make a record of your practice. In fact, many people find that keeping a practice log not only maintains the intention and motivation, but also enables them to acknowledge their efforts and progress in developing this new skill. On the opposite page, you will find a daily mindfulness practice log to record the details and observations of the different mindfulness exercises introduced in this chapter.

After recording the type and frequency of your practice for a week or so, you can review your diary. It can be helpful to hold a few questions in mind as you do this:

- What can you learn about your practice?

- Does this have any implications for your practice in the coming week(s)?

- Do you need to make any changes to develop your practice further?

- Are there practices that are easier than others, and if so can you be curious as to why?

- Is it worth persevering with those practices that are harder?

Key reflections

- Our minds are naturally restless

- Mindfulness involves learning to be more aware of the nature of the mind and being able to bring one's awareness into the present moment

- There are different types of mindfulness practice

- Mindfulness takes practice, and can be difficult or frustrating at times

	Mindful of sounds	Mindful body scan	Mindful breathing	Mindful walking	Mindful eating
Monday Time Length Reflections					
Tuesday Time Length Reflections					
Wednesday Time Length Reflections					
Thursday Time Length Reflections					
Friday Time Length Reflections					
Saturday Time Length Reflections					
Sunday Time Length Reflections					

9 Compassionate mind training – building the soothing system

Mindfulness can be a powerful approach to laying the foundation for a compassionate mind, and may in itself help move people towards the groundedness and stability of the soothing system. However, it can be difficult to regulate emotional difficulties when our threat system is powerful and dominant. This is where directly accessing and utilising the soothing system can help (see Chapter 2 for a reminder of this). In CFT, when helping people with emotions they find difficult or distressing, we sometimes refer to the process of 'bridging out' of the threat system into the soothing system; in other words, helping people move from a system dominated by the sympathetic nervous system (the fight/flight/freeze response), to one with good parasympathetic 'tone' (typically associated with states of calm and relaxation). You've already started some of this process with the mindfulness practices that were introduced in the previous chapter. In this chapter, we'll explore five further ways to do this:

- Body posture
- Breathing
- Facial expression
- Voice tone
- Memory and imagery

Body posture

Just as high divers or gymnasts will compose themselves by adopting an upright, grounded and confident body posture before engaging in their high dive or floor routine, so too is it important for us to find a helpful posture from which we can bridge in to access the soothing system. The way we hold our body can have a significant impact on our feelings, thoughts and behaviour. You might already have some intuitive knowledge of this, but we can experiment with it as you're reading this paragraph. Wherever you're sat at the moment, allow your body to slump completely in the chair, almost as if you had no bones to hold it up. Allow yourself to collapse in the stomach, and let your head drop forward. Hold this posture for 30 seconds or so, and notice how this leaves you feeling. Now, take a couple of deep breaths, and sit upright in the chair. Find a posture in which you feel comfortable, but alert, with your shoulders slightly back, chest open, and head upright. Hold this for 30 seconds.

What did you notice from this? When I take my clients through this, they often report feeling heavy, shut down, unmotivated or unenthusiastic with the former posture, and grounded, alert and stable with the latter. Although further studies are needed to support initial findings, it has been found that adopting confident postures is associated with increased feelings of power (Carney et al., 2010). Moreover, when our posture is hunched this inhibits our ability to breathe with the diaphragm, an important component of developing the type of breathing rhythm we'll be working on later in the chapter. Given this, it can be helpful to learn how to embody postures that are conducive to physiological (e.g. parasympathetic nervous system) and emotional states of groundedness, stability and safeness. Let's have a go at this with a short exercise.

Exercise: Developing a grounded, stable body posture

Start by standing up, with both feet close together. Imagine what would happen if someone were to push gently against your shoulder, or if you were on a moving bus or train but were unable to hold on to anything. Now think about the posture that you might adopt that would give you the best chance of retaining your balance in these situations. Often people find it helpful to try standing with their feet shoulder-width apart, with a little 'bounce' in the knees. Try this out. Maybe if someone were to give you a push on the shoulder now, what would happen?

Unlike the first posture, the second posture probably allows you to feel a bit more rooted so that you would remain stable and balanced, even if gently pushed. Now see if you can continue with the second, more grounded posture, with your spine long, your head at an alert position, looking forward (rather than down), and shoulders rolled back slightly so that the top of your chest is open and broad. Hold this posture for 30 seconds or so.

Now we're going to recreate this posture, but this time sitting on a chair. Gently lower yourself onto the chair, with your feet roughly shoulder-width apart. Allow your back (from the base upwards) to be supported by the back of the chair. Try to maintain your straight and alert head position. Gently allow your shoulders to drop a little, and move slightly backwards, keeping your chest in an open and confident position. Let your hands rest on your lap, and experiment with having your palms face down, or facing upwards. Maintain this posture for 30–60 seconds, mindfully noticing the sensations in your body.

What did it feel like to hold this type of posture? If you can, continue to practise this whenever you get the opportunity. Although it may feel unnatural at first, this will get easier to 'step into', and more comfortable with time and practice. Going forward, this will be the posture that we will embody to start all of our practices. You may want to begin practising this posture, particularly when noticing the presence of an emotion you're finding difficult, like anxiety or anger.

Soothing rhythm breathing

One of the main ways of strengthening our soothing system is through using the breath. Scientific studies have shown us that breathing in certain ways can have a significant impact on our physiology, helping to create an inner sense of grounding and stability.

How breathing can affect our body and mind

Breathing, just like the heart pumping blood around the body or the intestine digesting food, is one of our body's automatic processes that we don't need to think about or bring any effort to. However, unlike our heart and digestion, we are able to exert conscious control over our breathing when required. Moreover, when we do, this can have a direct impact on our nervous system, and therefore, our physiology. Given that our emotions and feelings – including those that cause us distress – are governed by physiology, it makes sense that learning to breathe in particular ways may be helpful in developing emotion regulation skills (Arch & Craske, 2006).

When we breathe in, our sympathetic nervous system is stimulated. When we breathe out, our parasympathetic system is stimulated. If you remember, the sympathetic nervous system is related to the threat system, whereas the parasympathetic nervous system is generally associated with the soothing system. Interestingly, scientists can measure the relative influence of our sympathetic and parasympathetic nervous systems in a number of ways, one of which is called *heart rate variability* (or HRV for short). HRV measures the time variation between heartbeats. So rather than the heart beating like a metronome, there are small variations. For example, if you had a heart rate of 60 beats per minute, it might be that the time between one heartbeat and the next is 1.15 seconds, but between that one and the following is 0.85 of a second. This is an entirely natural process, but overall, the greater the variation in time between heartbeats (described as having higher HRV), the more the parasympathetic system is asserting influence on the heart, and the rest of the body. The less variation there is in time between heartbeats (described as lower HRV), the more the sympathetic nervous system is asserting control, which is associated with fight/flight/freeze responses and related feelings (anger, anxiety). Many studies have found that lower levels of

HRV are associated with mental health problems like depression, social anxiety and OCD (Chalmers et al., 2014; Kemp et al., 2010), and emotion regulation problems in general (Williams et al., 2015). Interestingly, as the Williams et al. (2015) study was correlational, the opposite was also true – people with higher levels of heart rate variability (so, greater para-sympathetic influence on the body) had higher scores on various aspects of emotion regulation, such as emotion clarity and impulse control.

So, what does this all have to do with CFT, emotion regulation and breathing? Well, scientists have found that by practising certain types of breathing rhythm for just 12 minutes – typically slower, even and paced – HRV can increase (Lin et al., 2014). Studies have also found that, when comparing research participants undergoing therapy, it was those who regularly practised slower, paced breathing that had a greater increase in HRV and reduction in distress levels (e.g. depression symptoms; Caldwell & Steffen, 2018). We also know that practising breathing can actually support our new brains, by providing the physiological conditions that can lead to open, reflective and empathetic ways of thinking about ourselves and others. So, learning to breathe in particular ways can be an important starting point for developing your compassionate mind and managing emotions that you find difficult or distressing.

Learning to breathe in CFT

The use of the breath has been a core aspect of many ancient physical, mental and spiritual practices, such as meditation, yoga and tai chi. In CFT, we try to activate calmer physiological and emotional states by practising what we refer to as soothing rhythm breathing (SRB). The following exercise builds upon the mindful breathing practice (Chapter 8), but involves a particular breathing pace and rhythm, intended to stimulate your soothing system (parasympathetic nervous system), and over time, provide a balance for your threat system.

Exercise: Soothing rhythm breathing

Find somewhere quiet with a comfortable place to sit, taking some time to engage in the five preparation steps for practice (p. 115). These include finding a comfortable, upright posture, allowing your shoulders to open slightly, closing your eyes or if not, resting your gaze directly ahead of yourself. Begin by bringing your attention to your breathing, noticing the sensations that are present in your body as you breathe in and out. If you notice your attention becomes distracted, and moves away from your breath, just observe this and gently try to bring your attention back to your breath, without judging or criticising yourself.

Now, as you're holding your attention in the flow of your breath, gently try to bring a soothing, calming, breathing rhythm to your body. This is likely to be a slower and slightly deeper rhythm than your usual breathing pace, but one that feels comfortable to your body. If you can, try to breathe in a smooth, even way, with a similar amount of air going in or out of your body each second that you are breathing in or out. If you notice your attention moving away from the breath, or that you become distracted in any way, once you acknowledge this, gently bring your attention back to your breath, tuning back into its soothing quality.

See if you can imagine a sense of 'slowing down' as you breathe out. As your breathing slows down, it can be helpful to tune into your sense of groundedness and stability, for example by noticing your feet on the floor and/or legs on the chair. It can also be useful to try to bring a friendly facial expression, by softening your brow and your jaw, and allowing your lips to find a soft smile. Notice how it feels to hold this expression gently on your face, and if it brings a change to the experience of your breath. Try to pay attention to the physical sensations that are present as you're gently holding this calming breathing rhythm.

How did you get on with this exercise? What did you notice from doing it? As with many things that we try for the first time, there can be some difficulties that emerge, and the 'tips and hints' box below outlines some things to hold in mind that commonly make SRB practice difficult or tricky.

Tips and hints – difficulties with soothing rhythm breathing

If you find your mind wandering during the practice, try to use this as an opportunity to notice this mindfully and, in a non-judging way, gently bring your awareness back to your breathing rhythm.

If slowing down your breathing rhythm is difficult, take your time with this. Start where you feel comfortable, and practise this exercise for a while like this, before gently trying to slow your breathing a little bit. Often, if we take this in small steps, it feels more manageable.

Sometimes it's helpful to have a focus on the breath as it moves in through the nose, filling the lungs, and then following it back out through the nose on the out-breath. Or alternatively, just holding attention in the centre of the chest as it expands on the in-breath, and contracts on the out-breath.

Try not to worry if you don't feel immediately soothed or calm during the exercise – the most important thing is the intention and effort to try to generate a different physiological and psychological experience, that over time, and with practice, can leave the mind and body calmer, more still and grounded.

Slowing down

When we've had time to practise soothing breathing for a while, we might be ready to take another step. As we mentioned above, one way to help to bring balance to your physiology and help regulate your threat system is by practising deep, slow breathing. There is growing scientific evidence (e.g. Lin et al., 2014) that slowing down our breathing to approximately five or six breaths per minute, combined with an even, slightly deeper but smooth breathing rhythm, can lead to a helpful balance between your sympathetic and parasympathetic nervous systems. The exercise below may help with this.

Exercise: Learning to slow down – how to slow your breathing

Find a quiet and comfortable place for this exercise, and sit in an upright, relaxed posture. If you feel comfortable, close your eyes, or if not, rest your gaze directly ahead of yourself, with your head in an alert position. Begin by bringing your attention to your breathing in a mindful way. Notice the sensations present as you breathe in and out. If you notice your attention becomes distracted, and moves away from your breath, just observe this and gently try to bring your attention back to your breath, without judging or criticising yourself for this.

Now, as you're gently holding your attention in the flow of your breath, try to bring a soothing, calming breathing rhythm to your body. This is likely to be a slower, deeper rhythm than usual, but one that feels comfortable to your body. Try if you can to breathe in a smooth, even way. If you notice your attention moving away from your breath, or that you become distracted in any way, gently bring your attention back to your breath and tune back into its calming quality.

Once you find your own soothing rhythm breathing, see if you can slow your breathing down a little further. To start with, it can be helpful to count alongside your breathing, starting a little quicker, and slowing down over time. Here's an example:

Breathe in	1 - 2
Hold	1
Breathe out	1 - 2

Hold	1
Breathe in	1 - 2
Hold	1
Breathe out	1 - 2
Hold	1
Breathe in	1 - 2 - 3
Hold	1
Breathe out	1 - 2 - 3
Hold	1
Breathe in	1 - 2 - 3
Hold	1
Breathe out	1 - 2 - 3
Hold	1
Breathe in	1 - 2 - 3 - 4
Hold	1
Breathe out	1 - 2 - 3 - 4
Hold	1
Breathe in	1 - 2 - 3 - 4
Hold	1
Breathe out	1 - 2 - 3 - 4

Continue in this cycle, breathing in and out. Try to avoid a staccato breathing pattern (with short, sharp pauses with each count), but instead see if you can find a *smooth*, even breathing rhythm. Try to practise for 5 minutes or so, initially, and over time, gradually extend the duration of your practice.

Using technology to help

Smartphones can often support us with mindfulness and compassion practice. For example, you can record yourself (or someone else) reading the above exercise guidelines out loud or download audio clips of guided breathing rhythm work on to your phone to guide your practice (for example, see the 'resources' section at www.balancedminds.com). You can also download apps to your phone that can guide your practice, and set the rate of breathing per minute (for example, on the App Store, take a look at Breathing Zone or Calm). These apps are quite useful as they give a visual to guide your breathing rhythm, and sometimes people who experiment with using them find that it takes the pressure off the process of paced breathing.

Facial expression

People's facial expressions are often a window to their emotions and feelings. In fact, many leading scientists in the area of emotion research – all the way back to Charles Darwin – suggest that emotions show themselves through our facial expressions. We know that facial expressions have an impact on our own, and other people's, emotions. Consider the following example: imagine walking into a room of strangers – say a party or gathering where you don't know anyone – and feeling a bit anxious and self-conscious. What can someone in that room do (without speaking) that can help to reduce or calm your threat system? It's often a warm, friendly expression – in particular, a smile – that allows us to feel more at ease and welcome. We also now know that changing facial expression can affect our feelings. Although some researchers question the reliability of these results, a number of well-known experiments have shown that facial expressions are associated with different feelings and judgements. For example, in one study (Stracke et al., 1988), researchers asked a group of students to watch a cartoon while holding a chopstick in their mouths in a way that activated the same facial muscles as a smile, and another group of students to watch the same cartoon while holding the chopstick in a way that triggered the frown muscles. The former group (with smile facial muscles activated) reported that they found the cartoon to be funnier than the 'frown' group did. More recently, Kraft and Pressman (2012) found that smiling was associated with a lower heart rate during stress recovery.

Exercise: SRB with friendly facial expression

You can try out adding changes to your facial expression to your breathing rhythm practice. Get back into your stable, upright body posture, and gently reconnect to your soothing rhythm breathing. After a while gently bring a warm, friendly expression to your face – something that feels comfortable and natural to you. If it helps, briefly think of someone you're very fond of and allow your face to move into a natural expression reflecting your fondness of them. Just notice how it feels to hold this facial expression while breathing in a soothing rhythm, for 30 seconds or so. Now allow your face to return to a more neutral, non-smiling expression while continuing to hold your soothing rhythm breathing. Practise this for another 30 seconds or so. Then return to your friendly facial expression, and repeat this sequence – 30 seconds warm friendly facial expression, 30 seconds neutral, for a couple of rounds.

Voice tone and inner talk

It's likely that you have experience of the impact voice tone can have on our feelings. Let's do a short experiment on this. Imagine that later today, your partner or a family member is upset with you about something. Imagine them telling you about this with a voice tone that shows their anger, distress or upset. What do you notice happens if you just imagine their voice tone? Often here people get a quick flush through of a threat system reaction even though this incident hasn't happened (yet!). Equally, if you bring to mind your partner's or family member's kind, warm, caring or reassuring voice tone, saying something caring or supportive to you, this is likely to stimulate your soothing system, and you might have a quick flush of feeling calm, safe or content. It turns out that we can generate threat-based or soothing-based feelings internally, not only by what we say to ourselves (e.g. criticise ourselves, or reassure ourselves), but, more importantly, by how we talk to ourselves; whether we talk angrily, or with warmth and care. This is our inner voice tone. Many of the people I work with in therapy describe that when they are critical with themselves, this can come with quite hostile and angry inner voice tones, which in turn stimulate our threat system physiology and emotions, similar to how we feel when someone else uses this type of voice tone with us. It can be important then to create inner speech that is caring, reassuring and supportive. We can tie this into our breath work, and use certain words or phrases that can further 'boost the signal' and help us to connect with a great sense of calmness.

Exercise: Soothing rhythm breathing with inner speech and caring inner voice tone

Connect back with your upright, confident body posture, friendly facial expression, and soothing rhythm breathing. After 60 seconds or so, try saying to yourself (silently, in your own mind) the phrase 'body slowing down' each time you breathe out. If you can, practise saying this phrase really quickly, and see what this feels like; then try saying it more slowly, so that it stretches out almost as long as your out-breath. After a while of repeating this phrase slowly as you breathe out, try to add a warm, caring tone to these words in your mind. Imagine a voice tone that is similar to the one you might use when speaking to someone you deeply care for. You can alter the phrase if that helps, saying instead 'mind slowing down', again slowly across the out-breath. Continue with this for another couple of minutes, repeating the phrases in your mind with a warm, kind voice tone. As you bring this practice to a close, take a moment to sit quietly and let its effects 'sink in', without rushing yourself onto the next thing you have to do. Notice how your mind and body feel.

As with all of these practices, take a little time after each one to note down or reflect on the experience. Try not to race on to the next exercise, but rather, take your time to experiment and acclimatise to using language and voice tone to help yourself by practising this exercise a number of times.

Memory and imagery

In trying to activate your parasympathetic system with the previous exercises, we've also been providing the opportunity for you to become used to experiencing emotions related to the soothing system. If you remember from Chapter 2, emotions linked to the soothing system (e.g. calm, content) are important as they facilitate experiences of slowing down and resting, and are also experienced when we feel cared for and nurtured. This is similar to when distressed infants feel soothed and safe by drawing comfort from their parents' caring response (warm voice tone, interested and kind facial expression, soft touch etc.) – if they are lucky enough to have this sensitive response. As we discussed in Chapter 4, attachment theory focuses on how the quality of early relationships with carers shapes the child's emotional world (and ability to emotionally regulate), and their future relationships with themselves and others. Bowlby's ideas are important as they help us to understand how other people treat us, can have a significant impact on our ability to feel safe, content and secure. Unfortunately, not all of us have had, or have, experiences in life that make us familiar with these types of emotions and feelings; some people's experiences of others is associated with a sense of threat.

Although we can't go back in time and help people to have more reliable, caring and supportive relationships, we can engage in practices, in the here and now, that can bring us into greater contact with these feelings. By doing so, in effect we take our brain and body for a workout, allowing our physiology to become accustomed to these types of feelings. In turn, this can help us to manage emotions we find difficult when they turn up. We will try to do this in two ways: memory and imagery. Although we'll separate them out, the two have overlapping features.

(i) Memory

Memory can be a funny thing; we often remember things that we don't want to, and forget things that might be quite good to remember! What many of us realise though is that, when we focus on a particular memory, this can change the way we feel in the here and now. For example, if you were to focus on a time you felt very anxious, it's likely you'd start to feel a bit anxious now, even though the situation wasn't happening currently. Similarly, if you brought to mind a time that you were at your happiest or most excited, you might start to experience feelings of joy in the present moment. Given this insight, we can use memory as a way to stimulate the soothing system and feelings related to emotional safeness.

Exercise: Soothing memory

Take a few moments to engage in the five steps of preparation (p. 115), finding a comfortable and quiet place to sit, engaging in your upright, grounded body posture, soothing rhythm breathing, and friendly facial expression. Gently close your eyes, if you can. Allow your body to begin to slow down, finding a calming pace of breathing. Take a minute or two with this.

When you're ready, bring to mind a time when you felt calm, peaceful, or content. This might be a memory of lying on a beach or walking through a beautiful wood. It could be a time sat around a dinner table with friends or family. It could be a moment with your partner or child. Just allow yourself – gently and kindly – to bring a memory to mind that has the qualities of calming, peacefulness or contentment. Spend a minute or so connecting with this memory.

If you find it difficult to recall a memory, that's OK. It could be helpful just to spend a little while focusing on your soothing breathing, helping your body to slow down. Then when you're ready, try to bring a memory to mind.

When you have an outline of the memory in mind, spend a few moments trying to tune in to different aspects of it, as if it's happening again in the present. For example, see if you can notice where you are and what people or objects are around you. Then notice if there are sounds or smells adding to this experience of calming or soothing. Now, still with your soothing breathing, see if you can notice and pay attention to how this memory leaves you feeling now – just gently sitting with the memory and the feelings that emerge.

If your mind becomes distracted, by sounds or thoughts, just notice this and gently and kindly, bring your attention back to the memory. When you feel ready, return your focus to your breathing rhythm for 30 seconds, before finishing the exercise.

How was this exercise for you? Make a few notes, if that's useful, and consider how you could return to this memory more often if it was helpful for you.

(ii) Imagery

Memories can be a powerful way of stimulating feelings, but what happens if you don't have many soothing or calming memories to call upon? Or maybe you have had experiences like that, but because your threat system is so strong at the moment, it's hard to connect with the feelings associated with them. This is where imagery – and creating images – might come into effect.

It might be helpful to start by thinking about what imagery is, and what it isn't. From a psychological perspective, imagery refers to sensory information in the mind that does not have an external trigger. In that sense, we could see that memory is a type of imagery, in that it can be experienced in our minds but not be related to external cues. Sometimes when people hear about practising imagery, they can feel a little cynical about this: 'What's the point of doing imagery? It's not real, anyway.' Of course, this is true in the sense that imagined experiences are not tangible in the same way as our external world is. And certainly, we are not encouraging you to practise this to replace 'real' experiences. However, what we do know is that imagery can be a powerful way of bringing about emotional change, and in that sense, helpful in developing our compassionate mind. The diagram below can guide us to understand the effect of imagery.

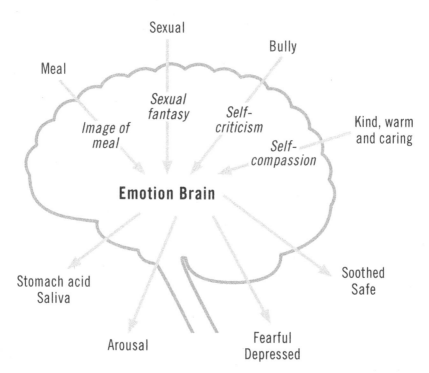

Diagram 1: How we respond to internal triggers in the same way as external triggers

Adapted from Gilbert, *The Compassionate Mind* (2009), reprinted with permission from Little, Brown Book Group.

1. Let's say you get home after a long day at work, absolutely starving. Luckily, your partner or flatmate has been really kind, and on the table is your favourite food. What do you think might happen in your body upon seeing and smelling the food? It's likely that you would start to salivate, and this happens because the sight and smell of the food stimulate a part of your brain (the pituitary gland), which in turn gets your body ready to digest the food. Now, take a moment, as you are reading this, to *imagine* your favourite food – imagine what it looks, smells and tastes like. What do you notice if you really pay attention to this image? Although there is no real food, the image of this can stimulate the same parts of our brain as seeing the real thing, and therefore leads to the same physiological response in the body.

2. Let's look at another example. Consider what happens in your body when you are with someone who you find very attractive, and things start to get a little steamy! Without going into too much detail, seeing someone who is attractive can stimulate parts of our brains, which in turn stimulate parts of our bodies, leading to arousal. However, imagining the same person, or any other person we find attractive and sexy, can do the same thing to our bodies – arousal. This, again, is because the imagined experience stimulates the same parts of our brain and body as the real, external experience.

3. Consider what it feels like being criticised or bullied by someone (for example, your boss or colleagues) over many months. How might that leave you feeling? Maybe a little low in mood, stressed, anxious or angry? We know this can happen because such experiences trigger our threat systems and the physiological processes linked to this (e.g. stress hormones). When this goes on over some time, it can leave us feeling anxious or low in mood. However, do we need a 'real' person to leave us feeling this way? Well no, because again we can criticise ourselves in our heads, and this can lead to low mood, increased stress and anxiety.

4. Finally, let's look at an example that links to compassion and the soothing system. Consider how it feels if you are surrounded by friends and
family who are kind, caring and compassionate to you. How might that
leave you feeling? Maybe a positive sense of safeness, or warm-feeling
connectedness? We know this can happen because when other people
treat us this way, this stimulates a variety of neurophysiological processes that give rise to the feeling of soothing and safeness. As you can
probably guess by now, we can stimulate this experience by using our
imagination and developing images of soothing and compassion that
can trigger our soothing system. This is not, of course, to say that these
images are replacements for real experiences of human connection, as
we are a social species after all. However, we can still use our minds to
generate images that have a soothing, calming effect on our brains, our
bodies, and therefore, our emotions.

In therapy, when we talk to our clients about imagery they can often
think that we are expecting them to create 3D, HDTV visual images, with
photo-like clarity. So, first up, it's important to clarify that this is not what
I'm expecting you to do in the following exercises! Imagery is usually
fleeting, transient and hazy. It is very rare to have stable, clear and vivid
imagery, so don't worry if you find this hard. The important thing is the
effort to bring an image to mind, and get a 'felt-sense' of what that is like.
Moreover, although when people discuss imagery they most commonly
refer to visual imagery, we can experience imagery in any of our sensory
domains – visual, auditory (sound), olfactory (smell), tactile (touch) and
taste.

Let's now have a go at practising imagery designed to stimulate your
soothing system by imagining a place that has certain qualities or associations related to the soothing system, and feelings of contentment,
peacefulness, soothing and safeness. The place could be 'real', in the
sense that you've been there and it exists in the real world, or it could be
somewhere entirely made up – a product of your own fantasy.

Exercise: Soothing system imagery – creating a calm place

Take a few moments to engage in the five steps of preparation for this practice (p. 115). So, find somewhere comfortable to sit where you will not be disturbed. Find a relaxed, upright posture and allow your eyes to close, if you can. Engage in your soothing rhythm breathing, allowing your body to slow down a little, with a sense of groundedness in the body as you breathe out. Spend a minute or two with this.

When you feel ready, allow your mind to move away from your breath, and slowly see if you can find a place in your mind that could give you the feeling of safeness, calmness or contentment. This place may be somewhere you have been before or somewhere completely 'made up'. Spend 60 seconds or so finding this place in your mind.

Try not to worry or get frustrated if no image comes to mind for a while, or if you find lots of different images appearing and struggle to pick one. Mindfully try to stay with your intention to allow an image to come to mind that feels safe, calming or soothing in some way, even if this is not fully formed.

When you do have an image of a place in your mind, spend a few moments mindfully paying attention to it. To start with, pay attention to whatever you can see in this place – this might be colours, shapes, or objects. Spend 30 seconds doing this. Next, notice if any sounds are present in this place, noticing the different qualities they may have, and how they contribute to you feeling calm and at ease. Spend 30 seconds doing this. Now, notice if there are any soothing or comforting smells present here and take a few moments to 'take these in'. Next, notice any physical sensations that are present – things that you might be able to touch or feel in your image, such as the warmth of the sun against your skin, or the feel of the grass or sand beneath your feet. Focus on this for 30 seconds. Spend some time becoming aware of how it feels for you to be in this place.

Maybe you can consider whether you are in your safe place on your own, or whether someone or something else (like an animal) is there with you. If you are on your own, consider who you might invite in to this image that would contribute to it feeling like a place of calmness and contentment. Consider how close or distant this person would be from you to help you feel at ease and safe.

As this is your own creation, imagine that somehow the place has an awareness of you. It welcomes you there and is happy to see you. It wants you to feel safe and calm. Notice how it feels to know that this place wants you to feel supported, secure and at ease.

Stay with this experience and the sensations and feelings it brings up for you for a while, if you can. Gradually bring this experience to a close, and open your eyes. Before moving on to your next activity, take a moment to become interested in the effects of your practice on your mind and your body.

If it helps, take some time to make some notes on what image(s) came to mind here. What was that exercise like for you? How did it leave you feeling? You might find it helpful to read through some of the suggestions in the 'top tips' box below about safe-place imagery.

Top tips – calm-place imagery

1. For some people, the word 'safe' can be a bit tricky and lead them to generate images of 'safety' rather than 'safeness'. A place linked to safety might be imagining (as one former client of mine did) being in a bunker with ten-feet-thick walls, with a force field around it that allows you to see out but no one to see in, and big guns on the outside. As you can see, this image is related to a sense of protection from threat, rather than the experience of calm and

being at ease. Safe places linked to safeness, on the other hand, are those that generate a sense of openness, curiosity, playfulness, and feelings of relaxation and being 'at ease'.

2.   If you find it difficult to find an image, spend some time looking online (e.g. Google images), or pay attention to your environment as you engage in your day-to-day activities. See if there are any places, objects or colours that contribute to your sense of feeling calm, content or peaceful. Following this, see if you can use these to guide your imagery.

3.   Be creative and try 'boosting the signal' of your image by stimulating your senses. For example, see what it feels like to practise this exercise while also having the smell of jasmine or lavender in the room, or soothing music in the background. Some people like to have something they can touch that has a calming or soothing texture to it, such as a semi-precious stone or piece of soft material.

Key reflections

- The soothing system – linked to the parasympathetic nervous system – is an important source of grounding, stability and regulation of the threat system

- It's possible to develop the soothing system through a variety of exercises – these include cultivating certain types of body posture, facial expression, voice tones, breathing rhythms and imagery

- There can be various blocks to experiencing this system, and it can take time to develop the emotions and physiology linked to it

10 Compassionate mind training – developing your compassionate self

If you remember, in the CFT approach we define compassion as 'a sensitivity to the suffering of self and others, with a commitment to try to alleviate and prevent it'; moreover, this definition contains *two psychologies*. The first one entails the ability to be sensitive to distress, to move towards it and engage with it. This, of course, may be quite difficult at times – and this is where the skills we developed in the last two chapters might help create the inner groundedness and stability to approach our difficult emotions. But remember, developing a compassionate mind isn't to move towards distress and then sink or drown in it – the second psychology involves the development of certain skills to help alleviate this distress. Building on skills that we've been working on in the previous chapters (mindfulness, soothing breathing, imagery), we will focus on how we can develop your 'compassionate self', to promote your ability to understand, approach and work with difficult emotions, and find helpful ways to regulate them.

Creating a compassionate mind

In Chapter 4, we discussed the idea of multiple versions of ourselves – different patterns that can show up and take over for some time. There are likely countless different versions that we can 'be', from angry, anxious, sad, and shameful, through to excited, prideful and so forth. The version of you, and the access you have to these different patterns, is likely to be guided by a mixture of your genes and experiences in life. Many of you will be reading this book because at least one of your emotions is either too 'loud' and dominant in your life, or is mostly absent or too 'quiet' when it turns up – when it would actually be helpful to experience it.

As we begin to build our skills in mindfulness and the soothing system, and have a bit more of a handle on some of the excesses of our threat system, we can spend more time thinking about, exploring and ultimately *choosing*, which type of pattern or version of ourselves we want to develop. In other words, having an awareness of our minds can give rise to the possibility of cultivating them in ways that serve us best. This is precisely what developing your compassionate mind involves.

It may be that some of you are lucky enough to have access to a compassionate self already, in which case this chapter could solidify this version of you, and help you direct this towards difficult emotions. However, for many others, while the seeds of compassion are inside you (as they are for all of us), they might be currently buried beneath the mud of your threat system, difficult emotions and tricky life experiences. The exercises in this chapter will allow these compassion seeds to grow.

Guided by the definition of compassion on the previous page, let's now look at the core qualities we need to cultivate our compassionate self.

Core qualities of the compassionate self

Take a moment to bring to mind someone you know in life who you see as compassionate. What qualities do they have? How do they show these qualities? Write a few of these down on a piece of paper. It might be that you list qualities like kindness, empathy, warmth, friendliness and patience. Think now about what qualities you would like to have if you could become a compassionate person. It doesn't matter if you feel you are a compassionate person or not, or whether you believe fully yet that you can be – just try your best to imagine what qualities you would embody that would show your compassionate nature to the world. Whichever qualities you've noticed, these can help to form the unique qualities of your compassionate self.

In addition to these, there are three core qualities that we are going to explore here. These are:

• Wisdom

- Caring-commitment
- Strength and courage

Wisdom

Wisdom in compassion is essential; in fact, compassion that is lacking wisdom can sometimes create suffering, rather than helping to alleviate it. Paul Gilbert gives a nice example of *unwise* compassion: imagine that you are walking along a river on a summer's day, and you see someone fall into the water, who appears to be drowning. In your 'compassionate', caring state, you run towards them and, *Baywatch*-style, dive into the river to save them. However, mid-dive, you realise: 'Sh*t, I can't swim!' While you have a caring intention here to save the person, without wisdom and an awareness that you can't swim, your compassionate action may result in more suffering, as it's likely you'll both end up drowning.

So, knowledge, insight and wisdom are crucial in and for compassion. As outlined in Chapters 2, 3 and 4, in CFT, wisdom entails an appreciation that we just find ourselves here, with a set of genes that we did not choose, and with a naturally tricky brain that easily gets us caught up in loops. This wisdom also includes an understanding that we are socially shaped – that we do not choose the environments we are born into, or many of the experiences we have in life, but that these play a significant role in shaping us into the person we are today. This insight allows us to appreciate that life is hard – that as part of being alive we will suffer, we will lose loved ones, experience rejection and setbacks, get ill and eventually die. We can also appreciate that while our emotions can cause us, and others, a lot of pain, we did not choose to have them, and that they too are likely to have been shaped by experiences in our life that we had little control over.

Wisdom in CFT is not a passive resignation to the realities of our lives; instead, it involves proactively taking responsibility to do what we can about these realities. This may include learning to step back from blaming and judging ourselves or others for the difficulties we or they face, or finding helpful responses to the difficult emotions we experience, or the situations that elicit them, in order to alleviate or reduce our distress. This wisdom is not only to understand, but also to work out what may help. It can arise from learning, previous experiences or in using our capacity for empathy and perspective-taking.

Caring-commitment

While wisdom is central to compassion, we do not want this to be applied in a cold or detached way. Compassion involves a commitment to noticing, engaging with and trying to alleviate distress, and often comes with warmth, kindness and a sense of caring, where possible. It is important to note here that kindness alone is not the hallmark of compassion. In fact, acting kindly can be associated with the desire to be liked by someone or to avoid being rejected. As outlined in Chapter 6, at the heart of compassion is the evolved motive to be *caring for*, the genuine commitment and intention to turn towards difficult emotions and distress, and find ways to regulate and alleviate these where possible.

Strength and courage

Compassion involves engaging with suffering, coming into contact with distress and threat system activation. Whether this involves being with a loved one who is dying from terminal illness, working through past traumatic experiences, or dealing with being rejected by someone, having strength and courage is crucial in dealing with any distressing emotions that emerge in these situations. To engage with suffering – to make contact with our threat system and not be overwhelmed by it – we need to have a sense of inner confidence, stability and groundedness. As mentioned in Chapter 6, if you consider international figures that are often labelled as compassionate, such as Nelson Mandela, they are described as strong or courageous. Courage and strength are to compassion what roots are to a tree; they allow us to remain grounded, to tolerate and even approach suffering without being blown over.

Now that we've spent some time thinking about the different qualities important for compassion, let's see how we can bring all of this together.

Cultivating the compassionate self

So, if your compassionate self is a type of pattern, self-identity or version of 'self', it's important to practise a number of exercises that help to cultivate this.

Using memory

You can develop your compassionate self by connecting with previous times in life you've embodied this pattern, or been this version of yourself. As we explored in the previous chapter, purposefully bringing types of memories to mind can trigger similar physiological reactions and states of mind in the here and now. Let's try this using the exercise below:

Exercise: Compassionate memory

Take a few moments to connect with the five steps of preparation for this practice (p. 115). Sit in an upright, comfortable position, allowing your shoulders to open slightly. Engage in your soothing rhythm breathing. Allow your breathing to slow a little, and gently rest your attention in the flow of breathing in, and breathing out. Stay with this for 60 seconds, or so. Allow your face to relax, and gently bring a warm or friendly expression to your face.

When you feel ready, bring to mind a memory of a time that you remember feeling compassion for another person, or perhaps, an animal. It might be a time that you offered help to someone who was struggling with a difficulty at work, or a friend having a difficult time in a relationship. It might be a time that you helped someone to carry their heavy bags on to the train, or when you looked after your poorly pet. Try to pick a memory in which the other person (or animal) wasn't in too much distress so as to not heat up your threat system too much.

Within this memory, try to remember what your compassionate intention was towards this other being – what did you want for them? Spend 30–60 seconds focusing on this, trying to hold that intention in mind.

Next, see if you can remember what your body language or facial expression was like. Consider how the way you were standing, the way you held your body, or the expression on your face conveyed your compassion and kindness towards the other. Notice if you can reconnect to that feeling now. Maybe you could try to remember the words you said, the tone of your voice, or what you did – again, just hold in mind all these characteristics, and how they conveyed your compassionate desire for this other being. Take some time to connect with each of these. If you can't remember these specifically, just try to imagine what facial expression, voice tone, words or actions you might have had, given your compassionate motivation towards this person.

Spend a couple more minutes focusing on the memory. When you are ready just let the memory fade, and come back to your breath again, before opening your eyes and coming back to the present moment.

What was this exercise like for you? Try to repeat it a number of times, either with the same memory or a different one, so that you get accustomed to this 'pattern' of the compassionate version of yourself.

Developing your compassionate self – acting techniques

A powerful way we can help you to develop your compassionate self is through using techniques that actors are taught and trained in. So, this next part of the book is going to give you a chance to tap into your inner Leonardo DiCaprio or Natalie Portman!

Some of you might be wondering what actors' training has to do with developing our compassionate self? Well, actors train to develop certain ways of being (thinking, feeling, behaving, moving, interacting and so forth) that best embody or represent the character they are portraying. Although some actors may have had shared experiences or share personal characteristics with the person they are portraying, many don't. Either way, it is through the practising of various skills, including but not exclusive to those involving memory, imagination, empathy and embodiment, that they find ways to connect with and 'step into' the person they are playing. They may spend time observing the type of character they are going to play, noticing body postures, facial expressions, tones of voice and movement.

Crucially, actors spend time creating the space to *be the person they want to be.* In this sense, it is similar to what we are doing together in this book – creating space for you to be the person you want to be, to develop a compassionate self as it is this part that has the skills, the motivation, and ability to help you manage difficult emotions when they emerge in life. For our purposes, we're going to start with how we can use imagery, memory and embodiment to help you with this. Remember you can find audio guides to these exercises in the 'resources' section of www.balancedminds.com.

Exercise: Compassionate self

Take a few moments to connect with the five steps of preparation for this practice (p. 115). Sit in an upright, confident yet comfortable position. Engage in your soothing rhythm breathing and friendly facial expression. Close your eyes, if you can. Allow your breathing to slow a little, and gently rest your attention in the flow of breathing in, and breathing out. Stay with this for 60 seconds or so.

Now, like an actor getting into a role, you are going to use your imagination to create an outline of a deeply compassionate version of yourself. So, for a moment, bring to mind the qualities you would have if this were the case. Remember it doesn't matter if you feel you actually are a deeply compassionate person, or not. The most important thing is just to hold in mind for a few moments what these qualities might be. Let's spend 30 seconds bringing these qualities to mind.

We are now going to focus on the three specific qualities of compassion that we have discussed earlier – caring-commitment, wisdom and strength.

To start with, let's focus on the quality of wisdom. There are many ways of thinking about what wisdom is, and sometimes it's described as the combination of knowledge plus experience. But an important source of wisdom for our compassionate self involves an understanding that we are all caught up in the flow of life, and just like other people, there is so much about ourselves we didn't choose. We didn't choose the genes we have, our gender or ethnicity. We didn't choose our parents, the family that we grew up in, or so many of the social circumstances that have influenced us in life. We didn't choose to have a brain that can get caught up in tricky self-critical or worry loops, or that can experience emotions which, at times, can be quite distressing – like anger, fear, sadness and shame. And of course, if we struggle with managing difficult emotions, this is unlikely to have been of our choosing either, and might actually be something we wish were different.

The wisdom of our compassionate self involves stepping back from self-blame and criticism of ourselves, and gives rise to an understanding that *this is not our fault*. But wisdom here is also linked to learning how to take responsibility for how our minds work, and for any difficulties that we have in managing our emotions or dealing with difficulties in life. This involves focusing on the desire to try to be the best we can, to cultivate something helpful and compassionate within us, both for ourselves and for other people.

Now, imagine that your compassionate self is strong, confident and grounded. This strength emerges from both the wisdom through which we can see the reality of life, and the commitment to do what we can about this. It involves the courage to face difficulties and tolerate the discomfort they bring, as well as bravery to confront our fears about change. Imagine that your compassionate self is strong and has inner confidence. Feel this connected to your upright body posture in your chair, the feet grounded on the floor and your steady breathing rhythm.

Consider what tone of voice you would use, how you might stand and walk. Sometimes it's helpful to imagine that like a strong tree with deep roots, or like a mountain, your compassionate self is grounded, stable and solid. It can be in the presence of difficult emotions but tolerate them. Spend a short time imagining how you would stand, what your posture would be like, as this strong, grounded person.

Finally, let's focus on the quality of commitment to care. Your compassionate self has a deep caring-commitment – this is partly linked to an appreciation that life can be very hard, and that we can all struggle with many things in life. So, given this, your compassionate self is motivated to be caring and committed to alleviating your own, and other people's, suffering. It also has a desire to contribute to your own, and other people's, well-being. Imagine how you would stand if you had a connection with this . . . consider what your facial expression, or your voice tone, might be like if you were deeply caring and committed to alleviating suffering. Focus here, if you can, on the intention to be helpful, not harmful. Spend 30–45 seconds imagining this.

Try to bring these qualities – strength, wisdom, caring-commitment – together, and like an actor getting into a role, imagine stepping into the shoes, body and mind of your compassionate self. How might you hold your posture? How would you stand as this strong, committed version of you? How might you speak, and what would your voice tone sound like? How would you think and feel? How would you respond to people as your compassionate self?

Now, imagine that you're walking along a street, in the body of your compassionate self. Imagine what your body posture would be like, what your eye gaze and head position would be. Consider what your facial expression and voice tone would be like, and how you would greet people as you meet them on the street. See if you can imagine seeing someone on the street who needs help – maybe an elderly person struggling to carry heavy bags, or someone who has fallen over and hurt themselves. As best you can, in the body of your compassionate self, imagine approaching this person and directing your compassion to them in a wise, supportive and caring way. Hold in mind your compassionate intention, your facial expression and your voice tone as you imagine this.

If it helps, imagine that you can see this version of you from the outside. How would you look? How would you move about and interact with people as this compassionate version of yourself? Again, don't worry if you don't feel that you have these qualities. Like an actor playing a character, just imagine what it would be like if you did.

Spend a couple more minutes allowing yourself to connect to your compassionate self. Take your time connecting with the different qualities. When you are ready, just let the image fade, and gently come back to the present time.

As discussed throughout these practice segments of the book, it can be helpful to make a few notes on your experience of this exercise. What did you connect with, or alternatively, find difficult, during this exercise? Sometimes it's useful to keep in mind the analogy of learning to drive a car – and how difficult it can be at first to coordinate pushing the right pedal, holding on to the steering wheel and not hitting things, checking your mirror, changing gears and so forth. At first, it can be hard to bring all of these together, but over time, they blend in a smooth way that feels far less burdensome. Similarly, the different aspects of the compassionate self can initially feel overwhelming, and hard to hold in mind at the same time. But with practice and training, these can come together in a way that feels more natural and accessible. Some recent research by colleagues of mine has found that two weeks of practising this exercise, along with things like soothing breathing (Chapter 9), led to significant reduction in self-criticism, shame and depression symptoms, and an increase in self-compassion, being open to compassion from others and having compassion for others (Matos et al., 2017).

Embodying your compassionate self – bringing the virtual into reality

So far in this chapter, we have thought about how we can use memory and imagination to develop your compassionate self. There is an emerging research evidence base that suggests spending time meditating on, or imagining, being compassionate can have a positive benefit on our mental health and well-being. However, in this book, we don't just want to stop there! Although helpful in itself, we don't want to leave you in a 'virtual' reality of the compassionate self, but rather, help you to bring this into your life in a meaningful way. We are now going to explore how to personify your compassionate version of yourself in your day-to-day life. In Chapters 15 and 16, and throughout Section Five (and the online material, accessible at https://overcoming.co.uk/715/resources-to-download), we will look at applying this more specifically in dealing with difficult emotions.

Exercise: Bringing your compassionate self into daily life

There are a number of steps to help you achieve this.

Step 1: Consider how you would actually be 'in the real world' as your compassionate self, given the images you brought to mind in the above exercises. For example, how would you engage in your daily-life tasks as your compassionate self? How would you be different? How would you move, walk, or stand? What would your facial expression or voice tone be like? How would you treat people?

See if you can practise this in your own home: doing your daily activities as if you were being this compassionate version of you. Really focus on your intention to try to embody being a compassionate person. This might initially seem a little strange. However, just like you might practise giving a speech in your bedroom before the 'real thing', rehearsing your compassionate self in this way can help enhance those qualities for when you are interacting with the 'real world'.

Step 2: Once you've practised some of this in your own space, see what it's like to take your compassionate self outdoors. For example, if you're actually walking down a local street, or you're in the supermarket, try to practise being your compassionate self. This might involve just focusing on your body posture, facial expression, eye gaze, or voice tone. Even if you only manage to remember to 'be' this version of you for 30 seconds, that is 30 seconds more of your compassionate self stored up in memory. It is through this practice that you can cultivate and get more familiar with the compassionate part of you.

Step 3: See if you can now bring this compassionate version to other people. Start with trying to express this compassionate version you've been practising by directing it towards others in a way that feels relatively easy. For example, maybe you could intend to be helpful or kind to someone – holding a door open for someone, expressing your gratitude to a friend or family member, doing something kind for someone. If you can, really try to focus on your *intention* to be this compassionate version of you as you're engaging in the action.

Step 4: After you've practised 'being' your compassionate self in easier scenarios, you might feel able to bring this version of you to something that is a little trickier. This might be 'bringing' your compassionate self to approach a difficult conversation with a work colleague or friend, or to a situation where someone else is struggling (maybe a friend who is unwell, or to a stranger in need of help).

Step 5: It's important to find ways to remember to practise your compassionate self. You may have the potential to be an outstanding runner (maybe there's a Usain Bolt version of you that could have been in the world), but if you don't spend time exercising and creating opportunities to run, then it's unlikely that you'll ever see this version of you come into the world. Take a moment to think about how you can remind yourself to practise being your compassionate self as often as possible. Here are a few ideas that others have found useful:

- Carry an object (like a stone, or a piece of jewellery or fabric) in your pocket so that each time you put your hand in, you are reminded to re-engage with your compassionate self

- Put reminders on your phone at various stages through the day, telling you to practise being your compassionate self

- Put a picture that is meaningful to you on your phone or laptop home screen, that can trigger your intention to be compassionate

Ideal compassionate other

Another way we can develop our compassionate mind is through using an image of a caring, compassionate 'other' that embodies qualities of compassion. We could think of this compassionate other as a compassionate friend, a compassionate companion, a compassionate mentor or any other name that feels meaningful to you. In this way, it builds nicely upon some of the ideas of attachment theory that we discussed in Chapter 4 (p. 60). For example, we can learn to seek this image when we need it (proximity seeking) to help us to manage our distress (safe haven) when something difficult has happened. But we can also use it to encourage and support us to move out into the world, try things out and pursue things that are important for us (secure base). Let's take a closer look at this.

Creating the compassionate ideal – what qualities would you want?

As we found out in Chapter 9, using imagery can impact our brains in the same way as experiencing something in real life. So, just as imagining your safe place can leave you feeling calm and at ease, or visualising your compassionate self can generate a sense of commitment, wisdom and strength, developing an image of a compassionate other can activate the experience of receiving compassion. To begin with, take a few moments to consider the qualities of compassion you would appreciate in another. It might be helpful to consider the following:

1. If you've experienced compassion from someone in the past, what qualities did that person have? How did they show their compassion to you? What personal characteristics or attributes – for example, kindness, warmth, non-judgement – did they have?

2. If you've seen someone show compassion to others (not you), what qualities did they have? How did they show this compassion?

3. If you were having a tough time, what qualities of compassion would you find helpful if someone was trying to help you with your struggle?

With the responses to the questions above in mind, it can be useful to consider what an image of a compassionate other (e.g. it's appearance, qualities and so on) might be like for you. Use the following questions to guide you.

What would you like your ideal caring, compassionate image/other to look like? Describe their physical appearance and facial expression (your image does not have to be human – it could be an animal or part of nature).

_____

_____

_____

_____

_____

How would you like your ideal compassionate other to sound? What tone of voice would they have?

_____

_____

How would you like your ideal compassionate other to relate to you? What would help you to sense their commitment and kindness to you?

_____

_____

_____

_____

_____

How would your compassionate other help you to manage your difficult emotions?

_____

_____

_____

_____

_____

Based on some of these reflections, let's now try out an imagery exercise to develop your compassionate other.

Exercise: Creating your ideal compassionate other

Take some time to engage in the five steps of preparation for this practice (p. 115), sitting in an upright, confident and comfortable position, allowing your shoulders to open up. Engage in your soothing rhythm breathing and friendly facial expression. Let your eyes close if this feels OK. Allow your breathing to slow a little, and gently rest your attention in the flow of breathing in, and breathing out. Stay with this for 60 seconds or so.

Spend a few moments thinking about the qualities you would value in an ideally compassionate other. Spend 30 seconds or so focusing on this. We're now going to focus on three specific qualities of compassion that we discussed previously – wisdom, strength, and caring-commitment.

Wisdom: Hold in mind that your compassionate other is wise and understanding. They have an understanding about the nature of human suffering, that we have 'tricky brains' that easily get caught up in loops, and emotions like anger, shame and sadness that can be very painful, that we did not choose to have. They will understand that much of what happens inside of us is 'not our fault', or our choosing. They will understand the difficulties we experience in life, and will never blame or criticise for this. However, they will also help us to take responsibility for the things we struggle with in life, like difficult emotions, and how to manage these helpfully. Take 30 seconds or so to hold this in mind.

Strength: Now take some time to imagine that your compassionate other is strong, courageous and grounded. They have a sense of authority and inner confidence – somehow you know that whatever difficulties or distress you experience, they will remain rooted and stable in the face of this, lending their strength to help you with your difficulties.

Caring-commitment: Your ideal compassionate other has a deep caring commitment to you. They are there to support and help you and see clearly into the nature of how hard life can be for you at times. They do not criticise you and want to help you to build compassion for yourself, and for other people.

See if a visual image of this compassionate other begins to form in your mind. What would your ideal compassionate other look like? Maybe you could consider whether they are old or young ... male or female ... short or tall. Remember, this image doesn't have to be someone you know; it can be an amalgamation of different people or an entirely created person that you've never met. Maybe your image isn't of a human being, but of an animal or part of nature. Spend 60 seconds or so visualising your ideal compassionate other, even if this is a fleeting image.

Now if you have an outline of an image, spend a moment focusing on the facial expression. Consider what the tone of their voice is, and how this somehow conveys a sense of their compassion towards you. If your image is of an animal or piece of nature, imagine what it would be like for either of these to have a facial expression or voice tone. Don't force this – go with what seems helpful for you. Just try to focus on this for 60 seconds or so.

Consider how your ideal compassionate other became compassionate – maybe they experienced pain and suffering but learned how to dedicate themselves to the compassionate path. They understand the reality that pain and suffering is part of life. Your compassionate other knows that we all just find ourselves here, with our tricky brains. They understand that our thoughts and feelings can run riot within us and that this is not our fault.

Your compassionate other has a deep wish for you to have compassion for your life. They are not judgemental or overwhelmed by what you feel. Your ideal compassionate other wants to be there just for you. They offer you their strength, care and wisdom. They have a deep desire to support you, to understand you.

What does it feel like, knowing that this ideal compassionate other is committed to supporting you? Allow yourself to receive the compassion from this being for a few moments, and see how that feels in your heart, your body, and your mind.

When you feel ready, gradually let this image fade and come back to the present moment, opening your eyes when you are ready. Take a few moments to absorb the effects of this practice, if any.

If it's helpful, make some notes on what this exercise was like. Maybe you can note down what your image looked like, what it sounded like. How did it feel to be in the presence of this image? As with the compassionate self exercise earlier in the chapter, it can take time to work on and develop this image, and it may well change over time from the image you start with.

Top tips – compassionate other

Although some people find developing their compassionate other very easy, for many it can be tricky. Here are some tips that might guide you:

1. Don't feel you have to go with the first image that comes to mind – play around and experiment with different ones until you find one that works best for you.

2. Creating images of someone you know in your life can be helpful to start with but remember, 'real people' can do 'real things' – that is, they can hurt us and let us down, and this could then impact upon how helpful your image is. If you do pick someone you know, it's probably most helpful for them to be someone you have a good, uncomplicated relationship with.

3. Having an image of someone compassionate but who has now passed away is a common choice for people. Although this might

be an effective choice, it's possible you will feel grief when you remember them. If so, it might make sense to create a different image of another being as it's likely that your feelings of sadness at the loss of this person might get in the way of the potential helpfulness of this image.

We'll return to the ideas and exercises in this chapter later in the book, to focus on directing our compassionate self to work with difficulties to do with regulating emotions. For now, though, see if you can set your intention at regularly practising being your compassionate self.

Key reflections

- You have multiple 'parts' of yourself, of which one is your compassionate self

- Like other parts, your compassionate part can be practised and strengthened through various memory and imagery exercises

- Two main practices to develop your compassionate mind here are the 'compassionate self', and the 'ideal compassionate other'

- Your compassionate self has some key qualities or attributes: wisdom, strength and caring-commitment

11 Fears, blocks and resistances to compassion

As we touched on in the previous chapters of this section, there can be various difficulties to developing our compassionate minds – whether that's in giving compassion to others or to ourselves, or in being open to receiving compassion from others. It turns out that compassion can be tricky for many reasons, and we refer to these as FBRs – the fears, blocks and resistances to compassion.

Fears of compassion are when we would like to be more compassionate, but are frightened that we may become weak, vulnerable or overly sensitive. For example, Clyde felt that becoming more compassionate to himself would connect him to feelings of sadness and grief about some of the difficult experiences he had had early in life (his parents died in a car crash, but he had never grieved for this loss). In comparison, Vicky felt that if she became more compassionate to others, this would make her vulnerable to their difficulties, and she could be taken advantage of by them (this had happened with a previous friend she had been kind towards). For her, compassion was linked to activating her threat system in an attempt to protect herself.

Blocks to compassion involve things that tend to get in the way of us being more compassionate in the world. So, this is not so much that we are scared of being more compassionate (although we may also be), but find that life is too busy, or certain things get in the way of being compassion (e.g. various life stresses, such as a relationship breakdown, physical health problem or financial problems).

Resistances to compassion are when we are not frightened of or blocked to compassion, but we just don't want to do it. For example, Kerry felt that she was undeserving of self-compassion because she had been unfaithful to her husband. In comparison, Scott was resistant to being compassionate to other people as he felt people should be strong and there were 'bad people out there' who had hurt him in the past. Of course, it might be that fears, blocks and resistances blend into each other. For example, it might be that a resistance actually turns out to be linked more to an underlying fear.

Misunderstandings about compassion

There can be some general misunderstandings about compassion, which can feed into fears, blocks and resistances. These include:

Compassion as 'weak': Often when I teach about CFT, or in my therapy sessions, the word compassion can trigger a common response: 'I don't like it, it's weak,' or 'I don't like the sound of that, it'll make me vulnerable.' Here, there are beliefs – often that have been learned over many years – that being compassionate to others makes you vulnerable, weak and able to be taken advantage of or hurt.

Compassion as niceness: A significant problem that we face with the word compassion is that it is synonymous with being nice or kind. Now, it's not to suggest that you can't be compassionate as well as being nice and kind. However, if we feel compassion *has to be* about being nice and kind, then it's likely we may compromise ourselves for the sake of others, or feel unable to move into the reality of how hard and distressing life can be.

Compassion as letting people/ourselves off the hook: For many people, being compassionate to ourselves (or others) would mean letting ourselves (or others) off the hook – or allowing ourselves (or others) to get away with mistakes or even making excuses.

There's a variety of ways that we can work with fears, blocks and resistances to compassion:

Tips and hints – how to manage fears, blocks and

resistances to compassion

- Remember the three system model, and see if you can notice when your threat system is coming online. When you notice this, rather than judging the experience, see if you can return to your soothing breathing or safe place image to help regulate the threat response, as a start

- It could be helpful to remember the idea of 'old brain–new brain' (Chapter 3). Are there any loops in the mind that are blocking your experience of compassion? If this is the case, see if you can be mindful of these loops, and try to step back and refocus on your intention to remain open to signals of care, as well as you can. If you notice a threat response emerging during this process, for example, anxiety or sadness, see if you can validate, and endure this experience, using your compassionate self

- Start where you can – with small steps. For example, see if you can notice and stay open to moments of others being kind or caring to you (e.g. this could be a shop assistant or a colleague). The key is not to ignore the small, day-to-day examples of this (e.g. someone holding a door open for you; someone smiling and wishing you a nice day). Being aware of kind gestures, however small, can help your mind become familiar with this experience

- See if you can start by connecting with some compassion towards this struggle you're having (with compassion). Bringing compassion to your experience of finding it hard to be compassionate might feel like a bit of a leap, but see if you can stick with it! Try your best to reflect on the reasons for why you're finding compassion tricky, without trying to push the discomfort away or getting annoyed with it or yourself

Paul Gilbert and colleagues (Gilbert et al., 2011) have conducted research on the fears of compassion, linked to the three flows of compassion (Chapter 6, p. 98): the fear of being compassionate to others, the fear of receiving compassion from others, and the fear of being compassionate to oneself. They found that higher scores on one 'flow' were related to higher fears on another flow – so greater concerns about being compassionate to others was related to greater fears of receiving compassion from others. And both of these, in turn, were related to greater fears of directing compassion to oneself. They also found that fear of compassion was associated with higher levels of stress, anxiety and depression symptoms. In many ways, this is not surprising. Given that we are a social species, and that our brains have evolved to be highly sensitive to, and needing of, the care, kindness and support of other people, it is no wonder that if this is blocked – and therefore we are disconnected from the soothing system – our threat systems are more likely to kick in and take over. This again highlights the importance of practising new patterns – those that will help to bring the soothing system online in our brain and body so that we can use this to regulate our threat systems and emotions that we find distressing or difficult to experience.

The compassionate ladder

Sometimes the difficulties with the compassionate mind training exercises in the previous chapters are specific – that is, some exercises are OK and quite helpful, but others are far more difficult. A useful way to manage some of the difficulties in experiencing compassion is by using the metaphor of the 'compassionate ladder'. When you struggle to engage with any of the exercises in the previous chapters of this section, or find that they stimulate unpleasant threat emotions (e.g. anxiety, sadness, anger), you can always move down the rungs of your compassionate ladder, choosing exercises that you find easier to engage with but that also help you to manage difficult feelings in turn. Here's an example: Dav found mindfulness, soothing breathing and safe place imagery straightforward, and very helpful in beginning to work with his difficult emotion (shame). However, when he moved on to developing his compassionate self, he found this very difficult. He felt undeserving of compassion, and found that this stirred up a feeling of anger and criticism towards himself. While noticing these feelings emerge during the exercise, we agreed that it would be helpful to manage some of these feelings by shifting to an exercise that was easier for him (soothing breathing and safe place imagery). He felt this helped to ground him again, regulated his threat system and, in turn, the anger and self-criticism he had begun to experience.

With ongoing practice, this approach to working with difficulties that emerge during CMT exercises can help you feel more secure and confident to move up the ladder again. If you do hit on problems during these exercises, try your best not to come off the ladder completely, remembering that you can also return to your mindfulness exercises as a way of grounding yourself into the here and now.

I've given just one example of what this ladder might look like in Figure 9 (opposite). The steps are roughly based on the order in which we have introduced practices in this book – you may or may not have these exercises in the same order. For example, it might be that the rungs of your 'ladder' are different to those illustrated in the diagram and that you want to reorder how high up (harder, maybe more difficult or activating of threat system) and low down (generally easier to connect with, practise and experience threat system regulation by doing) the practices are. It may be that you need other things to put at the lowest rungs of the ladder – for example, a stone or picture that you find grounding, or music or calming smells that help you to feel at ease and more relaxed.

Figure 9: The compassionate ladder

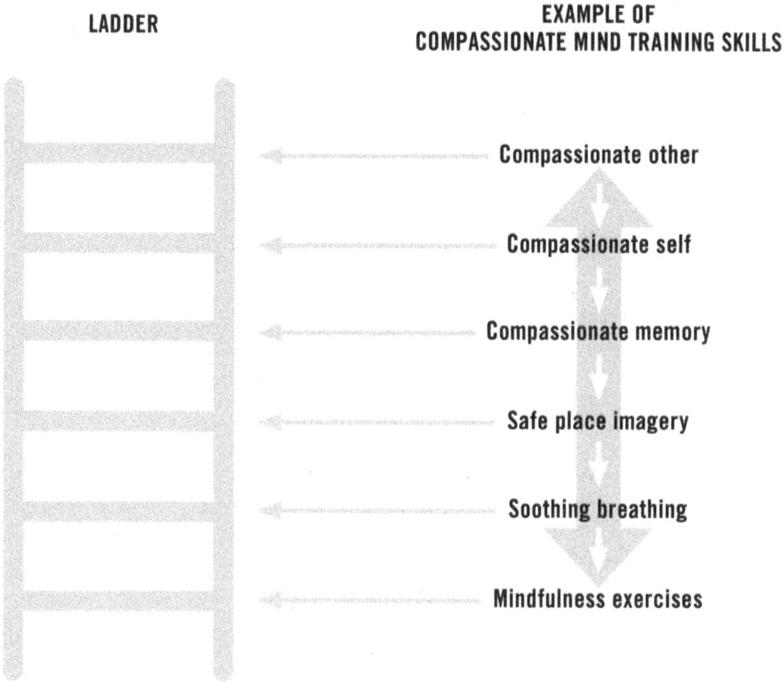

| LADDER | EXAMPLE OF COMPASSIONATE MIND TRAINING SKILLS |

Compassionate other

Compassionate self

Compassionate memory

Safe place imagery

Soothing breathing

Mindfulness exercises

Key reflections

- Developing compassion is not easy – many people find they hit upon difficulties when developing their skills in this area

- Difficulties with developing compassion can often involve fears, blocks or resistances

- Recognition that these exercises (and compassion more generally) are sometimes difficult can be helpful as a start for bringing compassion – but this time to the fact that we struggled with compassion in the first place

SECTION FOUR

Using your compassionate mind to manage your emotions – compassion-focused emotion regulation

In the previous section of the book, we spent some time practising a variety of compassionate mind skills. We're now going to focus on how we can bring these skills, and the understanding that you have developed throughout the book, and apply them in a more specific way to help you with regulating your emotions. We'll approach this by returning to the model we introduced earlier. If you remember, in Chapter 5 we discussed the concept of emotion regulation, and presented a model to outline different ways that people can struggle with emotions. In Figure 10 on the next page, we've expanded this model to include *helpful* ways to manage each of the emotion regulation steps. So, if you look at the figure, the central column guides the five main aspects of the emotion regulation process. On the left-hand side are some of the most common difficulties people have with managing these steps. On the right-hand side of the model are the more healthy or helpful ways that people can engage in each step.

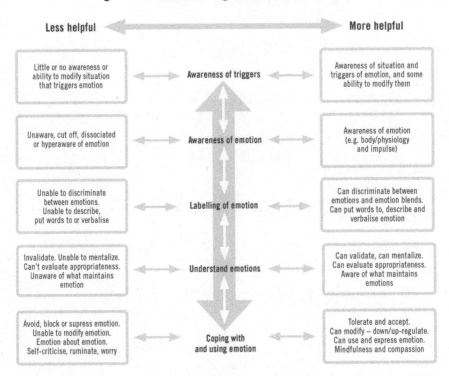

Figure 10: Emotion regulation model (ERM)

Let's explore this new aspect of the model with an example.

Example: Helpful emotion regulation

If you remember back to Chapter 5, we saw an example of how Kirsty struggled to regulate her emotions in various ways in the lead-up to giving a presentation. Looking at the model in Figure 10 above, we saw that her responses tracked the left-hand side of the diagram. To help explore the additional, healthy emotion regulation aspects of the model (right-hand side), let's take a look at how Simone approached a similar stressful situation. Simone also worked in a junior position at a large management consultancy firm. She too had been working on an important project with a team of colleagues, including her boss who was taking the lead. Similar to Kirsty, at the last moment her boss also had to pull out of giving the presentation, and like Kirsty, she also found public speaking anxiety-provoking.

1. Awareness of triggers

Upon finding out she would have to step in to do the presentation, Simone shared with her colleague that 'The heat's about to go up in the kitchen!' She was aware, given that she had little experience in giving presentations and how important it was for it to go well, that she was in for a tough few days. Although not feeling any strong emotions yet, her awareness that the situation could be emotionally activating led her to plan for how she could make the situation a bit better; this led her to approach a more experienced colleague later that day to get some tips and advice about how to give the presentation.

2. Awareness of emotion

As time passed, Simone noticed that she was feeling tension in her body – particularly in her stomach, chest and shoulders. She was aware of how her emotions were leading to worry about the presentation, and to wanting to avoid working on it.

3. Labelling of emotion

The day before the presentation, Simone had lunch with her colleague Kalil, who asked about how she was feeling. Simone was familiar with these feelings, as she'd had them many times before, and therefore described what had happened, and that she was feeling anxious. She also described feeling angry that her boss had pulled out at the last minute, and that she had only found out about this through his secretary.

4. Understanding of emotion

In talking to Kalil, Simone was able to articulate why it made sense she was feeling the way she was. She recognised it was understandable that this was an anxiety-provoking situation – after all, public speaking was something she'd always found difficult, and there was a lot riding on this presentation. She was able to validate the feelings she was having, including her sense of annoyance at her boss.

5. Coping with emotion

Given that she was able to notice, label and understand why she was feeling the way she was feeling, it may not be surprising that Simone also found helpful ways to cope with and manage her emotional experience. She spent some time practising skills she'd been working on with her therapist, including mindfully tolerating her feelings and using breathing and imagery exercises to help her stay grounded and present, rather than avoiding her emotions (as discussed in Chapters 8, 9 and 10, with a more in-depth explanation throughout the chapters in this section). Although challenging, she didn't try to suppress or block out her feelings, but instead, accepted that they would likely be present in the coming days. Knowing that, when struggling emotionally, she usually found it helpful to speak to friends, she arranged to have dinner with a good friend the day before the presentation. As she shared her experience, Simone not only received her friend's understanding and support but, by talking through this, she also decided that it was important to 'listen' to her anger. She recognised the validity to her anger, as her boss had landed her in a difficult situation with little notice and no explanation for why he'd done so, or acknowledgement of what impact this may have had on her. This led her to request a meeting with him so that she could voice these feelings in a productive yet assertive way.

Summary

If you compare the two, Simone's way of managing her emotions in this challenging situation is clearly very different from Kirsty's (Chapter 5). She was more able to engage in strategies and skills from the right-hand side of the emotion regulation model, and although she still found it a difficult and stressful time, was able to cope and ultimately, give an excellent presentation. So, in this following section of the book, we're going to take a chapter for each of the above steps, looking at how we can apply our compassionate mind skills to improve emotion regulation at each of the five stages. As you proceed, see if you can slow down, allowing time and space for your skills to develop, on each of these steps. As we'll be discussing how mindfulness and the 'compassionate self' skills can help in this process, it's important that you've already spent some time working on the skills training in Section Three.

12 Compassion-focused emotion regulation skills (CERS) – awareness of emotion triggers

So, let's start with the first step of the emotion regulation model. As much as we may like it to be different, life often brings stressful situations to our doorstep – arguments with friends, a family member's illness, difficulties at work, relationship break-ups. However, as we discussed in Chapter 5, some people find it difficult to predict the potential stress associated with an upcoming situation, struggle to stop a potentially emotionally distressing situation as it's happening, and/or find it difficult to modify stressful situations once they find themselves in them.

Emotion Regulation Model (ERM)

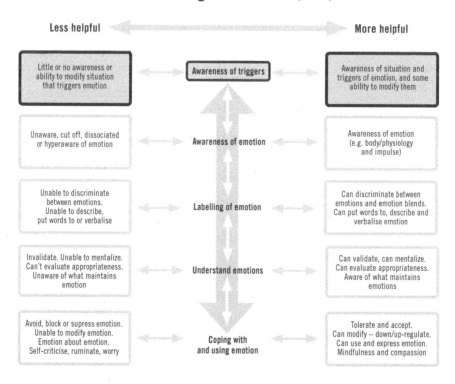

Less helpful ← → More helpful

Less helpful		More helpful
Little or no awareness or ability to modify situation that triggers emotion	**Awareness of triggers**	Awareness of situation and triggers of emotion, and some ability to modify them
Unaware, cut off, dissociated or hyperaware of emotion	**Awareness of emotion**	Awareness of emotion (e.g. body/physiology and impulse)
Unable to discriminate between emotions. Unable to describe, put words to or verbalise	**Labelling of emotion**	Can discriminate between emotions and emotion blends. Can put words to, describe and verbalise emotion
Invalidate. Unable to mentalize. Can't evaluate appropriateness. Unaware of what maintains emotion	**Understand emotions**	Can validate, can mentalize. Can evaluate appropriateness. Aware of what maintains emotions
Avoid, block or supress emotion. Unable to modify emotion. Emotion about emotion. Self-criticise, ruminate, worry	**Coping with and using emotion**	Tolerate and accept. Can modify – down/up-regulate. Can use and express emotion. Mindfulness and compassion

Here's a personal example that highlights how problems at this stage can lead to difficulties managing emotions. When I moved to London over a decade ago, I was working in a busy mental health hospital in an eastern part of the city called Tower Hamlets; it's fair to say my first week was a lovely but chaotic induction into life and work in a new city! Lots of new colleagues, IT systems to learn, meetings and patients to get my head around. For the first few nights, I stayed on a friend's sofa bed, as there had been a delay on the flat I was moving in to, so I wasn't getting much sleep. Eventually, I got the all-clear to move in on a Wednesday, but, being new to the job, I was reluctant to take the day off for the house move, and decided to move in during the evening after work. On Wednesday daytime, I was juggling meetings, phone calls with estate agents, arranging removal vans and attending ward rounds. I remember finding myself increasingly on edge, anxious and even annoyed with a few of my new colleagues, but I couldn't, for the life of me, work out why this was happening. After a long night of moving house, very little sleep, and a nightmare commute to work the next morning, I found myself snapping at a colleague when he joked about me being late for a team meeting. That same evening, talking to a friend, I felt clueless as to my feelings and reactions earlier in the day: 'Why did I snap at my colleague? Why am I feeling like this? I should be excited, I've just moved to a wonderful city and started a great new job!'

Looking back, how can we make sense of why this happened to me? Well, to start with you can probably see that I was under many time pressures, and had a number of important goals that I was trying to achieve (e.g. meeting new colleagues, learning new work systems, moving home and so on). However, by focusing attention and energy on one goal, this led to a blocking or thwarting of progress in another. In turn, this then led to greater arousal, tension and ultimately, an inability to regulate my emotions. Unfortunately, because of how many plates I was spinning, I was 'blind' to what was going on. Interestingly, when I spoke to my friend about it, they were incredulous – how did I *not* spot that this situation was so clearly stressful (in fact, they responded: 'Are you sure you're actually a psychologist, Chris?!'). As the saying goes, sometimes 'you can't see the wood for the trees'.

So, if I had to rerun this experience, what could I do differently? Well, there are many things of course, but in terms of this first step of the emotion regulation model, it would have been useful if I'd been aware of the *potential* of this situation being stressful on a general level, and that it was also likely to be creating goal conflicts and pulling me in different directions. If I had been aware of this, I could have started taking steps that might have been useful in managing my emotions more helpfully.

In this chapter, we're going to explore how can we improve awareness of emotional triggers. We'll break this down into three practice sub-steps:

1.   Developing attention and awareness to common (and individual) triggers of emotions

2.   Modifying triggers/situations that lead to emotions

3.   Selecting to engage in situations and events in a wise way

Let's take some time to look at each of these in turn.

1. Developing attention and awareness of triggers of difficult emotions

Identifying previous triggers to difficult emotions

In part, we're taught history at school to understand how and why things happened in the past, with the hope that this may help to bring a different, more informed approach to the 'now'. The same can go for managing our emotions. We can look back on our own history, observe the types of situation that previously triggered difficult emotions in us, and based on this, look out for similar situations in the present and future so that we can bring a wiser, more compassionate response to them. Let's use an initial exercise to try this out.

Exercise: Learning from the past

1. Take some time to think over occasions that you've found yourself struggling to manage difficult emotions in the past. If you can, try to find something that's happened relatively recently, so that it's nice and fresh in your mind, but not anything that was too overwhelming.

2. Identify what emotion you struggled with at this time – were you feeling angry, anxious, sad, ashamed? Or maybe something else?

3. See if you can identify what the trigger was to that difficult emotion. Was there a stimulating, threatening or tricky situation happening at the time? Maybe an argument, or disagreement with a friend? Perhaps a struggle at work, or in your personal life, in which something was getting in the way of your motive or goal (e.g. moving house, financial struggles, physical health concerns, or something you were trying to achieve)? Or was there something happening in your own mind – for example, painful memories, worry, rumination or self-criticism – that might have triggered this experience?

Take your time to reflect on this. If it helps, make a few notes for each of the points above. What have you learned about the triggers to your emotional experience?

Once you've done this, repeat the process of steps 1 to 3, but for different occasions in the past when you've struggled to manage an emotion. After you've run through a few, take a step back and look at what you've noted down. Are there any particular triggers that are similar, or overlap in some way? Are there any patterns to your triggers and emotional experiences and reactions? If so, is there a way to look out for these triggers if/when they show up in the future? A bit like you might check the forecast so as to take an umbrella if it's going to rain, having an awareness of the type of situation that can trigger emotional struggles can help you not to get drenched. It's also helpful to remember here (as we discussed in Chapter 2) that emotions are linked to our motives. So, when our motives are going well – for example, in our pursuit or something that we want to achieve – we tend to experience positive emotions. However, if our motives are blocked or thwarted, this typically triggers threat system emotions – for example, anxiety, frustration, irritation, and sometimes rage.

For some people, there aren't any particular or specific triggers to difficult emotions that are easily identifiable. In fact, emotional ups and downs can be linked to a whole range of things, including our diet, how much sleep we got the night before, hormonal changes through the month, or the picking up of a virus. Nonetheless, it may be helpful to keep an eye out for any patterns as time goes on. It might be useful to hold in mind some of the examples in Table 2 below, which highlight common stressful situations or triggers for difficult emotions.

Table 2: Common triggers for difficult emotions

Common triggers to difficult emotions	Tick if a trigger
Involving other people	
An argument with a friend	
An argument with a family member	
An argument with a colleague at work	
An argument with a stranger	
The beginning or end of a friendship	
The beginning or end of a romantic relationship	
Others showing too much or too little interest in you	
Others failing to appreciate your contribution/efforts	

Involving stressful situations	
Work stress	
Stress travelling to work	
Starting/leaving a job	
Financial problems	
Health concerns	
Moving house	
Blocks to something you wanted or were trying to achieve	
Things that happen in your own mind	
Negative thoughts or judgements about yourself (e.g. I'm an idiot/no good)	
Worrying or catastrophising about the future	
Bad or unpleasant memories	

Notice how many of the situations above are about being blocked, thwarted or disappointed in the pursuit of goals, desires, wants and wishes. So, while emotions may arise when we are in direct threat (e.g. fear), many of our emotions arise when we are blocked from things that we want. To compassionately manage your emotions, it can be helpful to recognise the types of situations that may trigger emotions, but also to identify if there aren't any obvious triggers. It's also helpful to hold in mind that sometimes it's the accumulation of stressful events that lead to us struggling with difficult emotions. A problem some people have is that they feel it's OK to feel distressed if there is one significant difficulty happening in life, but they may struggle to recognise that having lots of smaller struggles or moderate stress is still likely to create the context for difficult emotions. As the saying goes, it is 'the straw that broke the camel's back', although actually with accumulation in mind, it is recognising the million straws underneath the final one that are actually the issue.

Some people find it helpful to check in with other people that know them well, and show them the above table of triggers. They might help you to remember situations that triggered difficult emotions for you in the past, that you had forgotten about. It's also helpful to remember that this process can take time; in a sense, you are drawing a picture of something here (patterns of triggers to difficult emotions), but just like with any drawing or painting, it can take time to see what is being depicted.

Regardless of whether you were able to notice specific patterns, what can help you to start managing difficult emotions is to become more aware of the present moment triggers. Let's look at this below.

Increasing present-moment awareness

Chapter 8 introduced the idea of attention training and mindfulness, and discussed how these can be powerful ways of grounding awareness in the present moment and providing a bridge out of the threat system. Once you have spent some time developing mindful awareness, it can then be used in a variety of ways to help with this first step of emotion regulation. As mindfulness can help to bring greater awareness to our present-moment experiences, it can be useful as a way of noticing situations in the here and now that have the potential to trigger difficult emotions. One way of dividing this is between those that are external to us (i.e. in our environment), and those that arise inside of us (i.e. in our minds or our bodies). Let's take a look at this in more detail.

Awareness of external triggers to emotions

External triggers to difficult emotions are events or situations that occur in life and are often out of our control – for example, loss, moving home, challenges at work, a long commute, the weather and so on. They might also include people you are related to (e.g. your boss at work, or your partner or a family member), or strangers (for example, interacting with angry and aggressive people, or people who are very passive). Remember that it's often things that threaten us, that get in our way, or stop us from getting what we want (e.g. blocked motives) that can be related to emotions we find difficult to manage. Let's explore this in the below exercise.

Exercise: Increasing awareness of external triggers

Think about situations or events that you have going on in your life at the moment, or situations that are coming up in the next day or week(s) that may have the potential for triggering difficult emotions in you. Take a few minutes thinking about this. When you have one in mind, consider the following questions:

1. What is the potentially triggering situation?

_____

_____

2. What is it about the situation that is stressful or triggering for you? Hold in mind whether it is a direct threat (e.g. a critical boss) or being blocked or thwarted from something you want.

_____

_____

3. What emotion(s) is it triggering in you?

_____

_____

4. What can you do to be mindful of this situation when it happens?

_____

_____

If you can, come back to this exercise on a number of occasions (for example, once or twice a week); over time it can help improve your awareness of the type of external events and circumstances that may lead to emotional difficulties.

Awareness of internal triggers to difficult emotions

In Chapter 3 we explored the concept of loops in the mind – how our new-brain capacity for thinking (e.g. ruminating, worrying, self-criticism), imagining and self-monitoring can turn in on itself by stimulating old-brain emotions, and defensive behaviour. We discussed how many of us can get caught in particular types of thinking-feeling loops that can drive much of our distress. So, another way of looking at this is that certain loops in the mind may in themselves be the triggering 'situation' for difficult-to-manage emotions. The way we'll look at it here, linked to this step of the emotion regulation model, is to see how we can become aware of how our imagination, thinking and ability to plan can, if focused on potentially difficult situations in the future, cause us difficulties with emotions, even if we're not currently experiencing a difficult emotion.

Exercise: Noticing internal triggers to difficult emotions

To become more aware of internal triggers that may go on to trigger difficult emotions, take a look back at Chapter 3, and to the notes you made about the types of loops in the mind that you tend to get caught up in. Once you've done that, see if you can try out the following mindful steps:

1. *Remind yourself* to notice and pay attention to your own mind, and to what is passing through it. In particular, see what it's like to be aware of certain types of new brain activity that might, if they are frequent and locked in, lead to the triggering of old brain emotions like anger and anxiety (and potentially, 'loops in the mind' about something that hasn't happened yet).

2. *Ground yourself in the present moment.* Employ your mindful skills to ground yourself back into the here and now. It may help to do a short practice – 1 to 5 minutes of anchored mindful practice, for example a short mindfulness of breathing, sounds or body scan exercise. If you notice that your mind keeps returning to the future, or to patterns of thinking that may over time lead to difficult emotions if left to their own devices, use this as a gentle prompt to bring yourself back into the present moment. If these new brain thoughts or images are forming as you're in the middle of a particular activity (e.g. making dinner, walking to the train station), see if you can root your awareness back into the present moment of 'doing'. Focus on the slicing of the food you're preparing, the sound of water as you fill the pan to boil, the smell of the food as it's cooking in the oven. If you're walking, see if you can ground your attention in the sensory experiences of this – maybe noticing the sensation as your feet make contact with the ground, or noticing smells, colours or sounds around you.

3. *Notice when you become distracted.* At some stage, awareness is likely to move away from the anchor and be drawn into future worrying or some other distraction. When this happens, the key

is to not judge, blame or give yourself a hard time. Instead, notice the reactions you have about getting distracted (e.g. frustration, self-criticism), and with a type of kind awareness ('Oh, there I am criticising myself again') take this as an opportunity to gently bring your awareness back to the present moment. Remember, it doesn't matter if your mind wanders once, ten times or a hundred times – minds are designed to wander! Mindfulness involves noticing when our minds wander, and using this as an opportunity to ground ourselves back to the anchor, back to the present moment.

Just as with external triggers, over the next week or two, spend some time practising the above exercise. Try to see this as a way of *embracing and becoming familiar with your own mind* – to learn about it, to notice what it's like, how it functions, and how by being aware of these, this may help to reduce the likelihood of our minds getting caught in difficult emotion triggering loops. This can help you take important steps in developing mind awareness.

2. Modifying triggers/emotionally stimulating situations

If we are aware that a situation has occurred that may (over time) trigger distressing emotions and feelings, it can be helpful to consider what we do with this – how we can try to modify this wisely. It's important here to remember that this is not about avoiding emotions, or situations that may be emotionally distressing (such as an exam, or having a difficult conversation with someone who has upset us). It is about taking steps to alter or modify the course of a situation slightly so that we don't experience *unneeded* or *unnecessary* distress. It may be that for some people, taking responsibility for modifying triggers of difficult emotions may also give a sense of confidence, control and empowerment. Here's an example.

Tara came to therapy for help with feeling stressed at work. Although generally known as someone who was very calm, composed and emotionally balanced, in the past couple of months she had frequently lashed out at colleagues with anger and annoyance. On one occasion, she walked out of a meeting, swearing under her breath, slamming the door as she left. On another, she told a colleague who came to her for help, 'Why don't you fucking leave me alone to get on with my own job, instead of getting me to do yours all the time?' During therapy, some of the focus with Tara was on Step 1 of the emotion regulation model – helping her to notice and become aware of the triggers and situations that were associated with her angry outbursts. She worked as a social worker in a busy inner-city team, with a caseload of very distressed and, at times, risky clients. Her service was under a lot of financial pressures and was understaffed to boot. In fact, over the past year, her caseload had increased significantly, going up from fifty to over eighty, far more people to work with than advised. Tara started to make notes of when her anger bubbled over and noticed that this was often following team meetings where new clients were allocated to staff, even though she could see that all her colleagues were also overworked. She also noticed 'internal' thinking-feeling loops, particularly about her manager: 'She doesn't have a clue, look at how thoughtless she is handing out more and more work – we can't cope!' This led to increased anger and hostility towards management and the service itself.

Once Tara recognised these thinking-feeling cycles, she also spent time – through doing an imagery exercise and using the wisdom and strength of her compassionate self (Chapter 10) and directing this through writing (Chapter 19) – to consider how she could bring changes to the situations that would trigger her anger. Tara decided to organise a meeting with her boss to talk about the situation. Before the meeting, she practised being calm and assertive (rather than letting her anger guide her too much) by using her *soothing rhythm breathing (Chapter 9) and compassionate self imagery (Chapter 10). In the meeting, she described her recent struggles, and together with her boss, started to plan ways to manage the situation differently. They agreed that having a staff away day, with an external facilitator, might help the team to think creatively about how caseloads and other work demands could be better managed in the future. Although she still described feeling stressed, Tara felt much calmer, and less angry, following this meeting, and had some hope that things might change positively. And even though it turned out that it took a few months before her caseload started to reduce, Tara felt much better for being in contact with her emotions about this, and feeling more able to express these and get her needs met.*

To consider how to modify situations that might be causing unhelpful levels of emotional distress, it's useful to recruit the part of you that has relevant skills for this – your compassionate self. If you recall from Chapter 10, this version of you has certain qualities: commitment to care for your well-being, sensitivity to your distress, and a desire to do something about this; strength and grounding/emotional stability/steadiness to help you engage with difficulties without getting overwhelmed; and crucially, wisdom to understand how situations trigger our threat systems, and the ability to take perspective and discern helpful ways of managing emotionally triggering situations. Let's look at this.

Exercise: Using your compassionate mind to modify trigger situations

As you learned about and practised in Chapter 10, take a few minutes to get into your compassionate self, focusing on your body posture, facial expression, soothing rhythm breathing and sense of yourself slowing down and groundedness in your body (the five steps of preparation, p. 115).

Next, focus on your compassionate intention to address distress and suffering – to be helpful and supportive to yourself.

Bring to mind your core qualities of wisdom, strength and commitment. Feel your way into connecting with this part of you, remembering that your compassionate self will not try to avoid situations that have triggered distressing or difficult emotions, particularly when they are important for us to engage in (e.g. an upcoming interview or going on a date). Instead, our compassionate self is able to bring wisdom to how to work with situations that are distressing in a way that is supportive and most likely to facilitate you navigating it in a helpful way.

To engage in this exercise, you might want to consider whether there is a current, ongoing situation that is causing you distressing emotions, that you'd like to work through as an example. Or if you're not currently experiencing this type of situation, take some time to bring to mind one from the recent past, and use this as the example to hold in mind, even though it has passed now. With this in mind, take some time to consider each of the following questions:

- What does your compassionate self understand about how and why this situation is a trigger for distressing emotions (e.g. are these situations linked to disappointments, to feeling threatened or being blocked from a goal?). Is this a new trigger, or one that is typical and familiar to you?

- Standing back from the situation, are there ways you could think or behave that would either change some of the aspects that are triggering distressing emotions, or change your relationship to them? What might they be?

- As your compassionate self, what qualities and skills would you need to make these modifications?

- Is there anything else that could help you with this? For example, is there someone you could speak to who would help you in thinking through things and making the changes you need to make?

- What does the compassionate self know about what's helped in the past in similar types of activating situations?

- What might your compassionate self do if this was a good friend who was struggling with the same type of difficulty?

- What wisdom would your compassionate self bring to the situation? How would that leave you feeling?

Similar to the other exercises that we've done in this chapter, try not to see this exercise as something you would do only once. It can be useful to re-engage with your compassionate self for a number of occasions where difficult emotions are triggered. This has the benefit of helping you get used to approaching difficulties from a particular part of you, which will also come in useful later in the book.

Tips: Modifying triggering situations

- Speak to someone you trust or value. Ask them about the situation, and if they have any ideas about what might help

- Try to view awareness of emotionally triggering situations as an opportunity to engage with this from a different (compassionate) mind state. Maybe this is an opportunity to embody your wisdom, strength and commitment to support and help yourself and the difficult emotions you sometimes experience

- What have you noticed that other people have done in similar situations? If there is someone you respect and trust, what might they do?

- If you've experienced a similar situation in the past, was there anything that you did that was wise and helpful? Was there anything that you did that was unhelpful that could be avoided this time?

- Remember that your compassionate self is not 'all-knowing' but can wisely recognise that it might not have all the answers. For example, some situations *are* stressful and will trigger threat emotions. So, rather than changing the situation, or attempting not to experience threat emotions, it's more helpful to work with our inner reactions to them and try to engage with the part of us that will be supportive and helpful. We will address some of these points in Chapters 15 and 16, in Section Five, and throughout the online materials accessible at https://overcoming.co.uk/715/resources-to-download.

3. Wise selection of situations

A number of people find it hard to regulate their emotions because they struggle to *anticipate* how a future situation may trigger a particular emotion, and because of this, do not engage in wise steps that may modify the situation in a way that will help them to manage their emotions in a helpful way (Gross, 2015). This is often described as 'situation selection' and involves our capacity to select situations that are more likely to trigger the drive and soothing system and protect us from (or minimise) *unnecessary* contact with the threat system. It's important to emphasise the unnecessary here; I'm not suggesting that you should *avoid* any situation that you find is linked to difficult emotions for you, as this would not be a wise, helpful, or compassionate thing to do, but more likely a threat system-related 'avoidance' safety strategy. Instead, in this section we're going to focus on the idea of situation selection based on understanding ourselves, and wisely choosing not to enter or move towards distressing situations that are unnecessary or unneeded.

For example, if you're anxious about going to the dentist, it's not wise to avoid going for years and years, as this is likely to lead to a number of health problems, and a lot more pain (physical and financial) trying to fix your teeth. However, wisely choosing not to see an acquaintance who is very shaming, harsh and critical, and who often leaves you feeling anxious and low, may be a more helpful version of situation selection. Moreover, if you know that seeing certain friends, or engaging in certain activities (e.g. going to the cinema; swimming or reading a book) is very helpful in creating positive feelings in you, this might be something important to try to do more of. Many of us engage in situations or behaviours (e.g. excessive use of social media; eating certain foods) that we know may make us feel worse or unhappy; so, the point is not blaming ourselves for this but learning to live in a way that is conducive to your well-being.

The wisdom of your compassionate self is key here. Interestingly, research has found that older adults tend to be better at this type of emotion regulation strategy than younger people. For example, older people tend to spend less time with threat system-inducing material (e.g. negative videos and articles), and are more likely to pursue pleasurable situations than young people (Livingstone & Isaacowitz, 2015). Older adults are also more selective of the people they socialise with, which may indicate that they are more thoughtful about which type of people they will experience positive emotions with, and which would be less enjoyable (Carstensen et al., 1997).

Take a moment to think about your ability to select situations in a way that regulates your emotions wisely and healthily. Hold in mind the following questions:

- How able are you to select situations that leave you feeling the emotions of the threat system (e.g. anger, anxiety, shame)?

- How able are you to minimise unneeded contact with situations, experiences or people that stimulate the emotions of the threat system, and generally leave you feeling 'bad'?

- How able are you to select situations that leave you feeling the emotions of the drive system (e.g. excited, joyful or energised)?

- How able are you to move towards and maximise the frequency of situations, experiences or people who leave you feeling the emotions of the drive system?

- How able are you to select situations that leave you feeling the emotions of the soothing system (e.g. calm, content, connected)?

- How able are you to move towards and maximise the frequency of situations, experiences or people who leave you feeling the emotions of the soothing system?

Key to the above is to check in with your compassionate self to help clarify that the answers are not about avoidance, running away from, blocking or ignoring unpleasant emotions that are actually telling you something important (see Chapter 2 on the function of emotions). However, many of my patients find themselves 'out of shape' with the above answers – unable to manage and minimise situations linked to the threat system, and with difficulty making regular or healthy contact with the emotions of the drive and soothing system. Our work often involves helping them to bring greater *balance* to this, and a greater agency at this first stage of the emotion regulation model to navigate away from the threat system and towards the drive and soothing system emotions. Let's take a look at how you can find this healthier balance to your three emotion systems:

Exercise: Wise selection of situations

Take a few moments to prepare yourself for the practice, connecting with your body posture, facial expression and breathing rhythm outlined in Chapter 9. When you feel ready, bring to mind the image and qualities of your compassionate self – wisdom, strength and caring commitment.

From this part of you, consider the following questions:

- What situations do you have in the coming weeks that may trigger your threat, drive or soothing system emotions? If you look in your diary, can you spot potential difficulties that might arise in the next week or two?

- If there are upcoming situations that may trigger threat system emotions, is there something you can do to limit the impact of them, or stay away from them in a wise and non-avoidant way?

- If there is a lack of situations that are associated with drive system emotions, what can you do to increase these? What situations would these be? What situations could you engage in that you might get a sense of excitement, happiness or pleasure from?

- If there are infrequent opportunities to experience situations that may be linked with soothing system emotions, what can you do to increase these? What situations would these be? What situations could you engage in that might offer you a sense of calmness, contentment or caring connection?

Take some time to think about each of these. Make some notes on a piece of paper if it helps (some people find it helpful to keep a diary or notebook to record their reflections on these types of exercises). Sometimes people find it useful to return to these questions at the start of each week or month, looking forward and setting a wise, compassionate intention for the time to come.

Key reflections

Step 1 of the emotion regulation model focuses on *awareness of emotion triggers,* and in this chapter we have developed insights and skills about how:

- Being able to recognise how situations can affect our feelings is important in emotion regulation

- Predicting emotionally triggering situations, and wisely selecting to engage in situations that are likely to bring us into contact with emotions of the drive (excitement, joy) and soothing (calm, content) system, and minimise unneeded contact with those of the threat system (e.g. anger, anxiety), can be a useful, forward-looking emotion strategy

- Being aware of when a situation has triggered a particular emotion, and learning which types of situations typically activate difficult emotions, can help us effectively navigate our emotions

- Being able to modify an emotionally triggering situation when we are 'in it' can help to minimise the experience of negative emotions such as anxiety or anger, or enable us to better tolerate them without getting overwhelmed

13 Compassion-focused emotion regulation skills (CERS) – awareness of emotions

While it's helpful to become more aware of, and able to modify, situations that trigger difficult emotions, it's also important to be aware of emotions themselves once they've been triggered. As a comparison, although I may know that chopping vegetables could be a situation in which I could cut my finger, if I *don't notice* that I've actually cut my finger when chopping vegetables, then it's unlikely that I'll do anything helpful for the bleeding. As we explored in Chapter 5, some people find it difficult to notice or track signs that they are experiencing a particular emotion. Just like with not noticing if we've cut ourselves, if we are unaware of the signs of emotion when they're triggered, this is likely to make regulating them particularly difficult. So, in this chapter, we're going to explore the second step of the emotion regulation model (Figure 11, overleaf), *awareness of emotions*.

There are a many different personal examples I could give for this type of emotion regulation problem. Just a couple of weeks ago, at the end of a long, hard day at work, I received an email from someone, criticising me for not delivering on a task they expected me to have completed by then. I left my office, went home, and shortly after walking in the front door, my wife asked whether we should go out to eat that night. Without thinking, I responded in an abrupt, curt way with her: 'I don't know, whatever you want,' which then led to a mini-argument. Now, looking back, while I was aware that the situation (receiving the email) had been unpleasant, I hadn't tracked how this had triggered an angry response in me. I was *unaware* of how my heart rate had increased, how I was holding my shoulders and arms more tightly. I wasn't aware that I had an urge not to speak and be left alone in my angry thoughts. I

Figure 11: Emotion regulation model (ERM) – awareness of emotions

Less helpful		More helpful
Little or no awareness or ability to modify situation that triggers emotion	**Awareness of triggers**	Awareness of situation and triggers of emotion, and some ability to modify them
Unaware, cut off, dissociated or hyperaware of emotion	**Awareness of emotion**	Awareness of emotion (e.g. body/physiology and impulse)
Unable to discriminate between emotions. Unable to describe, put words to or verbalise	**Labelling of emotion**	Can discriminate between emotions and emotion blends. Can put words to, describe and verbalise emotion
Invalidate. Unable to mentalize. Can't evaluate appropriateness. Unaware of what maintains emotion	**Understand emotions**	Can validate, can mentalize. Can evaluate appropriateness. Aware of what maintains emotions
Avoid, block or supress emotion. Unable to modify emotion. Emotion about emotion. Self-criticise, ruminate, worry	**Coping with and using emotion**	Tolerate and accept. Can modify – down/up-regulate. Can use and express emotion. Mindfulness and compassion

didn't notice the ruminating thoughts playing through my mind about the person who had emailed me: 'How dare he criticise me for that – he knows I've had so much on recently,' and 'What's he been doing with this anyway, how come he hasn't helped?' Partly because I wasn't tracking these changes inside me (which could be accurately described as anger), I wasn't able to regulate this emotion, and instead took it out on my wife, who was completely innocent and simply asked me a general question about the evening!

Now clearly there might be many more helpful things I could have done here. To start with, it would have been useful to be more aware and mindful of my own emotional temperature – to track that I'd been stimulated into my threat system. This might have included noticing the tension in my stomach, muscles and jaw; the swirling, angry rumination in my mind, blaming the person who had emailed me; how my attention kept on returning narrowly to the email, reading it over and over again. If I'd noticed this, I might have been able to slow myself down a little, maybe through my breathing rhythm or some imagery, and had the intention not to carry the heat home with me that then got transferred to the disagreement with my wife. Greater awareness of my emotional state might have also helped me to forewarn my wife, letting her know that I was feeling angry, and that I was struggling to work out how to react best to the email. Unfortunately, when we are blind to our emotions as I was, we are more likely to act them out in unhelpful ways. For me, my lack of awareness of my 'emotional temperature', meant that I carried extra heat home with me from work in a way that then caused further problems.

So, in this chapter, we're going to look at how to become more aware of the emotions that we're experiencing.

Emotion patterns

Emotions tend to show up with a particular *shape* or *pattern*. The type of shape or pattern might differ between emotions (for example, the shape of anger and joy are normally quite different), and depending on the trigger, the context, and a host of other factors, the shape of the same emotion might be quite different from day to day. For example, while anger might show up with a similar pattern most days, there can be a big difference between the anger that gives rise to shouting and aggression, and the anger that is experienced but not expressed (for example, passive aggression).

In this chapter, we're going to look at the different patterns that emotions come in, and practise how we can become more aware of these. In the compassionate mind approach, we say that *emotions shape the mind and body,* and we can see some of the different features of emotions in Figure 12 on the next page (see also Chapter 1 for further discussion). These features include changes to what we are paying attention to, the content or process of our thinking, our behaviour or urges, physiological changes in our body, changes to our motives, and the images in our minds.

Figure 12: Emotion 'features'

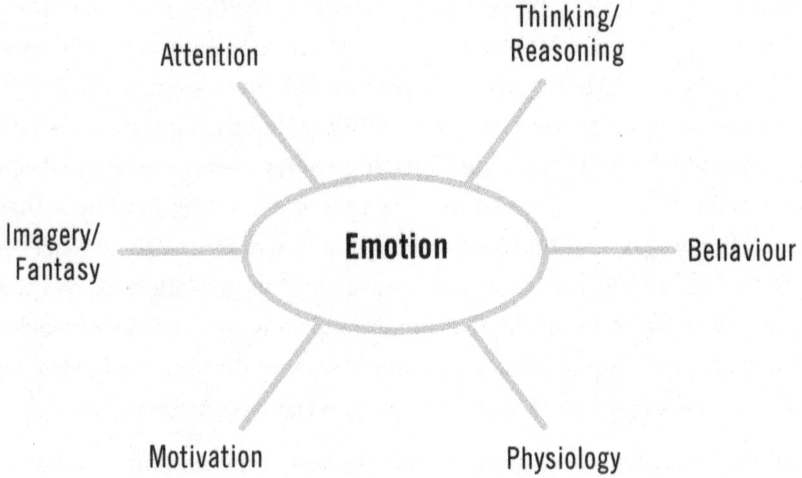

Thinking/
Reasoning

Attention

Imagery/
Fantasy

Emotion

Behaviour

Motivation

Physiology

Let's look at how this might work. When an emotion is triggered (you may not at this stage be able to label what emotion that is), it tends to show up with certain features, for example:

Physiology	You may notice certain changes in your body – for example, heart beating faster, sweaty palms or tension in your stomach. This is because, when an emotion is triggered, it comes with a pattern of physiological changes that not only precipitate the emotion itself but prepare the body to take action of some type.
Behaviour and impulses	Given the physiological changes in your body, you may also be aware that your body has an urge or impulse to engage in a certain action, or that you have already engaged in a particular behaviour or action. For example, the desire to move away or flee a situation, to slam a door or shout. You may also become aware of other ways that emotions express themselves, for example, in your facial expression or voice tone.

Motivation	You may feel motivated to avoid harm, to challenge or compete in some way, or to connect or care for someone or something.
Thinking	You may notice that your thinking takes on a particular type of content (e.g. 'How dare he do that,' or 'I can't cope, I need to get away'), or that its focus changes (e.g. worry about events coming up, replaying events from the past).
Imagery	You may notice certain images playing through your mind, for example, linked to the worst-case scenario, or images related to past memories.
Attention	It may be that you can notice that your attention has changed, maybe becoming broader, narrower or focused on a particular thing (e.g. a person, an event).

So, when an emotion 'turns up', with various features or clusters of characteristics, healthy emotion regulation is likely to involve an awareness that this emotional pattern has been triggered. Unfortunately, as we saw in Chapter 5, many of us can struggle to notice the various signs that a particular emotion has been triggered, and instead feel cut off or dissociated from the emotion. So, a little like being colour-blind, the features of the emotion may be present, but we are unable to perceive them clearly. Of course, if this is the case, we might miss out important information that the emotion is conveying about what is happening to us, and therefore, be unable to take helpful steps to manage a given situation. So, let's take a look at what might help here.

Awareness of emotion

It can be useful to start with to reflect on which aspects or features of emotions you are able to notice or be aware of. When I'm working with my patients who are experiencing difficult emotions, we'll often take time with them to explore the different features they can detect. For example, we'd spend time seeing if they can locate where this feeling shows up in the body. While this will be different for each of us, anxiety is often experienced in the stomach and chest, whereas anger can be around the top of the chest, shoulders, neck and jaw. Sadness can show with a heavy feeling in the chest or stomach. There have been various studies looking at this, including a recent, very well-known one (Nummenmaa et al., 2014). In this study, the researchers showed participants emotionally stimulating material (e.g. short stories, movies) and then asked them to colour in an outline of a body, showing where they would feel an emotion strongly, and where they would experience a lack of or decreased activation in the body. On average, across the participants, they were able to develop the below graphic that graphically represents how people (on average) tend to experience basic (e.g. anger, sadness, happiness) and complex (e.g. shame, pride) emotions.

Figure 13: Location of emotions in the body (with darker and lighter areas representing where participants located emotions).

(NB: as this diagram is best seen in colour, you can view this by searching online for 'map of emotions in the body'.)

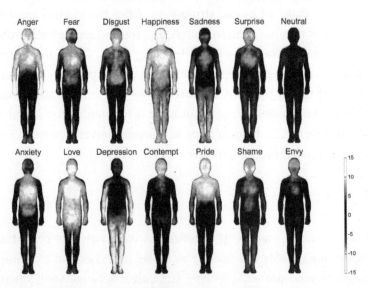

Image used with permission from Dr Lauri Nummenmaa, *Bodily maps of emotions*, PNAS

This type of image can be useful as a guide for exploring where emotions show up in the body. In fact, you might find it helpful to explore whether these patterns of activation are similar to what you experience for each of these emotions (we will come back to looking at this in more detail in the coming pages).

In my clinical work, I might explore with my clients what urge, impulse or behaviour comes with the emotion – for example, anxiety often comes with a desire to move away or flee, whereas anger can bring a desire to confront, stick up for ourselves, shout, throw or hit. And as we explored in Chapter 2, these emotions often show themselves in patterns of thinking in stereotyped ways – for example, worry with anxiety, rumination with anger. For some people this can be difficult, as they identify a physical sensation, but rather than associating it with an emotion that could be made sense of, they conclude instead that it is indicative of there being something physically wrong with them.

Take some time to look through Table 3 on the next page, and see if you can map out the different patterns of some of your emotions. You'll see an example that was already completed by Jess, a previous colleague of mine who was keen to look at her own emotional awareness. If you find it difficult to do this 'cold' (i.e. not connected to the emotion you're focusing on in the table), take a few moments to recall a time that you felt that particular emotion and, with that in mind, see if you can answer the questions.

Table 3: Emotion awareness chart – Jess's example

Emotion	How easy is it to notice this emotion once triggered?	What tends to trigger this emotion (e.g. situations, own feelings)?	Where does it show up in my body?	If it were to grow, which parts of my body does it move in to?	What does it feel like in my body (e.g. pleasant or unpleasant; light or heavy)?	What is the impulse in my body? What does my body want to do?	What happens to my thinking? What thoughts or images come to mind?	What do I pay attention to when feeling this emotion?
Anger	Very easy	Unfair treatment	Shoulders and jaw	Arms and hands	Strong, energising	To approach people, to shout	Someone saying sorry to me	People's mistakes
Anxiety	Difficult	New people or situations	Maybe stomach	Not sure	Unpleasant but hard to feel	Not sure	Blank – can't think	Not sure
Sadness	Hard	Feeling alone and loss	My head	Heart and stomach	Heavy and unpleasant	Cry	Images of being on own	Not having a relationship
Shame	Very easy	My own needs/feeling	Stomach	Shoulders and chest	Very, very unpleasant	Curl up, hide, disappear	People criticising me	Other people
Joy	Easy	Seeing close friends	Legs and arms	Not sure, but feel need to move	Very nice, energising	Move, do things, see people	Thoughts about good/ fun things	Pleasure and doing things
Contentment	Hard	Lie-ins, weekends	Not sure	Not sure	Nice I think but not sure	Not sure	Not sure	Not sure

Emotion awareness chart

Emotion	How easy is it to notice this emotion once triggered?	What tends to trigger this emotion (e.g. situations, own feelings)?	Where does it show up in my body?	If it were to grow, which parts of my body does it move in to?	What does it feel like in my body (e.g. pleasant or unpleasant; light or heavy)?	What is the impulse in my body? What does my body want to do?	What happens to my thinking? What thoughts or images come to mind?	What do I pay attention to when feeling this emotion?
Anger								
Anxiety								
Sadness								
Shame								
Joy								
Contentment								

Don't worry if you found it hard to recognise the pattern of your emotions. And remember, sometimes we will experience an emotion following something that's happened (e.g. being rejected or stood up on a date), but other times there may be no obvious trigger and the emotion may be related to non-consciously accessible things, such as changes in our hormones, our diet or even feeling tired. And moreover, sometimes the emotions we struggle with are secondary. For example, Keith was in a meeting at work, and was asked a question about a project he was leading on but that he couldn't remember the answer to. In the moment, he experienced anxiety, which was unpleasant but manageable. However, after the meeting he started to beat himself up; 'Everyone saw you didn't know – they'll all think you're useless and a waste of time.' This, in turn, triggered a powerful shame response, and Keith described feeling beaten down, inferior and like he wanted to hide away.

Recognising emotions and the way they shape and pattern your physiology, urges, and thinking is a skill, and like many other things in life, you can develop it with practice. Interestingly, when people do spend time completing this exercise, they often notice how varied and rainbow-like their emotions are. They have their own ways of thinking, patterns in the body and action-desires. No wonder tracking them can be tricky! But if we slow down and reflect on exercises like this it will help us to become more familiar with their different textures, and then over time we can become more mindful and aware of them when they show up in us. One way we can explore this is through further development and honing of mindfulness skills.

Mindfulness of emotion

Utilising your attention and mindfulness skills can help you in becoming more familiar with the different features of emotions. As we discovered earlier in the book (Chapter 8), mindfulness involves intentionally paying attention to the present-moment activity of our mind and bodies in a non-judgemental way. Cultivating mindful awareness can help us to become more familiar with the different features of emotion as they arise in our mind and body, and rather than having threat-system reactions to this (e.g. trying to avoid or ruminate about why we are experiencing it), we can instead observe it as it passes through our awareness. Let's explore how to develop your skills in this area.

Exercise: Mindfulness of emotions – noticing their shape and pattern

Take a moment to find a comfortable, upright position in your seat, with your shoulders dropped, and chest open and relaxed. If you find it helpful, gently close your eyes. Take a few moments to ground your mind in the present moment, noticing the sensations in your body as you breathe in and out. Now, take a few minutes to become aware of what emotion or feelings you're currently experiencing. See if you can:

- Notice where this turns up in the body (e.g. a particular area, multiple areas at one time, or shifting over time to different regions of the body)

- What is your body posture like in the presence of this emotion?

- Are your muscles tense or relaxed?

- Notice what your facial expression is like

- Notice the quality of the feeling – pleasant, unpleasant or neutral

- Notice the intensity of the feeling. Is it mild, moderate or strong? What is the energy of the feeling like?

- Recognise what the urge is in your body, given the presence of this emotion

- Silently name, if you're able to, what the feeling is (e.g. 'here is anger' or 'anxious')

- Notice any thoughts that come with the emotion – this could be images

Continue to hold mindful awareness to this feeling. If you notice your mind getting pulled into judgements, or that it's getting dragged elsewhere, notice this and gently bring your awareness to focusing on the above aspects of the emotion. Notice what it's like to observe different emotions (sensations, feelings, thoughts, images, urges) emerge, linger and then transition. Whether these emotions are unpleasant, neutral or pleasant, just stay in the position of *observer* of your experience – being curious and open to whatever shows up.

If you notice yourself getting caught up in new brain judgements or stories about what you're feeling, or feel the urge to move away from or block certain aspects of the emotion you are experiencing, try to remain in the observer position. Remember, although we may have the urge to react to our emotions in this way, mindfulness helps us to notice these urges, and recognise them for just that – urges. So, if you can, have the kind intention of just being in the presence of these reactions, holding in mind that mindfulness helps us to take a position of non-reactivity. From this accepting, observing position, gently bring your awareness back to whatever emotion is currently patterning through you. Take another minute or two with this.

Now see if you can pull back a little; try to observe yourself doing this exercise. Become aware of your mind exploring your body, and what feelings and emotions you are experiencing. Notice what it's like to be mindful of this, to be an observer of your own experience. Just spend a minute or two holding this 'awareness of being aware' position.

Finally, you might notice that the initial emotion you were paying attention to has now been replaced by something else. And that in a few more moments, something else will arise. As the observer, try to maintain this awareness of the emergence of emotions, noticing what they feel like when they are present, and then as they begin to fade. Allow this process to repeat again, and again, and again.

Continue this for 5 minutes or so, before bringing awareness back into the room and opening your eyes if they were closed.

If you found aspects of the above exercise difficult, this might offer you a motivation to practise it regularly over the coming days and weeks. Sometimes people find this exercise difficult because there wasn't a strong emotion activated in them at the time. Noticing whatever emotion or feeling is present, and the intensity and shape it comes in, is what is important here, even if the feeling is boredom, emptiness, nothingness or any other subtle emotional experience. So, you don't need a strong emotion to practice being curious and mindful. However, it can also be helpful if you found it difficult to connect with feelings or emotions, to deliberately 'trigger' an emotion to pay mindful attention to it. To do this, it might be helpful to return to one of the emotion-triggering situations that you identified in Chapter 12. Spend a few minutes placing yourself back in the situation (if it's happened already), or imagining being in a situation that is coming up shortly, and then use that as the backdrop of the mindfulness of emotion exercise you've just tried, spending time again on each of the questions.

Continue practising the exercises in this chapter, honing your ability to notice the shape and patterns of your emotions when they're triggered. Try to hold any difficulties or blocks you have with any of the exercises with open curiosity, kindness and compassion to yourself – returning to the compassionate mind skills and practices of Section Three.

Key reflections

Step 2 of the emotion regulation model focused on *awareness of emotion*, and in this chapter, we have developed insights and skills linked to how:

- Emotions come with a particular pattern or shape, texturing our physiology, attention, thinking and actions

- The pattern of emotion features can differ significantly between emotions (e.g. sadness and joy), but also within emotions (e.g. types of anger, such as irritation or frustration)

- Learning the shape and pattern of emotions – especially through mindfulness – can help to improve emotion regulation skills at this step

14 Compassion-focused emotion regulation skills (CERS) – labelling emotions

As we discussed in Chapter 5, words can be an imprecise tool for describing emotions. A former client of mine put this succinctly as 'using a black and white camera to capture colour'. For some people who have difficulties in this area, it can feel like there's not even a camera in the first place. Although most languages have a broad and rich lexicon to describe different emotions, using words to describe feelings can have limitations. While this may limit all of us from precisely describing our inner emotional world, some people experience a greater deficit in this area. As we discussed in Chapter 5, some (although by no means all) people who find it difficult to name and label their emotions may struggle with alexithymia. If you remember, *alexithymia* is a Greek word that means 'without words for emotions', and describes difficulties in identifying, describing, understanding and expressing emotions.

Whether this emerges out of alexithymia or other processes, researchers have found that difficulties in identifying and discriminating emotions are associated with higher levels of mental distress, and decreased emotion regulation abilities (Pandey et al., 2011). So, in this chapter, we're going to explore how to develop skills at the third step of the emotion regulation model (see Figure 14, opposite).

I can remember a clear example of a struggle I've had with this third step of the emotion regulation process. About eight years ago I went for an interview for a job I was really keen to get; it was a promotion, and would involve working in a great organisation and to make it better, the pay was much more than I was earning at that time. I revised thoroughly before the interview, and on the day felt that I'd given a good reflection of myself, and why I'd be suitable for their service. As I was going to meet my

Figure 14: Emotion regulation model (ERM) – labelling of emotion

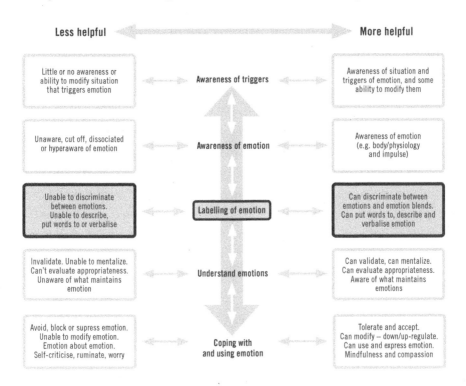

wife for a drink and something to eat that evening, I received a call from the manager of the service. She told me that I'd given a good interview, but that they were concerned I didn't have enough specific experience for the post, and that instead, they'd given it to an internal candidate. When I met my wife and told her about it, she asked me how I was feeling, and I found myself really struggling to be specific. I responded by saying I felt 'pretty crap', and 'low', but couldn't say anything further. When my wife asked again later in the evening, I again struggled to describe what I was feeling and ended up changing the subject and talking about what we were going to eat. Looking back on it the next day, I realised that I was aware of the tone of my feelings (they were very unpleasant), but that I was unable to voice or express them clearly. With hindsight, I can recognise that I felt sad, defeated and ashamed about not getting the job. But I can also see that I was feeling angry, particularly because I'd put a lot of work in and it felt like they had always intended to give the position to an internal candidate. There might have been many reasons why I'd struggled to put words to my emotions that evening; certainly I was struggling with many different, strong feelings at the same time, and this was making it difficult for me to separate them. Maybe the feeling I'd let my wife down by not getting the job (so a sense of shame) was shutting me down to describing other emotions. But I'm also aware that experiencing certain emotions – anger in particular – can make it harder for me to be clear about my feelings and emotions. It's almost as if anger clouds or muddies my emotional waters. I'm also aware that there are reasons why this might be, and in particular, that my own experiences growing up as a child make this a particularly tricky emotion to regulate.

But why is all of this important? Well, distinguishing between emotions (especially negative emotions), and being able to name and label emotions accurately, is an integral part of the emotion regulation process. For example, studies have found that people who are able to discriminate between negative emotions are up to 50 per cent less likely to retaliate in an aggressive way to someone who has hurt them (Pond et al., 2012), and consume 40 per cent less alcohol when stressed (Kashdan et al., 2010). In terms of labelling emotions, experimenters at the University of California found that when participants had to describe their feelings while engaging in a scary task (approaching a tarantula!), they had a reduced physiological reaction to stress compared to people who just approached the spider but didn't verbalise their feelings (Kircanski et al., 2012). Other studies have also found similar results in different emotionally stimulating scenarios (e.g. anxiety about public speaking), suggesting that when we use language to describe our emotional experience, this seems to reduce activation in areas of the brain associated with emotion (e.g. amygdala) and physiological responses in the body.

So, in this chapter, we're going to explore different ways to help label your emotions, put words to them and distinguish between blends of different emotions.

Present moment labelling

Let's start with practising putting words to what's going on for us at the moment.

Exercise: Present moment emotion labelling

The purpose of this exercise is to help you become familiar with noticing and naming your feelings in the present moment. It's quite simple, but it may take a while to find the words to describe your feelings. If this is the case, take a look at the list of emotion descriptors in Table 4 (p. 221) which may help you with this. Take your time with this – don't rush!

- At the moment, I am feeling . . .

- At the moment, this emotion is like . . .

Try to repeat this in the coming hours or across the rest of the day. If it helps, take a few notes so that you can look back on this later in the day or week. Do you feel the same way over many hours, or do your emotions change?

Some people find it helpful to set a reminder on their phone or diary so that they are prompted with these same questions throughout a day or week. It can be that, through doing this, you can get more practised at noticing, recognising and naming your feelings, even ones that are hard to describe.

One way to start getting more practised (and confident) with labelling your feelings is to use a diary or notebook to help you record your experience. This is how to do it: over the next week, see if you can set your intention to 'check in' and make a regular recording of your feelings throughout the day. For example, after a difficult meeting with your boss or supervisor, or before going out to meet some new friends. As this is happening – or shortly afterwards – write down in a notebook, in your diary or on your smartphone, what your primary feeling(s) are. Use the guidelines below to help.

Exercise: Emotion daily review

Towards the end of your day, find a piece of paper or use your smartphone, and take a moment to look back over the day. Think about the different things you did: work, meetings, phone calls, meeting friends, exercise. Make two columns, and in the first, write down some of these (don't worry about listing them all, pick four or five).

Consider which emotions you felt during these specific parts of the day. In column two, in line with the event from the day, write down the emotion or feeling you experienced. Here's an example of one that Jalal – a client of mine who struggled with his emotions – made:

Event	Emotion
Big meeting with senior management	Anxiety, tension
Lunch with a new colleague	Anxiety
Discussion with my son about his poor school marks	Anger, irritation, anxiety
Doing work emails after dinner	Anxiety, apprehension

Although Jalal found this hard to start with, over a number of weeks he became more able to describe his feelings. He began to notice the important nuances between different types of similar feelings (e.g. irritation and annoyance compared to apprehension), and that emotions typically turn up together, and can easily blend and fuse.

It's also worth noting that for some people, it's not so easy to link a specific emotion to a particular situation; instead, it can seem like every or 'all' emotions at the same time. For example, Tessa described conversations with her husband in which she'd feel angry, anxious, sad and ashamed all at the same time. If you notice something similar to this, it can be useful to note down which was the most intense, or the one that was most frequent during the situation.

As we've been discussing in this chapter, some people can find it difficult to name any feelings or emotions when they review their day. If this is the case, don't despair – it's worth returning to the exercise on present moment emotion labelling (p. 217) and take some more time practising that. It may also be that this is difficult because it's hard to separate out feelings, and we'll return to this later in the chapter, and also in the online material about 'too little' emotion that accompanies this book (see https://overcoming.co.uk/715/resources-to-download).

Range of emotional experience

As we discussed in Chapter 1, there are many different ways of classifying emotions, and different ideas around how and why so many emotions exist. One way of looking at our emotions is by considering primary or basic emotions, and emotions or feelings that are commonly associated with them (i.e. alternative words used for a particular emotion). Take a look at Table 4 (p. 221) to see what we mean here. As you'll see, at the top of the column a 'major' emotion is listed, and underneath it, emotions or feelings that are associated with it. It turns out that there are many different ways of describing a broadly similar emotional state; for example, under 'anger' we might describe feeling irritated, annoyed, frustrated and so on.

This table isn't meant to be exhaustive (for example, key emotions like surprise, shame, envy and jealousy are not included), but a helpful way of clustering emotions and feelings a bit like a family. With this table in mind, take some time to work through the different scenarios below. Remember, it's not that there is a right or wrong way to feel in a particular situation; for example, while being criticised by someone may leave one person feeling angry, it could leave another feeling anxious.

1. You're at work in a meeting with your boss and a number of colleagues. Your boss is giving feedback on recent outcomes, and mentions you for particular praise, highlighting your hard work, creativity and teamwork. Which emotions might you experience at this moment?

2. You're at work in a meeting with your boss and a number of colleagues. Your boss is giving feedback on recent outcomes, and openly criticises you, highlighting how everyone else in the team appears to have far outperformed you, and that you are letting people down. Which emotions might you experience at this moment?

3. You say yes to going on a date with someone who has liked you for a long time, but you're unsure whether you see them as just a friend, or potentially something more. Which emotions might you experience?

4. You go on a date with someone that you have liked for a long time, although you're unsure whether they reciprocate your feelings, whether they see you more as a friend or are only going on the date so as not to hurt your feelings. Which emotions might you experience?

5. In two days you're going on a holiday with a group of your best friends. Which emotions might you experience?

6. You see on Facebook that a group of your best friends has gone away for the weekend together, without inviting you along. Which emotions might you experience?

Table 4: Emotions and their 'family tree'

Anger	Anxiety	Sadness	Disgust	Joy	Calm	Safe
Irritated	Scared	Disappointed	Revulsion	Excitement	Peaceful	Content
Frustrated	Fearful	Sorrowful	Distasteful	Energetic	Relaxed	Secure
Annoyed	Terrified	Distressed	Abhorrent	Lively	Tranquil	Warm
Cross	Agitated	Despair	Repugnant	Enthusiastic	Laid-back	
Furious	Tense	Despondent		Eager	Serene	
Raging	On edge	Remorseful				

You can continue to explore your emotions in this way, but rather than using these types of questions, turn to TV, film and books as the scene-setter. For example, the next time that you're watching a movie, use your empathy to imagine what emotions you might experience if you were in a character's place. Similarly, when reading a book or a story in a newspaper, try to put yourself in the shoes of the lead character, and use the above emotion list to explore your feelings. If the table doesn't include the emotions you might feel, add to it! Keep on practising this, helping yourself develop your emotional vocabulary and range.

If you want, you can also re-look at the earlier scenarios, but this time holding in mind self-conscious emotions. Self-conscious emotions – such as shame, guilt, embarrassment, pride, and envy – are generally understood to emerge later than primary emotions (e.g. anger, sadness, fear, joy), and require new brain competencies such as self-reflection, theory of mind and so on. Which of these emotions can you imagine experiencing in the above situations? We will come back to look at one of these self-conscious emotions (shame) in a lot more detail in Chapter 16e.

How often do you experience different emotions?

To help understand your emotional world further, take a look at Table 5. You'll see that it lists the same emotions (and emotion 'relations') as Table 4. However, this time there is space next to each emotion. In this space, see if you can mark (or do so on a piece of paper) how often you experience each emotion, with 0 = never, 1 = rarely, 2 = sometimes, and 3 = almost all the time. If it helps, use the time frame of the previous month as a reference for thinking about this.

What did you discover from this? Did you notice whether particular emotions turn up in your life more often than others? Are some emotions rarely experienced? For some of us, we might notice that there is a 'go to' emotion that tends to turn up commonly in life, regardless of whether it's

Table 5: Rating the frequency of emotions and their 'family tree'

Anger	Anxiety	Sadness	Disgust	Joy	Relaxed	Safe	
Irritated	Scared	Disappointed	Revulsion	Excitement	Peaceful	Content	
Frustrated	Fearful	Sorrowful	Distasteful	Energetic	Calm	Secure	
Annoyed	Terrified	Distressed	Abhorrent	Lively	Tranquil	Warm	
Cross	Agitated	Despair	Repugnant	Enthusiastic	Laid-back		
Raging	Tense	Despondent		Eager	Serene		
Furious	On edge	Remorseful					

Scoring system: 0 = never, 1 = rarely, 2 = sometimes, 3 = almost all the time a useful or appropriate emotion for the situation. So, learning to notice, label and experience a range of different emotions, and familiarising ourselves with their particular shape and pattern, is an important part of healthy emotion regulation. We're going to come back and explore how our compassionate minds can help us to up-regulate (increase the experience) certain emotions in the additional online material, accessible at https://overcoming.co.uk/715/resources-to-download.

Memory and emotion labelling

Another way of approaching this is to use a memory of an emotionally stimulating experience. Let's give this a try.

Exercise: Labelling emotional memories

Find a comfortable and quiet place to sit. Take a few minutes to bring to mind a recent time in which you felt stressed or upset in some way. Allow this memory to form in your mind. Start by recalling where you were, whether there was anyone else around you, and what was happening. As you do this, try to stay in a curious mind – so the idea is not for you to remember in a way that takes you back into the feelings too strongly, but allows you to reflect on and explore them.

Now spend some time focusing on the different aspects of feelings we have been exploring. Let's start with what you noticed in your body. Where did you notice the feeling? What was the feeling urging your body to do? What were you thinking? What was going through your mind? And if you behaved as the emotion wanted you to, what would you do?

Given this, spend a few moments bringing to mind words that would describe this feeling. Taking your time, holding in mind the situation, and the feeling in your body, gently repeat the phrase, 'I was feeling . . .' adding in the word(s) that might describe your emotion.

When you feel ready, allow the memory to fade. If it's helpful, spend a few moments connecting to your soothing breathing, letting yourself slow down and feel grounded in the present moment.

How did you find that exercise? What was it like to use memory as an opportunity to practise labelling your feelings? It might be useful to practice regularly with different memories. If you found it difficult to find a word for the feeling you had, take a look back at the list of words in Table 4 (p. 221) for some ideas.

Discriminating between emotions

Many people use general labels to describe how they're feeling. Take a moment to think about it. When someone asks you (or you ask someone else) how you're feeling, what are your common responses? 'I'm fine', 'Not too bad', 'I'm grand'?, 'Not great', or 'Could be better'? While these convey information about our feelings in a simple and brief way, they can hide so much of what is going on for us. Let's look at this with the example of Jennifer.

Jennifer came to therapy because her partner suggested she needed to. In our initial sessions, she was very quiet, made little eye contact, and gave minimal elaboration on how she was feeling, and what struggles she was experiencing. Over a number of sessions, her most common response to being asked how she was feeling was 'Not great.' When I tried to explore this feeling further, to find out what it meant, Jennifer would typically shrug her shoulders, look at me in a blank way, and just repeat, 'Not great.' Although it took some time, practice of compassionate mind skills (to help her feel more grounded, 'present focused' and able to access an open, reflective new brain; see Section Three) and persistent exploration, we were able to help Jennifer become more skilful at differentiating and discriminating between generic descriptions (e.g. 'Not great') and more nuanced descriptions of her feelings. Figure 15 highlights what we uncovered – the emotions and feelings that sat *underneath* her phrase, 'Not great.'

Figure 15: What lies underneath initial descriptions of how we're feeling

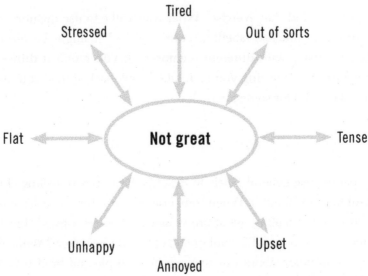

So, for Jennifer, there was a considerable amount of feeling underneath 'Not great' – in fact, it turned out that it was because she was feeling so many, mixed and conflicting emotions, that she found it difficult or too confusing to separate them out, let alone name them.

Recognising mixed feelings

While it's useful to learn about and name specific emotions (e.g. anger, anxiety, sadness), just like with Jennifer, the reality is that emotions are often experienced or arise in blends. Many of our experiences and relationships involve multiple emotional reactions. For example, on a first date, we may feel a mix of excitement and anxiety – or even boredom and disgust if things don't go very well! We may love and feel angry towards our parents, or our partner. We may respect and hold our boss or colleagues in high esteem, and feel angry or anxious about comments they make about us, at the same time. It's important to recognise that having mixed, or seemingly opposite feelings in the same situation or towards the same person are completely normal. To help understand about the blends of emotions you might experience, take a look at the exercise on the next page, and spend some time reflecting on some of the situations, people, relationships or memories that bring up mixed feelings in you.

Continue to practise this labelling exercise in the coming weeks. Sometimes this is an eye-opener in helping us recognise how often our emotional worlds are about blends, rather than a singular emotional experience. It might also be that you begin to notice that certain situations tend to trigger mixed emotional responses, or certain emotions tend to turn up alongside others (e.g. anger and anxiety). This knowledge can lead to insight and wisdom about your inner emotional world, helping you to label and describe more clearly what you're feeling, and to learn how to communicate this in a helpful way to others. We will develop some of these ideas further later in the book, in particular in Chapter 16d (multiple emotional selves) and Chapter 16e (shame).

Many of the skills we've explored in this chapter relate to mindfulness (see Chapter 8), in that by paying attention to what is happening we begin to know the subtlety of our feelings and emotions. It's a bit like listening to music; when we start *really* paying attention closely to what we are listening to, we begin to make distinctions between different kinds of instruments, rhythms, beats or melodies. Similarly, with food, mindfulness helps us to pay close attention to what we are eating, and we can notice different textures, scents and flavours that, when we are rushing through it, we might have missed. Mindfulness then is a way of beginning to notice the subtleties of the textures of our experience, that there are common 'colours' or patterns of emotions, some in the background, some in the foreground. Some emotions block out others, and sometimes we have to bring attention to focus on those emotions that we might be hiding from or trying not to notice. We'll return to some of these ideas in Chapter 16b and Chapter 16d.

Exercise: Labelling mixed emotions

Things I have mixed feelings about (e.g. a person, situation, memory)	Type of emotions or feelings I experience (list different ones)	Emotion that I experience most powerfully or clearly in this situation	Emotions I don't experience at this time (list)	Emotions I would least like to feel or even try to avoid

Key reflections

Step 3 of the emotion regulation model focuses on the *labelling of emotions*, and in this chapter, we have developed insights and skills linked to how:

- Putting words to feelings can help to regulate them

- Emotions and feelings often come in blends – this is a common and 'normal' experience

- It takes practice to learn how to notice and discriminate between different feelings

15 Compassion-focused emotion regulation skills (CERS) – understanding emotions

In Chapters 12, 13 and 14, we explored difficulties at the first three steps of the emotion regulation model. However, it's also possible that we face no particular challenges at these steps: for example, we may have an awareness of triggers of our emotions, can notice emotions as they arise inside us, and are able to put accurate labels to whatever our feelings might be. However, we might still struggle to understand *why* we're feeling the way we feel. In fact, many of the people I see for therapy struggle to comprehend and validate their emotional experiences, particularly when these emotions are powerful or painful. So, in this chapter, we'll look at Step 4 of the emotion regulation model (Figure 16) and how to develop skills in this step of the emotion regulation model.

Here's an example of a difficulty I recently had with this step of emotion regulation. On my way home after giving a talk on compassion to the general public, I was stopped by a charity fundraiser. They were raising money for a mental health charity and wanted me to sign up to regular monthly payments. I politely said that I couldn't stop, but that I worked in the mental health field, and respected the charity they worked for, and their attempts to raise money for it. Not taking 'no' for an answer, the charity worker blocked my path as I tried to carry on walking, and went on to tell me that I was a hypocrite for working in the area while not contributing to the charity. As calmly as I could, I tried to explain that I already contributed every month to various charities, including a mental health one. At hearing this, he rolled his eyes, put on a sarcastic voice tone and said: 'Sure, that's convenient isn't it – why don't you just carry on walking you selfish *******.' At that moment, I lost my cool; I told him (not very politely) to leave me alone, and that he was a disgrace

Figure 16: Emotion regulation model (ERM) – understanding emotions

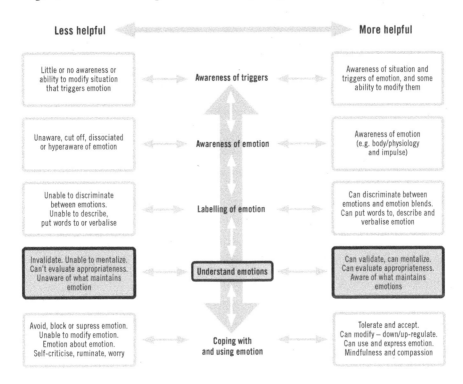

Less helpful		More helpful
Little or no awareness or ability to modify situation that triggers emotion	Awareness of triggers	Awareness of situation and triggers of emotion, and some ability to modify them
Unaware, cut off, dissociated or hyperaware of emotion	Awareness of emotion	Awareness of emotion (e.g. body/physiology and impulse)
Unable to discriminate between emotions. Unable to describe, put words to or verbalise	Labelling of emotion	Can discriminate between emotions and emotion blends. Can put words to, describe and verbalise emotion
Invalidate. Unable to mentalize. Can't evaluate appropriateness. Unaware of what maintains emotion	Understand emotions	Can validate, can mentalize. Can evaluate appropriateness. Aware of what maintains emotions
Avoid, block or supress emotion. Unable to modify emotion. Emotion about emotion. Self-criticise, ruminate, worry	Coping with and using emotion	Tolerate and accept. Can modify – down/up-regulate. Can use and express emotion. Mindfulness and compassion

for acting like he was. My voice was so loud that a few people in the street turned to look. I stomped off past him, thinking about all the other angry things I should have told him, and imagining going back and carrying on arguing with him. As I got home, I started to think about my response. 'What the hell, I just gave a talk on compassion, and then I go and do that? What sort of person does that make me – a complete fraud.' I also started to think differently about the person who I had argued with: 'Poor chap was just trying to raise money for a good cause after all, and had probably been out there all day,' and 'I really shouldn't have got angry there, that was not the right thing at all.'

In this example, there are various aspects of the emotion regulation process I struggled with. Notice how, after having lost my temper, unintentionally I started to engage in *unhelpful responses*. I started invalidating my emotions and experience (telling myself I shouldn't have got angry), rather than being curious about how and why I did. I ended up fighting with it and having a negative view of myself as a fraud, rather than trying to understand and work with the emotion itself. To make matters worse, for the rest of the evening I veered from angry rumination (at the worker) to shame-based rumination (at myself for how I reacted). I was aware that I was remaining stuck in anger and shame, and saw that my ongoing emotional reaction was further indication that I was a 'compassion-fraud'. Let's look at this more closely.

One of the difficulties that can emerge at this stage of the emotion regulation process is our reaction to emotions when they arise. In my case, I invalidated my experience, feeling it was unacceptable and indicative of 'wrongness'. In turn, this blocked me from being curious as to why it made sense that I became angry in the first place. This then led to the experience of shame (the sense of myself as a fraud), which kept me locked further into my threat-based emotional distress. When we fight our emotional experiences, by directing shame and anger at ourselves, essentially our threat system is activated.

In comparison, it's likely a number of things could have helped me in this situation; first, it would have been helpful for me to slow down, as I was heated up into my threat system in a way that led me to respond unhelpfully to the charity worker. But sometimes we do get captured by our emotions 'in the moment', and may have to focus instead on what is helpful in regulating them after they have been triggered. So, in hindsight, if I'd been able to take a few minutes to engage in my grounded body posture, soothing breathing and access my compassionate mind, I'd have been able to validate why I felt like I did, as it's horrible to be accused of lying in the way I had been. I'd have been able to see why I'd become angry, but also started to think about what I would need that would help me to manage the feelings I'd been left with after this encounter. I might also have been able to shift into imagining why the charity worker had reacted in the way he had; for example, it could be useful to imagine what sort of day he might have had, standing in the heat, having many people ignore him or actually lie to him about already being a member of the charity.

So, in this chapter, we'll explore how to turn towards ourselves and our difficult emotions with understanding and empathy. We'll explore this in two stages that are relevant to this fourth step of the emotion regulation model.

1: Validate

It's common for people to *invalidate* their emotions. Invalidation means that we see something as not valid or 'legitimate', and discredit or discount it. In terms of our emotions, this involves a perception that the emotion is somehow incorrect, or even wrong, or is not fitting or appropriate given the situation that led to it. A client once said to me: 'I shouldn't be feeling sad, I shouldn't be crying – nothing that bad has happened for me to feel like this.' Although unintended, when we invalidate our emotions, we create a threat system response to ourselves and our experiences. Essentially, we are telling ourselves: 'You shouldn't be feeling like this, there's something wrong with you.' Some of you may have had an experience of other people doing this to you – for example, someone telling you to 'stop getting so angry'. Mostly, this type of invalidating response, whether directed from ourselves or others, is an attack on an already heated threat system, and only serves to turn the temperature up, rather than cool it down.

Validating our feelings involves connecting with the *reality of them*, of what led to them. It involves appreciating and recognising why we're feeling what we're feeling, and whether the emotion or our reaction during it was helpful. Let's see what we can do to help using our compassionate mind. To start with, see if you can bring to mind a recent time when you invalidated your emotions. When you have an example, try the exercise overleaf.

Exercise: Using the compassionate self to validate emotions

Find a quiet place to sit in an upright, comfortable but alert posture. Take a few moments to engage in your soothing rhythm breathing, allowing your body and mind to slow down as you breathe out. When you feel ready, bring to mind the qualities of your compassionate self:

- Wisdom – that we all just find ourselves here, caught in the flow of life and shaped by things that we often didn't choose. You understand that we've been bestowed emotions, some of which can be very painful to experience and difficult to manage. While this is not our fault, wisdom here involves learning how to react helpfully to them

- Strength – hold in mind that this version of you (linked to your body posture, breathing rhythm and intention) is confident, grounded and stable. It can tolerate being in the presence of difficult emotions

- Commitment – try to hold in mind that this version of you intends to address distress and suffering, and do what it can to be supportive and caring to yourself when you experience difficult emotions

When you feel connected to this part of you, take some time to explore the following steps:

1. Start with trying to validate your initial invalidation. Given the wisdom of your compassionate self, maybe you can hold in mind that it's understandable that we often invalidate our emotions. It might be that you can have an appreciation of the reasons why you might invalidate your emotions – for example, maybe this is something that others have told or taught you about emotions, or perhaps it's because you found it difficult to understand or accept your emotions in the past.

2. Now, see if you can gently move on to recognising the original emotions you felt, and directing some understanding of why you

felt the way you did in the first place. Although formulaic at first, it may be that you can complete the following sentence, naming the emotion and the situation as appropriate:

'I can see why I was feeling . . . . . because the situation with . . . . . is a difficult one'

or

'It makes sense that I felt . . . . . as this was a tricky situation to deal with'

3. Try to remember that our emotions have important evolved functions – that they emerged to do certain things to help us manage important motives or situations that could affect our well-being (and if it helps, take a look back to p. 27 which outlines some of these).

4. Given the pattern of responses that emotions come with (see pp. 203–5), can you also validate how you responded or acted when you were experiencing the emotion? Is it possible to see that sometimes we shout or threaten people when we get angry, or get tearful when we're sad? That emotions come with a range of responses, and that even if you're not proud of your response, that it's likely other people have also responded in similar ways when they've experienced the same emotion you struggled with?

5. Although you may wish that you hadn't experienced the emotion, it can be useful to remember that you didn't choose to be able to experience it. Hold in mind that you – like me and everyone else – didn't decide to have emotions in the first place; that we just find ourselves with a body and brain capable of experiencing emotions, but that we are not the architect of this.

6. It can be useful to hold in mind that the emotion you experienced is likely to have been triggered by something, and that conversely if you hadn't experienced the triggering situation, you wouldn't have experienced the emotion in the first place. This type of perspective-taking can help us to recognise our emotional experience was the result of a cause-and-effect process.

7. Think of a friend who has been struggling with distressing emotions recently – maybe someone who has been quite anxious, sad or angry. Given that you're connected to your wise, strong and caring version of yourself, consider how you might see your friend's emotional struggles as valid and understandable. Can you then redirect these insights towards your experience?

8. Finish with focusing on your compassionate intention about this emotion and situation going forward. From your compassionate self, really focus on your desire to mindfully notice times that you start to invalidate your emotional experiences. Really focus on your wise, committed intention as the compassionate self: What are you going to do regarding this emotion, and your tendency to invalidate it, in the coming days and weeks? What would help you to step back from invalidating your emotions? What will help you in trying to validate your feelings?

If you've been invalidating your experiences for many years, it might take some practice to step out of this automatic or habitual response, and consciously do something quite different. If you find this exercise difficult, it can be useful to notice what this is about; is it just alien for you to take this validating approach? Or in trying to do so can you notice that your threat system is activated? If it's the latter, it might be helpful to recognise what the threat is. For example, one of my clients told me: 'I don't deserve to have my feelings validated,' whereas someone else told me 'I'm worried that if I validate my feelings, I might feel very sad about how hard life is,' or 'Just be accepting in a way that says it doesn't matter or let me off the hook.' Validation is not about whether the emotions are good or bad, but how we can understand them and how best to deal with them once they have arisen. This turned out to be a helpful reflection for my clients and helped them return to their compassionate mind skills (Section Three) and recognise that they were experiencing threat emotions about validating threat emotions! We'll return to how to work with this in the next chapter, and also in Section Five. But for now, it can be helpful to recognise this process and bring compassion to yourself that this is hard and might take some time to work through.

Receiving validation from someone else

As pointed out at various stages of the book, our brain and body have evolved to be highly sensitive to the care, sensitivity and warmth of other people. It can be useful while holding this in mind, to consider how we can use other people to help validate our feelings. We can do this in three steps.

Step 1 – Turning to the kindness, care and concern of others

It can be useful to consider who you could deliberately turn to, to seek validation and support from. Make a few notes on a piece of paper, but in particular, think about people you know (friends, family, colleagues, neighbours) who have the qualities that you will find helpful – people who are sensitive, empathetic and caring towards you. When you have the opportunity, see if you can deliberately open up to them about something you've been recently feeling emotional about. Nothing major to start with as you are experimenting and testing things out. See what it feels like to allow their validation and concern for you to land. Afterwards, make a few notes about how this went, how it left you feeling, and what you can learn from it.

As you try this exercise, it's worth noting what feelings arise if you feel you don't get the response (validation) you'd like to from others; commonly, this might be disappointment, sadness or anger. Remember, emotional difficulties often arise when we are blocked or thwarted from something that we want. If this was the case, it's actually an opportunity to bring your compassionate mind skills to these emotions, validating the distress and bringing a compassionate, understanding response to this – after all, it's understandable to feel upset or disappointed when we don't get what we'd like. But it might also be helpful to consider how you might address this with the person who you feel let down by. How might you let this person know that you were hoping for validation from them? If – as your compassionate self – you could talk to the person about your feelings, what would it say? How would it (your compassionate self) bring this up? It might also be worth looking at Chapter 16c which discusses how to assert our needs to others.

If you're not seeing this person for a while, or able to speak to them on the phone, try the below exercise instead:

Exercise: Using memory and imagination to validate your feelings

Take a few moments to connect with your soothing breathing, upright body posture and friendly facial expression. When you're ready, bring to mind a memory of a time when you felt distressed, but felt validated by someone else. See if you can remember where you were, who the person was, where they were in relation to you. Take some time to focus on what this person did to validate your emotion(s). Maybe you can remember:

- What their facial expression was like, and how this conveyed their validation

- What was their voice tone like? How did this help you feel understood and validated?

- Was there something they said that helped you to feel your emotions were valid?

- Was there something else they did that showed their validation of your distress?

If it's hard to bring a clear memory to mind, take some time to imagine what this person might say, if they heard about the difficult emotion you'd been experiencing recently. Imagine what their facial expression and voice tone would be like. Notice the experience of receiving the validation and support from this person, noticing how this leaves you feeling, or any blocks and resistances.

Step 2 – Validation from your compassionate other

In Chapter 10 we spent some time developing an image of your 'compassionate other'. While generating this image can be a powerful experience in itself, it's also useful to consider how we can 'put them to work' to help with managing and regulating your emotions.

Exercise: Validation of emotion from the image of your compassionate other

Sit in an upright but comfortable position. Engage in the usual steps to prepare for a practice – body posture, facial expression, soothing breathing rhythm (p. 115). Now bring to mind the image of your compassionate other that you developed in Chapter 10 (p. 164). Take your time imagining their facial expression, voice tone and qualities of compassion for you – caring-commitment, wisdom and strength (take your time to explore and connect with these).

Now, bring to mind an emotional experience that you've been struggling with recently (you can use the same example as in the previous exercise). Holding this difficult emotion in mind, and the situation in which it arose, refocus back on to the image of your compassionate other:

- Given their wisdom and caring intention towards you, what would they understand about why you were experiencing this emotion? How would they make sense of it?

- How might they be able to validate your experience? What might they say about this? What do they understand about why you experienced this emotion?

- See if you can pay attention to their facial expression, voice tone and wise, caring intention, and what happens when you open to imagining your compassionate other relating to you in a caring, understanding way. What's it like for you to experience this type of supportive, compassionate validation?

After you've finished the exercise – make some notes or write your answers to the questions on some paper or your smartphone. What was that exercise like? What was helpful? How was it for you to receive validation and understanding from your compassionate other? If it was difficult to receive acceptance, validation and understanding from them, try to be curious to these blocks or resistances. Why might this be happening? If it's useful, return to Chapter 11 and take some time to re-explore some of the key difficulties in being open to compassion.

2: Mentalizing and understanding our emotions

Mentalizing is a term popularised by the work of British psychologists Peter Fonagy and Anthony Bateman. The term refers to the ability to pay attention to, and understand the mental states (for example, thoughts, feelings, desires and actions) of other people, as well as our own – that is, to be able to look at our own emotions, feelings, and actions and understand them in the context of our desires, needs, thinking and beliefs. If you remember, in Chapter 5 we described mentalizing as the ability to see ourselves from the 'outside', and other people from the 'inside'. So, while we may learn to notice and identify emotions as they arise, a significant difficulty for many people involves *understanding why they are feeling as they are*. One client once told me: 'I can tell you that I'm feeling angry, where it turns up in my body and what it feels like, but I don't really know *why* I'm feeling like this.'

Now, as has been said throughout the book, when you're looking for causes of emotion, remember they are often complex and difficult. We know for example that certain medications can affect our emotions, as can our hormones, a lack of sleep, and viruses. Research has even found that the health of our guts can change our emotional lives! So, some of the causes of our emotions may be unconscious to us. It's essential therefore to hold in mind that we won't always be able to know or understand what has triggered a difficult emotion – and in fact, straining too hard to 'find' a cause can actually cause more threat system activation, and exacerbate the emotion that we're trying to understand. Nonetheless, the psychological dimension of emotions is often a crucial aspect that we can learn more about.

Let's look at an example of this. Georgina came to therapy as she had been struggling in her relationship with Sue. She felt that Sue was passive and submissive with her, and was unhappy that Sue did not seem to be as animated, active and engaged in the relationship as she was. When we discussed this, Georgina found it very difficult to understand why Sue was behaving the way she was, particularly because when they first started seeing each other things seemed to be very different, exciting and fun. Added to this, Georgina described having become quite angry and demanding with Sue, something that confused her as she described herself as a 'laid-back and happy' person. As time went on in therapy, it turned out that Sue was having a very stressful time at work, and her mum had recently been diagnosed with terminal cancer.

When looking at the emotion regulation model, Georgina recognised that she could do aspects of the first three stages that we outlined in Chapters 12 to 14. She was aware of the situation that triggered her feelings (Sue acting in a submissive way), could notice emotions as they arose in her (particularly in how they influenced her body and the types of thoughts she was having about Sue), and she was able to label the emotions she was having (anger, disappointment). However, she found it exceptionally difficult to understand and reflect on what was happening in this situation, why Sue was feeling and reacting as she did, and why she (Georgina) was responding in the way that she was (e.g. with anger and making demands, rather than her usual calm, laid-back personality). As we progressed through our sessions and focused more on building her skills in this area, Georgina was able to appreciate that events happening in Sue's life were influencing her emotions and behaviour, and this had an impact on the relationship. Moreover, Georgina was able to self-mentalise; in other words, she understood why, unable to make sense of Sue's disengaged behaviour, she interpreted this as indicating rejection and lack of interest towards her. In turn, she could see how this had activated her threat system, leading to feelings of fear and anger, and defensive patterns of behaviour (becoming controlling and demanding).

This type of mentalizing is an important quality of our new brain (Chapter 3), and when harnessed, can help to bring perspective about the complexity of our own, and other people's, motives, emotions, needs and so forth. It can form an essential step in wisely regulating our emotions, and we can practise developing our skills here in combination with using our compassionate mind training skills. Let's look at this with an exercise. Before starting, bring an emotion to mind that you struggled with recently – one that you had been finding difficult to understand or work out why you'd experienced it.

Exercise: Mentalizing from the compassionate self

Find a quiet place to sit in an upright, comfortable but alert posture. Take a few moments to engage in your soothing rhythm breathing, allowing your body and mind to slow down as you breathe out. When you feel ready, bring to mind the qualities of your compassionate self – wisdom, strength and commitment. When you feel connected to this part of you, take the following steps:

Bring an emotion to mind that you struggled with recently. Name the emotion in your mind and the situation that led to it.

1. Recall what inner reactions you had in the presence of the emotion. What happened to your thinking? What were you paying attention to? What urges did your body have?

2. What was the motive that was linked to this emotion? Was it about protecting yourself or someone else? Were you trying to avoid something unpleasant? Were you pursuing or wanting something that might have been pleasant? Or maybe feeling frustrated and thwarted, or anxious and worried; or even feeling overexcited when trying to sleep!

3. Given the situation that triggered this emotional reaction, what ideas come to mind about why this might have been the case? Given what your motive was, or urge in your body, is there a way of seeing how this makes sense that you reacted with this emotion?

4. Given the wisdom of your compassionate self, see if you can connect with a sense that your emotional reaction (whatever it was) was not your fault. You didn't choose to have emotions – these were designed for you, not by you. Remember that emotions were designed through evolution to be fast-acting responses to help us meet specific goals or needs.

5. Given your social shaping and previous life experiences, is there a way of understanding why this situation led to this difficult emotional experience?

As with many of the skills we've been exploring in the past few chapters, take your time with these practices and exercises. Try them out, reflect, then repeat. It can be helpful to start with checking out some of your thoughts and reflections from this exercise with a friend or family member unconnected to the difficulty you were experiencing, and see if they can help you to reflect on and mentalise about the struggle.

3. Listening to what our emotions are telling us – the wisdom of emotions

Some cultures tend to hold negative ideas about emotions, and this idea has certainly been reflected through history and literature. Many of the Greek philosophers, writing approximately 2,500 years ago, saw emotions as 'lower' parts of the soul, and the non-emotional as 'intellectual', and for the Stoics, emotions were sometimes viewed as mistaken value judgements. And from Shakespeare (e.g. *King Lear* or *Romeo and Juliet*) to comic books (e.g. the Hulk), emotions are often depicted in literature as the cause of pain, suffering and destruction. Given this, it might seem strange to consider that emotions hold a type of *wisdom*. However, looked at another way (and as we discussed in Chapter 2), it's likely that emotions evolved to do exactly this – to provide information that might help us navigate situations in our environment. The flush of anger when we've been belittled or transgressed; the flush of fear in the presence of danger, and sadness upon experiencing loss or failure. Key here though is how able we are to *listen* to what these emotions are telling us about what is happening, so that we can respond (and even regulate our response) in a way that is helpful for our and others' well-being. Over time this can lead to a wisdom of emotion – and gets to the heart of why wisdom is sometimes described as a combination of knowledge *plus* experience.

But to gain access to the wisdom of emotions, we might need to strengthen our ability to listen and reflect on what they're telling us. This is particularly the case when what the emotions are telling us is unpleasant, aversive or even scary. When we are in high threat system activation, we are more likely to become submerged in emotion, or want to avoid or push away from it. However, with the help of your compassionate mind skills, we can start to learn from our emotions.

As ever, it's useful to try to listen to emotions from a position of stability and groundedness. To help with this, take some time to work through the below exercise, and the questions/prompts to help you explore your emotions in this way.

Exercise: Listening to the wisdom of emotions

Find a quiet place to sit in an upright, comfortable but alert posture. Take a few moments to engage in your soothing rhythm breathing, allowing your body and mind to slow down as you breathe out. When you feel ready, bring to mind the qualities of your compassionate self – wisdom, strength and commitment. When you feel connected to this part of you, take the following steps:

1. Bring an emotion to mind that you struggled with recently. Name the emotion in your mind and the situation that led to it.

2. Recall what inner reactions you had in the presence of the emotion. What happened to your thinking? What were you paying attention to? What did your body want to do?

3. Given this pattern of emotional reaction, try to listen to the wisdom of this emotion. Consider the following questions:

   • How might this emotion be trying to help you, given the situation?

   • If the emotion could speak, what is it trying to tell you about what has just happened?

   • What is it asking you to address, or suggesting might need to be done (e.g. to challenge an injustice; to reconnect following a loss)?

4. Sometimes an emotion can hold wisdom, but overheat in such a way that it urges us to engage in actions or judgements that are unhelpful and unwise. If you notice that this is happening, turn back to the support, groundedness and strength of your compassionate self. Connect with your posture, soothing rhythm breathing and compassionate intention. Once anchored in this way, return to the questions above, tuning back into what your emotion is telling you.

Take some time making notes on what emerged from this exercise. Was there anything that you learned from this? If you can, try to use this approach as often as you can, and in particular, when you notice you find difficulty with an emotion or when you experience distress in the presence of an emotion. As outlined in Chapter 2, on a fundamental level we can see wisdom exists in all of our emotions:

Fear/Anxiety	Signals potential danger and motivates us to engage in a protective response (e.g. to move, or run away).
Anger	Signals a potential threat to us or others. It may also indicate a block to our goals, or an injustice. It can energise and motivate us to stand up for ourselves and others, and to challenge, be assertive or fight.
Disgust	Signals something noxious or toxic and motivates us to stay away from or expel (e.g. be sick) this (e.g. rotten food, other substances).
Sadness	Signals a loss of some type, and the need for reconnection or recovery of what was lost. This could be the loss of a loved one (e.g. through death) or temporary disconnection (e.g. the child being left for the first day at school). It can also emerge following a failure or setback (e.g. loss of money or a setback at work).
Happiness/Joy	Signals that something is valued or important to us, and moves us towards pursuing goals with rewarding outcomes.
Shame	Signals that our behaviour or actions may lead to rejection or being outcast by others, and motivates us to engage in behaviours to ensure our belonging/that we won't be rejected (e.g. by paying attention to others' responses, or appeasing them).
Guilt	Signals that our behaviour or actions have brought harm to others (or ourselves). It connects us to a type of empathy and motivates us to repair the harm caused, or prevent it from happening in the future.

Although the above are generalisations, they can be a useful starting point in guiding us to why we are experiencing a particular emotion. Of course, various things like our lived experiences and social shaping will influence this – for example, what triggers an angry response in me may trigger an anxious response in you, and vice versa.

As we're at the understanding emotions step of the emotion regulation model, we'll return to how to use the wisdom of emotions to engage in helpful action/expression in Chapter 16c. We'll also look at how to work with common blocks to listening to the wisdom of emotions (e.g. our inability to tolerate emotions; shame and self-criticism) in Chapters 16a and 16e.

4. Recognition of, and working with, what maintains difficult emotions

Some people are able to validate their emotions and to take an under-standing, empathetic and mentalizing stance towards them. What can trip them up is not being able to track factors that maintain a difficult emotion once it's triggered. As we discussed in Chapter 1, one of the key features of emotions relates to their duration – how long they last, and how long they take to settle. So, while some emotions show up briefly for a few moments before being replaced by something else, others tend to show up for longer – often because certain things keep them activated inside us. There are also certain things that tend to help emotions settle, and those that stir them up and keep them going.

As we've done at various stages throughout this book, one way that we can divide things that maintain difficult emotions is by considering those that are 'external' (i.e. they arise or exist outside of us) and those that are 'internal' (i.e. those that arise inside us). Of course, this is an artificial distinction, but in Table 6 overleaf there are some examples of common factors that can maintain difficult emotions

Table 6: Internal and external maintainers of emotion

Internal maintainers of emotion	External maintainers of emotion
Worry	Critical others
Rumination	Technology (e.g. social media, TV)
Self-criticism	Stressful job
Experiential avoidance	Sedentary activities (e.g. TV, computer games)
Justification (e.g. 'I have every right to stay angry, it was their fault')	Poor diet
Fear (e.g. if I let go of the emotion I might miss a threat, or get hurt in some way)	Poor sleep
Self-identity (e.g. 'This is just the person I am')	Substances (e.g. caffeine, alcohol or drugs)

Take some time to think about what might keep your difficult emotions going. If it helps, take a piece of paper and write down some notes. Are they mostly internal or external factors?

Working with internal maintainers: We'll touch back in on some further ways of working with internal factors in the next chapter, which looks at Step 5 of the emotion regulation model, 'coping with emotions'. In particular, the subchapters on tolerating and accepting emotions (Chapter 16a) and working with shame and self-criticism (Chapter 16e) may be particularly helpful. If you found that there were particular thoughts (e.g. a sense of being 'justified' to feel like this), Chapter 19 helps to explore how we can work with this in a helpful, compassionate way.

However, given the skills you learned in Section Three, particularly linked to mindfulness, it may be that you can use these skills to begin to work with many of the internal 'maintainers' of your emotions. For example, mindfulness can really support us when our new brain capacity for rumination, worry or self-criticism starts getting in on the act. When we become aware that it's 'loops in the mind' that are partly contributing to the longer duration of our difficult emotions, we can begin to learn how to notice these, step back and live more in the present moment. It might be useful here to turn back to Chapter 3 and take some time to reconnect with these ideas, and some of the ways to become more aware of these loops. It's often also helpful here to engage in more regular practice of some of the mindfulness exercises that we introduced in Chapter 8, as these tend to have knock-on, beneficial effects in helping us be more present in the here and now.

Working with external maintainers: In terms of some of the external 'maintainers' of your difficult emotions, it's likely that there are also a variety of things that you can do instead. For example, if you recognise that a poor sleep routine contributes to anxiety or anger persisting, it might be helpful to search online for some guidance to sleep hygiene (e.g. https://www.nhs.uk/Livewell/insomnia/Pages/bedtimeritual.aspx). In contrast, if you realise that too much time spent on social media is contributing to you feeling sad or lonely, it might be helpful to try a period of abstinence or reduced use of the internet (ironically, there are lots of good online guides to this!). It's surprising how many of us fail to recognise how things like diet, sleep (too much or too little), exercise (too much or too little), use of substances or physical illness can have a significant impact on our emotions, and crucially, our ability to regulate our emotions in a helpful, consistent way. It's useful then to take some time to reflect on these, and consider whether there are general health-related changes that could be useful to engage in alongside some of the other work you're doing with this book.

Key reflections

Step 4 of the emotion regulation model focuses on *understanding emotions*, and in this chapter we have developed insights and skills linked to how:

- We can commonly struggle to understand why we feel, think or act in a particular way, and invalidate our experiences

- Validation involves meeting our emotional experiences as legitimate and understandable

- It can be useful to learn how to take perspective about our experience with difficult emotions – to understand what has led to them, what factors can influence them, and what sits underneath them

- We can use our compassionate mind skills to facilitate validation, empathy and understanding of our difficult emotions

- It's helpful to notice if certain things keep difficult emotions going for you, and if so, to learn to address these so that emotions can arise and fall in a healthy way

16 Compassion–focused emotion regulation skills (CERS) – coping with and using emotions

Although we may be able to notice, validate and understand our emotions, this doesn't mean that we'll be able to cope with them, or use them effectively, once they show up. For many, emotions bring with them pain and distress and can feel overwhelming. Our inner world – our mind, our body, our sense of self – can be a difficult place to reside or rest in, if we're in the presence of powerful threat-focused and distressing emotions. In fact, this becomes so averse for some of us that we have to engage in defensive responses to manage these feelings. For example, we may try to fight the emotion off, block it, or to avoid feeling or experiencing it in the first place. Drink, drugs and distraction are typical ways of trying to cope with painful feelings for some people. We can also experience emotions in response to our emotions, which can make it hard to manage the initial difficult feeling. For example, we can feel angry about feeling anxious, anxious about feeling sad, angry, anxious or sad about feeling sad, and shame in response to any of our emotions. In fact, the combinations go on and on! Unfortunately, this creates an inner sense of stress and conflict and, ultimately, as the saying goes, *what we resist, persists*.

So instead of turning down the heat on a boiling pan of water, which might be our initial intention, trying to block, suppress or get rid of difficult feelings tends to increase the heat instead. While our threat responses are designed to help us avoid harm, and can do this quite successfully in the external world (for example, by avoiding a dangerous dog or a dark alleyway), using this same approach to avoid internal 'threats', like emotions, isn't always effective or helpful. It can be helpful then to look at aspects of the fifth step of our emotion regulation model (Figure 17 below) to see what might be useful instead.

Figure 17: Emotion regulation model (ERM) – coping with and using emotion

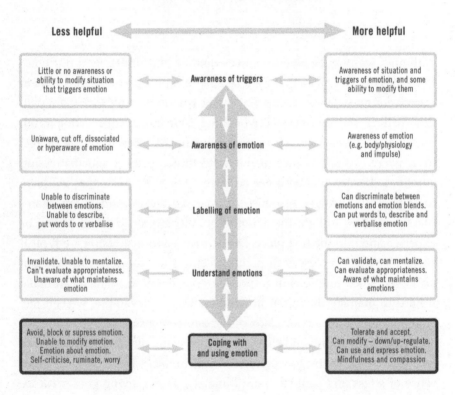

Here's a personal reflection of when I struggled with this step of the emotion regulation model. I remember as a child playing in a football tournament, and at the end of the week there was a penalty competition to see who, out of the players who had won a smaller penalty competition for their age group earlier in the week, would be crowned the winner across all the age groups. As one of the youngest there, I was due to compete against older boys, in front of all the people who were there at the camp (over a hundred). On the Thursday evening, my parents asked how I was feeling about the shoot-out the next day, and although I was very anxious, I instead told them I was 'OK'. That night, I remember not being able to sleep and worrying about if I was going to mess up and make a fool of myself in front of everyone. I kept trying to block out the emotion by watching TV and reading a comic, and kept my feelings to myself. All of Friday morning I worried about the competition in the afternoon. I remember getting increasingly panicky; so much so that I made an excuse and said that I'd injured myself and couldn't take part. Afterwards, I felt deeply ashamed of my anxiety – I thought I was *weak* for not taking part and letting my anxiety control me.

While it's understandable that many children (and adults) feel anxious about this type of performance-related situation, my response to feeling anxious only contributed to further difficulties. By avoiding the anxiety-provoking situation, pushing my anxiety away and not seeking help, I not only missed out on the shoot-out but also laid the path towards self-criticism and shame.

So, in the last step of the emotion regulation model, we're going to take a look at how your compassionate mind may help you to directly cope with difficult emotions, once they've been triggered. There are a number of key skills to this step of emotion regulation, and so we're going to break it down across five subchapters to make them more manageable:

a. Tolerating and accepting difficult emotions

b. Modifying the intensity of emotions

c. Using and expressing emotions

d. Working with multiple emotional 'selves'

e. Managing shame and self-criticism

Unfortunately, there isn't an exact science or formula for when it's helpful to tolerate and accept emotions, when to use and express them, or when to try to change their intensity – and of course, sometimes it involves a mixture of these! But this is where your compassionate self comes in – to help to guide you on this, with wisdom, and to help you make the best choice you can.

16a   Coping with emotions – tolerating and accepting

As we discussed in Chapter 2, like other animals, we have an evolved threat system that helps us navigate danger in the world. Many people have heard of the fight-flight system (a part of the threat response), which involves our capacity to engage in aggression or fighting as a way to deal with threats or to flee, avoid or move away from potential causes of harm. Although these behavioural strategies can be helpful, if they become generalised as ways to deal with our emotions and feelings, this can become problematic.

There is an increasing scientific literature highlighting that persistent attempts to avoid or fight off unpleasant emotions, feelings, images, memories or thoughts can actually lead to greater mental and physical distress (e.g. Aldao et al., 2010). This phenomenon was referred to by Freud as unconscious defence mechanisms, and more recently, as *experiential avoidance* (Hayes et al., 1996), where we have a threat-based response to our own experiences and engage in defensive responses to try to escape them. While understandable – if you think about it, avoidance of pain is a key motive for all animals – wise compassion may help us to take a different response to this instead. This is where using *tolerance and acceptance* of difficult emotions comes in.

Tolerating difficult emotions

One of the main difficulties people have with emotions is when they are too intense – that is, the emotion turns up with the volume set at the maximum when a midway mark would be more helpful. When our emotions are 'too loud', they can become the 'captain of the ship' – so we can end up lashing out, blaming and making life unpleasant for others (anger), get panicky or so fearful we avoid important situations and experiences (anxiety) or become overwhelmed with distress and pain with loss or absence (sadness). So, it's not that these emotions are wrong or bad, but more that they turn up with such potency that we are unable to use them helpfully. Although we will return to this theme in Chapter 16c, one way to start working with emotions when they are very intense is to learn how to tolerate them – to be in their presence but remain grounded, stable and anchored. When we're able to do this regularly, we learn that the volume of an emotion tends to turn down a bit. But it's not just that tolerance is helpful when an emotion is 'loud'; for some of us, emotions (whether generally or specific ones, such as anger or sadness) are so unpleasant or scary that we feel overwhelmed in their presence, no matter how strong they turn up.

As we found in Chapter 6, distress tolerance is a key aspect of the first psychology of compassion – the ability to move towards and engage with distress and suffering. Rather than being soft, compassion often involves strength and courage, enabling us to stay in the presence of something unpleasant (like difficult emotions), and not engage in unhelpful patterns of threat system-based behaviours (e.g. rumination, self-criticism). Of course, compassion is more than just staying in the presence of something distressing for its own sake – it involves having an active intention and motivation to alleviate our difficulties in some way, with wisdom and understanding. However, if we're unable to tolerate our emotions, then it becomes more difficult to do something helpful with them.

It's likely that you've had many experiences of tolerating an emotion, particularly if you have a clear goal in mind. For example, tolerating anxiety during a driving test, so that you'll have the freedom to get to places on your own, or tolerating feeling angry at a comment your boss has made, so that you won't jeopardise your chances at an upcoming promotion.

Just like any other ability, we can build skills in tolerating difficult emotions. In fact, we've already started doing this in Section Three. In this chapter, we're going to take some of the skills you learned in that section (e.g. mindfulness, body posture) and apply them further in learning how to tolerate emotions.

Mindfulness

There's a lot of research showing that practising mindfulness can improve emotion regulation skills (Roemer et al., 2015). Keep in mind that mindfulness really is about being aware of where your attention is, what your mind is focusing on, rather than just being on automatic pilot. There are a number of ways that mindfulness can help with difficult emotions. For example, mindfulness may help us notice unhelpful (although understandable) attempts to avoid difficult emotions, and become more familiar with our own bodies, minds, and habitual threat-based reactions, such as avoidance, suppression or blocking. So, as we've mentioned previously, mindfulness creates the potential for a mind-mindedness – an ability for us to become more aware of how our minds work, how they engage with difficult emotions, and the patterns of responses that we're likely to have practised over many months and years.

However, mindfulness can also help us to 'be with' the experience of an emotion – for example, the physical sensations in the body, whether it feels pleasurable or unpleasant, the urges or impulses that come with the feeling, along with patterns of thoughts (e.g. self-criticism, rumination, worry). Mindfulness can help us to approach and make contact with difficult, 'hot' feelings without being swept away by them. Let's look at a specific way of using mindfulness to help with this.

Exercise: Mindfulness of emotion – distress tolerance

Settle into your compassionate self posture in your chair, with your feet on the floor and an upright body posture. If you feel comfortable, close your eyes, and let your breathing slow down (approximately five to six breaths a minute if you can) with the out-breath being focused on slowing and settling into body grounding. Gently bring your awareness into the present moment, initially by paying attention to the sensation of breathing. After 30 seconds or so, slowly bring your attention to how you are feeling at the moment. Whatever feelings or emotions are present at the moment – or that arise during this practice – begin to notice what they are. It doesn't matter if these feelings are pleasant, unpleasant or neutral in tone – or whether they are strong or weak in intensity. Just notice the sensation that arises in your body with them, stepping back from judgements or thoughts about whether they should or shouldn't be there, or whether they feel distressing or not. Allow your thoughts and judgements – like leaves passing by on a stream – to gently move through your mind, and see if you can bring your awareness back to being with the experience of the feeling itself.

Notice where the emotion shows itself in your body, and the physical sensations it brings with it. Hold awareness gently to this, noticing the sensations that emerge with this feeling, where it's located in the body, or over time, where it moves to in the body. Remember you're in the observer position rather than trying to change anything about this experience – even if this is unpleasant – and simply allow yourself to experience the feeling in your body as it is.

If you feel you're getting pulled into or overwhelmed by the emotion, take a step back, grounding yourself back into the breath, the sounds around you, or in the sensations of contact of your body with the chair/floor. When ready, come back gently to noticing the feeling. It is often helpful to name or label in your mind the emotion you're experiencing – for example, 'this feels like sadness' or just 'sadness', or 'I'm feeling angry' or just 'anger'. The more you switch into noticing and describing from the observer position the less you are likely to be pulled into the maelstrom or flow of the emotion. At other times, people find it helpful to imagine 'breathing into the emotion', and with the in-breath, imagine creating space in the body for the emotion to 'be'.

You may also notice a whole range of thoughts arising which are telling you about what you can and cannot cope with, such as 'this is too much, I can't cope with this' or 'I should be able to be better with this' and so forth. This is a monitoring narrative, and here it's useful to note it but again just move back into observer position. If we keep telling ourselves that this is too much and we can't cope then, of course, that's going to make it more difficult to cope. But if we allow ourselves to develop the courage and strength to cope then over time, it's more likely that we'll learn how to do this.

As times goes on, see if you can notice if and when your mind becomes distracted from this focus on your feeling and emotion. It might be that your mind wanders to something else (e.g. something happening later today, or a memory), or that it's distracted by sounds, or something else happening in your environment. You might also notice judgements forming about the emotion itself – for example, asking if it's right or wrong, or experiencing concerns about it becoming overwhelming. See if you can notice these as understandable reactions that your threat system has, but imagine that, like leaves on a stream, or clouds in the sky, these thoughts and concerns can gently pass by, and then bring your awareness back to the sensation of the emotion in your body. You're not trying to fight off or push away from the feeling. Rather, you are trying as best you can to shift your attention into observing it as it shows up in your body, and how it brings along with it a whole range of thoughts and memories. Holding your observing attention here, you may notice that there is the pattern of how emotions show up in the body. Try to remain curious to this, and not get caught up in commentary or judgement. Continue with this process for another minute or two, and when you feel ready, bring the exercise to a close.

Take a few moments to reflect on this exercise, making a few notes on a piece of paper or on your smartphone. What did you learn from this? What happened to the emotion as you held mindful awareness to it in this way? Through further practice, how might this exercise help to develop your skills in tolerating emotions?

Stability of mind and body

Section Three explored how we can hold, tolerate and regulate the threat system by learning how to bridge from this to the soothing system. So, by engaging in your body posture, sense of grounding and breathing rhythm, we can practise how using this can help us to be in the presence of difficult feelings. It's important here to remember that this isn't about using the soothing system to soothe away difficult feelings, but rather, how we can use the parasympathetic system and sense of grounding and stability to help us tolerate the distress these feelings can bring. Let's look at how we can practise this.

Exercise: Distress tolerance – soothing breathing

Find a comfortable posture in your chair, with your feet on the floor, and an upright body posture. If it's helpful, close your eyes. Notice the sensations that are present as you breathe in and out. If you notice your attention wandering, just observe this and gently try to bring your attention back to your breath, without judging or criticising yourself for this distraction.

Now, as you're holding your attention in the flow of your in and out-breath, gently try to bring a soothing or calming breathing rhythm to your body. This will be a slower and deeper rhythm than usual (if possible, around six breaths per minute), but one that feels comfortable to your body. Try if you can to breathe in a smooth, even way. If you notice your attention moving away from your breath, or that you become distracted in any way, gently bring your attention back to your breath and tune back into the calming or soothing quality of your breathing rhythm. See if you can imagine a sense of 'slowing down' as you breathe out. It can also be helpful, as you breathe out, to connect to a sense of groundedness by noticing your feet on the floor. See if you can also notice your facial expression and try to soften your facial muscles, bringing a comfortable, friendly smile to your face. Notice how it feels to gently hold this expression on your face, and if it brings a change to the experience of maintaining your breathing rhythm.

Slowly bring your attention to a memory of a difficult emotion that you experienced recently. Try not to bring the most painful emotion, but one that you found difficult to manage at the time. It can be helpful to hold the situation in mind – where you were, who was present, and what triggered your emotion. See if you can bring this feeling into focus, noticing where it shows up in the body, the intensity of the sensation or unpleasant thoughts or urges that came with it. As you're doing this, try to remain connected to your soothing rhythm breathing. Check your posture, adjusting yourself back into an upright, confident posture and a friendly facial expression if you've noticed they've slipped away. If it helps, gently (and with a kind voice tone) repeat the phrase 'mind slowing down' or 'body slowing down' each time you breathe out.

Continue to hold the difficult emotion in mind alongside your breathing rhythm for another minute or two, before ending the exercise.

Take a few moments to reflect on this exercise, making a few notes on a piece of paper or on your smartphone. What did you learn from this? Through further practice, how might this exercise help you to tolerate difficult emotions?

Compassionate intention

Developing the compassionate self is also a powerful way to support yourself in tolerating emotions. As you might remember, this version of you draws upon mindfulness, soothing breathing, and body focus (e.g. posture, facial expression). But it also brings a specific intention and focus on core qualities of the compassionate version of you: strength, commitment and wisdom to understand what is being tolerated, and why this is helpful. Let's take a look at this in an exercise (if needed, return to Chapter 10 first to refresh yourself on the ideas of the compassionate self, before continuing here).

Exercise: Compassionate self – supporting distress tolerance

Take a few moments to engage with the five steps of preparation, as outlined on p. 115. When you've settled into a comfortable, upright posture on the chair, start by engaging in your soothing rhythm breathing. As you feel ready, connect with your compassionate self – your caring-commitment, wisdom, and in particular, your strength and courage (Chapter 10). Imagine stepping into the shoes of this version of you – how you might stand, what your facial expression and voice tone would be like, what your intention would be towards difficult emotions. Take a minute or two to connect with this.

When you feel ready, bring to mind an emotion that you find difficult to manage. If it helps, bring to mind a recent situation in which you struggled to manage this emotion. Spend a few moments looking through the eyes of your compassionate self at this difficult emotional experience/memory, as if you are watching it on a TV screen.

Focus back now on the qualities of your compassionate self.

Strength: Your compassionate self is strong, grounded and stable. Connect with your body posture and breathing rhythm. Imagine, like an ancient tree with deep roots, your compassionate self can stand in the presence of difficult emotions, just like a tree can tolerate the wind and rain.

Commitment: Hold in mind your compassionate intention – to engage in things that are difficult and find ways of being supportive and helpful to yourself, and where possible, reducing or alleviating distress. Remember that you are not on your own – your compassionate self is there to support you, to help you tolerate difficult feelings.

Wisdom: Your compassionate self understands that emotions are difficult for many of us to manage. It recognises that we didn't choose to experience these, nor struggle with them, but that these pass over time and we can only do our best.

If you feel yourself getting overwhelmed by this emotional memory, reconnect with your breathing and embodiment of your compassionate self. When you feel ready, bring yourself back to connect with the emotion you struggled with. Focus on just learning to be in the presence of this feeling, but from a perspective of security and groundedness that your compassionate self gives you. Notice what happens to the intensity of the fear or concerns about experiencing this emotion. Continue with this for another minute or two before finishing the exercise.

Take a few moments to reflect on this exercise, making a few notes on a piece of paper or on your smartphone. What did you learn from this? Through further practice, how might compassionate intention help you to tolerate difficult emotions?

As we've done throughout this and previous sections, it's important to practise these exercises as often as you can. The more practice you put in, the more likely that the next time a difficult emotion turns up, you'll be able to tolerate it and remain grounded.

Accepting difficult emotions

Alongside the intensity of emotions, another common difficulty for people relates to struggles about how long they seem to last – that it seems to take a long time for difficult emotions to settle, for us to recover after they've turned up. There can be many reasons for this, but the main difficulty relates to the understandable but unwise efforts we engage in to not feel a particular emotion, that unfortunately contributes to the emotion lasting longer. As we discussed in Chapter 15, if we try to respond to our difficult emotions from the threat system – particularly responses like avoidance, suppression, rumination, worry and self-criticism – this becomes akin to trying to put out a fire by bringing more fire. So alongside tolerating, it's also helpful to see if we can step back from our threat system response to them, and instead, try to accept emotions we find difficult or unpleasant.

In my experience, we can have a variety of concerns about accepting difficult emotions. Sometimes this is about the word 'acceptance' itself, which brings with it ideas of being passive, giving up or resigning ourselves to something. Acceptance in the way we'll focus on here is very different from these connotations. The fact is, once something has happened, it's happened; you cannot go back a second, minute, hour, day or year and undo something, no matter how much you might like to. In that sense, compassion here can help us to recognise that, although difficult and although there are often understandable reasons why it's difficult to accept something, there is ultimately no other choice than to accept what's happened. Anything else only gets in the way of reality and prevents us from doing what we can *now*.

Let's imagine you slip on the pavement and twist your ankle. The most important thing here is for you to recognise what happened, and then pay attention to what's going to help you to manage this (e.g. seek medical help, rest your ankle and so forth). Thoughts about how this shouldn't have happened, or anger at yourself that you slipped because you were carelessly checking your phone rather than looking at where you were going, are no help whatsoever; in fact, they're likely to make you feel worse – understandable though it is to think like this. A key issue here involves shifting from blaming to taking responsibility, which we have talked about so much. Blaming and shaming ourselves often leads us to get into a fight with ourselves, and can lead to us bringing threat system (self-blame, rumination, anger) to try to manage an experience that has already triggered our threat system (ankle pain).

So, given that it can be hard to step back from blaming, rumination and anger, what helps us to move towards acceptance? Well, one way is drawing upon the qualities of your compassionate self: wisdom to recognise that resisting something that is already present is unlikely to help; strength to tolerate and 'be with' the distress that some emotions elicit; and commitment to be supportive and helpful to oneself and to try to alleviate distress that can be alleviated. Acceptance doesn't mean passively going along with what is difficult, but, rather, using wisdom to recognise that what has triggered our feelings (and their intensity) is in part outside of our control, and influenced by a number of factors such as our learning history, conditioning, and environmental triggers. Accepting doesn't mean that we're not going to try to work on changing what is causing our difficult emotions; it doesn't mean that we collude with or passively go along with a situation, relationship or experience, without trying to change it, particularly if it is clear that these are unhealthy or bad for us in some way. Rather, in the moment, it guides us to try to 'be with' our experience, tolerating and accepting it as it is.

Compassionate acceptance

If you have a splinter in your finger, it's important to accept that it's going to hurt – spending your time trying to make it not hurt would be futile. However, you wouldn't just want to leave the splinter there, but instead, find a way to remove it. As Paul Gilbert notes, we can accept that we are feeling depressed (rather than shaming ourselves for this or getting caught in denial), but that wouldn't stop us from seeking treatment for depression. Let's try an exercise to help with the process of accepting difficult emotions using your compassionate self.

Exercise: Compassionate acceptance of difficult emotions

Take some time to engage in the five steps of preparation, as outlined on p. 115. Find a comfortable place to sit, and connect with your soothing rhythm breathing, grounded body posture, and friendly facial expression. Connect with your compassionate self (Chapter 10), and in particular its wisdom, strength and commitment. Take your time to feel your way into this. When you feel ready, work through each of the attributes outlined below. If, at any time, you feel overwhelmed, remember to ground yourself in mindful awareness of your body, soothing breathing and body posture, as a way of helping you to regulate your threat system.

Now bring to mind an emotion you find difficult to accept, or a time recently that you struggled to manage your emotions (take 30 seconds or so to do this). With this emotion or memory in mind, let's take each of the attributes of your compassionate self, in turn, to help with the process of acceptance.

Wisdom: As your compassionate self, you understand that we didn't choose to experience emotions and that although they can be unpleasant and, at times, painful, they evolved to help protect us and help us navigate the world. The wisdom of your compassionate self also recognises that the way emotions function for you has been shaped by many things in your life, most of which you had no control over. So, there is a non-personalised, 'no shame and no blame' acceptance of the nature of emotions.

Take 30 seconds to reconnect with your soothing breathing . . .

Strength: Drawing upon the tolerance exercise we practised earlier in this chapter (p. 257), while holding in mind an emotion that you find difficult, also bring to mind that your compassionate self is strong, grounded and stable. Notice your upright body posture, soothing breathing and sense of inner stability; that just like an anchored ship, the wind may blow and waves crash, but you can remain secure in the face of whatever emotion you struggle with.

Take 30 seconds to reconnect with your soothing breathing . . .

Commitment: Also hold in mind that your compassionate self is caring, supportive and helpful. It recognises that emotions can be very distressing, painful and unpleasant at times, and wants to be supportive and caring to that part of you that struggles in the face of them. It will do its best to support you in turning towards and accepting emotions, even when they are distressing, just as you might support a friend who is experiencing an emotional difficulty.

Take some time with each of the above qualities, using them to help you with accepting whatever emotion is troubling you.

You might also spend some time considering the following questions as a guide to helping the acceptance process:

- What qualities of your compassionate self would help you accept this difficult emotion? Really focus on what would be helpful

- What skills might you have learned from this book that could help you accept, and not fight or become overly caught up in this emotion (e.g. mindfulness, soothing breathing, imagery)?

- What can you do if you find this difficult? What would your compassionate self want to say to you in these difficult moments?

As you finish this practice and take some time to reflect on it, it's important to remember that you can tailor or adapt this to fit what will work best for you. The above exercise is just an outline – you may find that it's useful to reorder the steps or to emphasise one part more than another. Remember that your compassionate self will help you with this, and will be there to support you if you hit any bumps in the road with these exercises.

Working with 'emotions about emotion'

In Chapter 5, I introduced the idea of how emotions about other emotions seem to be a particular quirk of human beings, and can contribute to many of the difficulties we face when trying to manage distressing emotions wisely. We can experience emotions (e.g. anger, fear or shame) about other emotions (e.g. anger, fear, sadness, joy, calmness), or may find that certain difficult emotions emerge as a result or consequence of an initial emotion (for example, feeling anxious and shaky after feeling and expressing anger).

It's worth taking a look back at p. 77 to see what you learned about whether you have difficulties with emotion about emotion. Once you've done that, consider exploring the steps we've taken together in this chapter, but applying them to this instead. It's also useful here to focus on other steps of the emotion regulation model – for example, our ability to notice, label and discriminate between emotions, emotion blends and mixed feelings (Chapter 14). It might also be helpful to consider why you experience the secondary emotion, rather than just being able to stay with the initial emotional reaction you had. Sometimes this is linked to what we've learned in life – for example, that sadness is weak, or that anger is dangerous. Here, it might be that we can return to what we learned about and practised in Chapter 15, taking time to try to understand and reflect on these secondary emotional reactions. If you'd like to work in more depth with emotions about emotion, take a look through some of the following chapters, in particular those on multiple selves (Chapter 16d) and shame (Chapter 16e).

Key reflections

Step 5 of the emotion regulation model focuses on *coping with and expressing emotions*. In this subchapter, we have developed insights and skills linked to how:

- Many people try to stay away from unpleasant feelings and emotion. This is sometimes referred to as experiential avoidance

- Although it's understandable (due to our threat system's motivation to keep you safe) to try to avoid something painful and unpleasant, this often 'keeps the threat going' (essentially, what we resist, persists)

- Learning to accept and tolerate our difficult feelings can lead to a reduction in fear about them, and an increased ability to engage with life more fully

- Learning to tolerate and accept emotions can reduce the likelihood that we have 'emotions about emotions' (e.g. fear of our anger or sadness)

- Tolerance and acceptance doesn't mean that we passively 'put up with' or resign ourselves to difficult situations, but rather, we can wisely, intentionally choose to 'be with' our feelings so as to explore them, and have more freedom and choice as to how to deal with them

16b Modifying the intensity of emotions

Many people feel they lack control of their emotions. One client of mine used to like using weather analogies to describe her emotions. The first time I met her, she told me: 'I sometimes feel I've got more chance of controlling the weather than I do my emotions.' Another session she told me of her distress and powerlessness in the face of strong emotions: 'Some days, it feels like no matter what I wear or how good my umbrella is, I'm still going to get soaked.' It's impossible to control our emotions fully – and in fact, by trying to control those from the threat system we may make it more likely that we struggle with them. However, like dressing appropriately for different temperatures and types of weather, we can learn how to modify some aspects of our emotional experiences in a way that is wise and helpful.

If you remember, in Chapter 1 we used the analogy of emotions as a story, i.e. having certain processes, such as a start, middle and end. For emotions, these include what triggers them, how frequent they are, their intensity, duration and settling processes. Part of emotion regulation involves how we can work with these different aspects of the emotion 'story' in a way that gives rise to helpful emotion regulation. Of course, you've already started this process. For example, on the first step of the emotion regulation model, you learned how to select situations that made it less likely that you unnecessarily encountered threat emotions (thus changing both triggers to emotions, and the frequency of experiencing them), and started to increase contact with situations that may stimulate positive emotions.

In the second step of the model, you learned that by becoming more aware of the patterns of emotions as they showed up in your body, you were less likely to engage in avoidance. In step three of the model, you learned that labelling and discriminating the nuances between emotions was associated with more helpful emotion regulation strategies. Finally, in step four of the model, you learned that validation and empathy for our difficult emotions could help to reduce threat system reactions to them.

In this chapter, we're going to look at another way we can alter our experience of difficult emotions – by altering their intensity.

Modifying the intensity of emotions

Emotions can show up in different volumes. Some are subtle, barely perceptible and operating like quiet music in the background of our lives. Others are like standing at the front row of a thrash metal music gig – loud, overpowering and overwhelming.

The first thing when bringing awareness to the intensity of our emotions is to see if we can put this in context. An important context to start with is an awareness of what is currently going on in your life. For example, if you are being bullied by your boss or colleagues, it's probably a good thing that your emotions are intense, as they are trying to help to navigate a challenging situation. If you were numb or shut down to this experience (i.e. it was still stressing your body, but you were cut off from the emotional or psychological consequences), this might not be a good thing, as you're unlikely to be getting sufficient information, signals or energy to bring a change to the situation. If a loved one has just passed away or ended their relationship with you, it's likely that you'll feel intensely sad; again, this would be entirely appropriate given the circumstances. However, if you feel intense emotion in situations that you usually wouldn't, or have a sense that this is at a level that is not fitting or appropriate for the circumstances, it may be helpful to do something about this. For example, experiencing intense anger and frustration while waiting in a small queue at the supermarket, or intense anxiety when talking to a good friend. Equally, if you don't experience certain emotions in situations in which they could be quite useful (e.g. no contentment and peacefulness while lying on a beautiful beach, or no anger when someone mistreats you or a loved one), it might be useful to know how to 'dial up' the intensity level.

We can also look back in time and have an understanding about what might have influenced the intensity of our emotions (see Chapter 4). For example, if you've grown up in a home in which both of your parents were quite introverted and quiet, and who held a philosophy that children 'should be seen but not heard', it might be that your emotional intensity range is set quite low. In comparison, if you were raised in a home or culture in which emotions (e.g. love, affection, warmth) are valued and expected, it might be that your emotions are set at the higher end of the intensity barometer. The reflective point here is that we don't choose the intensity of our emotions; rather, we just find ourselves with emotions that turn up with a type of intensity range that may be fine or may lead to problems in various ways. However, this doesn't mean that we can't learn how to bring changes to them that might be helpful for our own, and other people's, well-being.

Decreasing the intensity of emotions

Let's start with looking at how to reduce the intensity of emotions, sometimes referred to as downregulating emotions. One of the key areas to focus upon when we experience intense emotions is how we can use the body and mind to help navigate these experiences. Here are some ideas:

Grounding techniques: There are many ways to ground or stabilise ourselves when we feel we're being dragged into the depths of intense emotions. Here are some that might help:

1.   <u>Posture</u> – as you're reading this now, take a moment to become aware of your posture in the chair. Now take a moment to adjust this, sitting for a moment with your feet firmly on the floor, about shoulder width apart. Sit in an upright, confident position, lengthening your spine slightly. Allow your shoulders to open and drop slightly. See if you can remain in this position for a minute, and then go back

to adopting the posture you were in previously, embodying this for 30 seconds, noticing any differences. Now, move back into the grounded, upright posture again, and see if you can maintain this for a number of minutes. See what it's like to allow a slight smile or friendly expression to come to your face (p. 137, Chapter 9).

This process – being aware of current posture, and then shifting to one that represents stability, groundedness and confidence – can be quite a powerful way of helping to bring down the intensity of an emotion by a notch or two.

2.   '5-4-3-2-1 grounding' – another grounding technique that's particularly helpful when emotions start to nudge high up on the thermometer is called '5-4-3-2-1'. This is a relatively simple approach helping us to ground through the five senses. Start at 5, and count down to 1, but following this guide:

5 – To start with, wherever you are, take a few moments to look around, and notice (maybe name these inside your mind) five things that you can see.

4 – Next, notice four things that you can feel. So that might be the contact between your feet and the floor, or your body and the chair. It could be the sensations of clothes against your skin, or the temperature of the room you're in.

3 – Wherever you are, become aware of three things that you can hear. Label what these are inside your mind.

2 – Focus now on trying to notice two things you can smell. Don't worry if you find this difficult, it might be that it's difficult to notice two different things, but the attempt to do this with a kind intention is helpful in itself.

1 – Finally, focus on one thing that you can taste. This could be to notice whatever taste is currently in your mouth (this could range from a strong sense of something to a subtle taste). Sometimes it's helpful to take a quick sip of water, juice or coffee, or bite a small piece of food, and just pay attention to what that tastes like.

These exercises are not about avoiding or trying to get rid of a strong emotion; rather, it's about helping you to slow down and ground yourself in the here and now and create a little space around a strong feeling.

Mindfulness: One of the insights that mindfulness practice helps to unfold is that our experiences – sensations, urges, thoughts, feelings and emotions – are just that, experiences. They begin, they are 'felt', and at some stage, they end. Nothing is permanent, everything stops at some stage. Mindfulness can give rise not just to awareness and the ability to notice and label emotions, but also that we can be 'non-reactive' to inner experiences. So even if an emotion has turned up with high intensity, we can learn to observe it, and label it but not get caught up in what it's urging us to do, nor the pattern it's trying to grip us in (e.g. rumination, worry, trying to suppress it or block it out). Once we start relating to our inner experiences in this way, it's common for some of the intensity of these experiences to drop off.

It can be helpful here to return to Chapter 8, and spend some more time practising some of the mindfulness exercises, as these will help you over time to relate to intense emotions differently. You may also find the 'mindfulness of emotions' exercises on p. 211 helpful.

Soothing Rhythm Breathing: As we explored throughout Chapter 9, the rhythm, pace and various other qualities of breathing can have a significant effect in engaging the physiology of the soothing system, and in particular, the parasympathetic nervous system. Turn back to this chapter, and reacquaint yourself with these exercises, perhaps making a commitment to practise them when outside of strong emotions, so that when needed, they can be available for you when the intensity rises. As with learning to swim, it's good to start in the shallow end, and then as you become more confident over time, move into the deeper, more choppy waters of the sea.

Do some writing: Sometimes when we're caught up with the intensity of an emotion, it's useful to stay connected to this, but 'be with it' in a different modality. One of the difficulties with intense emotions is that when they turn up, their patterns bring with them various sensations, thoughts, images, urges and so forth, and when we are in direct contact with these, we can lose the 'wood for the trees', and find it difficult to gain perspective or space from the experience of the emotion. In effect, we 'become' the emotion. The act of writing can help us engage in these experiences differently.

The key here is taking some time – maybe 5 or 10 minutes – to allow yourself to 'write' as the emotion that you're experiencing. So, if it's anger, allow the angry part of you free rein to put pen to paper and express what it's feeling, why it's feeling as it is, what thoughts, urges or desires it has. As best as you can, don't overthink this; just let the pen flow.

Afterwards, see how writing has impacted upon the intensity of your feelings. Do you notice any changes? If so, what are they? How might you use this in the future to regulate intense emotions?

Engaging in your compassionate image: In Chapter 10 we looked at how to develop an image of a compassionate other – someone (or thing) that is wise, strong and caring towards us. If you've spent some time practising this exercise, it can be a powerful way of helping you when experiencing intense emotions. It may be worth noting that if you're in the flow of intense emotions and you haven't practised this exercise much before, it might not be the most helpful time to start when you're struggling in this way. If you can, take some time when you're feeling more settled to start developing this image, and then sometime in the future, with practice, it may be a helpful strategy to turn to when you experience intense emotions.

If you do try this exercise to help reduce the intensity of an emotion, make some notes afterwards about what the experience was like. Did the exercise help? If so, what was it about the exercise – and the image itself – that was helpful? How could you remember to turn to this again in the future?

Physical activity: Many people I know swear by the power of physical exercise as a helpful strategy in dealing with intense emotions. Its likely part of this effect is through physiological changes associated with certain types of exercise, but similar to writing, it may be that physical exercise helps to 'switch' the channel that we are operating in, helping us to moderate and move from overly intense emotions. It's worth thinking about what type of exercise is most helpful for you; while some people need high-octane, cardiovascular exercise (e.g. running or a spinning class), others find that those involving slower, more deliberate body movement (e.g. yoga, tai chi) are more beneficial. It's worth trying out a variety of things, and seeing what works for you.

Talking with a friend: While the above strategies may be done alone, it's also useful to hold in mind the three system model that we discussed in Chapter 2, and how we learned about the potent role that other people can have in triggering our soothing system, and reducing distress. If you have someone in life that you feel comfortable with – a good friend who has attributes that are helpful when life gets a bit tricky – it may be useful to approach them for support. Consider, before you do, what you're going to speak to them about, and what you'd like help with. It might be that sometimes we know we just need a 'listening ear', whereas at other times we need advice, support or direction.

Using the new brain – reasoning and appraisal: There's been lots of research highlighting how certain ways of thinking about our emotions – and the situations that lead to them – can have a powerful impact upon exacerbating emotional distress (see Chapter 3). Similarly, we also know there are patterns of thinking that can have a beneficial impact in reducing the intensity of emotions. This can involve helping you to have a new approach – a new way of looking at your emotions and the situations that caused them. One common way to support yourself here is to recognise when you might be getting caught in threat system-based 'loops in the mind' about an emotion or situation, and trying instead to find more helpful, supportive or empathic ways of reflecting upon your feelings. To explore this in more detail, it might be helpful to take time to read through Chapter 20 on 'compassionate thinking'.

Accepting emotions: Although it may seem counter-intuitive, learning to accept emotions may help to decrease their intensity. One reason for this is that, if they are already present, if we try to stop or get rid of them, that's bringing the threat system to manage an emotion that may already have you in the threat system. Acceptance doesn't mean passive resignation; rather, it's how to be wisely alongside something that is already present. We discussed this approach previously (Chapter 16a), and it may be worth returning to reread it to support you with how this can help you to reduce the intensity of emotions. As you do this, it may be helpful to note that there can also be a subtle contradiction here, between acceptance of emotions in and of itself, and accepting emotions for the purpose of reducing emotional intensity.

Increasing the intensity of emotions

It's not just 'high intensity' emotional experiences that we need to consider modifying. For some people, problems arise from finding it hard to 'feel' emotions – that they turn up quietly, like a whisper or a delicate touch. As we discussed earlier in the chapter, this might be fine in some contexts and situations, but not so helpful in others. If you recognise that your emotional intensity is set low, and would like to experience stronger feelings at times, start by taking a moment to think about what might get in the way of higher emotion intensity. What factors may contribute to this for you? Has it always been like this, or is this a more recent experience for you?

One way to increase the intensity of emotions is to become more aware of (and ultimately, try to reduce the influence of) what's blocking them. Interestingly, we've already explored some of these in previous steps of the emotion regulation model, but these include:

- Invalidating the feeling – feeling that the emotion is somehow wrong or inappropriate

- Lack of familiarity of the emotion – like when first riding a bike or driving a car, if we've had little experience with certain emotions, we may feel unfamiliar with their shape, and unconfident in how we 'wear' them when they show up

- Fear of the emotion, or consequences of the emotion

- Shame – a sense that there is something wrong or flawed with us if we experience the emotion, or experience the emotion at a more intense level. We may also be concerned that other people would think negatively of us for experiencing this emotion more intensely. We will turn to work with this in Chapter 16e

Imagination: As we've explored through this book (e.g. p. 140), imagery can have a powerful effect on our physiology and emotions. Given this, we can use it as a way to 'turn up' the intensity of feelings. Let's explore this together.

Exercise: Turning up the volume of emotional intensity

Sit in a comfortable but upright, confident posture. Take a few moments to orientate yourself to the present moment and connect with your soothing rhythm breathing. When you feel settled, begin by bringing an emotion to mind that you would like to experience more intensely – for example, anger or excitement.

When you have an emotion in mind, take some time to think of a time recently when you've experienced this emotion at a lowish intensity level. Bring that situation back into mind, noticing where you were, and what you were doing. Try to remember what had happened that triggered your emotion in the first place.

Now, with this in mind, imagine the intensity of your emotion as a scale. So, if '0' was no emotion at all, and '10' was the most anyone could ever experience that emotion, make a note of where you would land on that scale. If your emotion intensity was at level '2', see if you can now imagine allowing the intensity to grow in you, to expand so that the setting 'level' was a bit higher (e.g. '5'). Just like turning up the volume on a stereo, imagine turning up the volume of this emotion.

If you could turn the volume up a bit, how might that feel in your body? Where would you notice the feelings showing up more? Where would the energy of the emotion want to flow in the body? If the emotion was at a higher level, what might you want to do? What would you say, or be thinking? If you were back in the original situation that triggered this emotion, how might you have responded differently if the intensity of the feeling had been higher?

Take some time with this, mindfully exploring whatever sensations, experiences or thoughts emerge as you're doing it. If you feel the volume is getting too high for you, remember that you can dial it down a little too, noticing your grounded posture, soothing breathing and ability to tolerate and be in the presence of difficult sensations.

If you can, make a few notes about your experience of this. What did you notice? What was it like to try to increase the intensity of an emotion like this? Key with this exercise is to go slowly and to go where it feels OK. Remember, it's fine for these exercises to stretch us, but not to overwhelm – so take small steps, allowing your body to acclimatise to this imaginal process. As you become more confident with repeated practice of this, try to imagine increasing the intensity scale.

Using writing: If you find imagery difficult, then it might be useful to use writing instead. Here's a guide on what you can try.

Exercise: Using writing to increase emotional intensity

Get a piece of paper and a pen. Bring to mind again the emotion and situation that you used in the imagery exercise above. Like before, take some time to bring the situation back to mind, remembering what had happened, who else was there, and what (low-intensity) feeling this triggered.

Now, with this in mind, see if you can take 5 minutes to write about this situation, but doing this from the perspective of the emotion. So, although it might seem a little strange, you are trying to write as the emotion would write about things. For example, if it was a situation in which you experienced low levels of excitement, write from the perspective of excitement, but excitement at a higher level of volume or intensity. Don't worry if it doesn't feel 'real', or if you wouldn't actually respond like this in real life. Instead, focus on writing this 'as if', like a character in a novel who could experience the emotion at a more intense level.

If this was the case, if this emotion had been at a higher intensity, how would you have felt in your body? What would your body have wanted to do? What might you have been thinking about? How might you have responded to other people around you? What would you have said to them?

After you've finished writing, take some time to reread what you've written. How does it feel reading this back? If you can, take some time to repeat this exercise, either using the same situation, or a different one that was linked to the same, low-intensity emotion.

Developing your skills further – online material

If having read and worked through this chapter, you feel there is more you'd like to work on in changing the intensity of your emotions, there is good news for you! There are some free to access, online chapters that I've created with precisely this in mind. The focus of these extra chapters is on the concepts of:

1.   *Too much emotion:* This is when we struggle with an emotion that turns up too often, too powerfully, or for too long, and which we feel unable to down-regulate in a helpful way.

2.   *Too little emotion:* When we struggle with an emotion because it turns up too infrequently, or too quietly when triggered, or over which we have little ability to experience or express (or more generally, 'up-regulate') in a way that would be helpful to us or others if we could.

These online chapters will look at specific emotions that we can experience 'too much' or 'too little' – anger, anxiety and sadness. They can be accessed for free here: https://overcoming.co.uk/715/resources-to-download

Key reflections

- Emotions can occur at different levels of intensity
- Sometimes their volume can be set too high, and it can be useful to find ways of reducing the intensity
- Sometimes an emotion arises with low intensity in situations where it could be helpful for it to turn up more powerfully
- There are a variety of ways to modify the intensity of emotions

16c Coping with emotions – expressing emotions and assertiveness

As we discussed earlier in this book, emotions evolved to offer us helpful responses in particular situations or contexts. For example, anxiety evolved to detect threats, and move us away from things that were potentially dangerous, whereas sadness signals the need to support and connect, often following some sort of loss. However, expressing and using emotions can be very difficult for many of us. For some, this is because they were never taught how to express feelings, and have not had good examples or role models of people expressing emotions in a consistent, helpful and constructive way. Other people may have learned that expressing emotions brings on threat emotions. For example, TJ was told by his father that expressing sadness was a sign of weakness and 'unmanliness', and on one occasion, at TJ's grandmother's funeral, he hit TJ for crying. As TJ became an adult, he struggled to express his feelings, and in particular, felt anxious when a new partner asked him to express his feelings (in particular, of sadness, fear and vulnerability) to her. In therapy, TJ realised that given his experiences growing up, expressing emotions (and particularly sadness and distress) had been associated with anxiety and shame (threat-based feelings).

Recall that the threat system evolved to detect threats, activate the body for defensive actions and thereby keep us safe. Above all else, the threat system is concerned with our safety even at the expense of causing us all kinds of other problems. One of my clients once told me that his threat system told him 'don't say anything – keep it to yourself' as only 'bad things happen when you show your feelings'. It's very understandable then that some of us have learned this way of approaching our emotions. However, non-expression of emotion can have its own unintended consequences

– for example, it can prevent us from receiving care and reconnecting with people (e.g. blocked sadness), or being able to stick up for ourselves when others are treating us unkindly or unfairly (e.g. blocked anger). Moreover, repressed/suppressed emotions can often lead to emotional eruptions, when habitual blocking strategies become overwhelmed.

Let's reflect in more detail about how this works for you. Take a moment to think about what lies within your threat system (i.e. what your concerns are) about expressing emotion. Is this something that you feel comfortable with in general? Or maybe there are some emotions that you feel comfortable with expressing, but others that are tricky? If you do struggle to express your emotions at times, is there a way of understanding why this might be? What fears or concerns might be linked to this, and where might you have learned that expressing emotions is threatening in some way?

There are usually two types of concern about expressing emotions, feelings or desires:

1. What will it mean about me? (E.g. I'll become weak, selfish, vulnerable or overwhelmed.)

2. What will others think about me (and how they will treat me) as a consequence of expressing my emotions? (E.g. They will criticise, not like or reject me.)

Now, these concerns can be for both positive and negative emotions. Think of certain positive emotions you might be fearful of expressing. Maybe you're worried about expressing your pleasure about certain kinds of music, in case other people don't share your tastes? Or expressing certain desires that you worry other people might not share with you. As with so much in our experience of emotion, it's not just *what* we feel, it's also how we *express* what we feel that's important. Keep in mind that one of the functions of emotions that Darwin recognised and argued for is that they are sources of social information to other people. So, when others can see the emotion in you (for example, by how this influences your facial expression, body posture, voice tone and so on), this can help them to understand you – what you're feeling, what you want, and how they might best respond to you. If, for whatever reason, you're not able to do this, it can make it harder for other people to understand you and meet your needs or concerns. Given then that emotions are a powerful source of communication and information for others (in fact, that was one of Darwin's original ideas about how and why they evolved), it's important to give thought to how you express them and how you talk about them. The more mindful and in tune you are with them, the greater the chances you will be able to express them in a way that is going to be helpful to you rather than just in some raw unprocessed way.

Exercise: Exploring difficulties with emotional expression

Let's see if we can take this a step further. Take a few minutes to consider and answer the following questions:

- Think about the emotion you find most difficult to express to others. Which emotion(s) is this, and what is your fear about expressing this emotion?

- How do you usually deal with this fear/concern (e.g. keep things to yourself/avoid others/put up a facade)?

- Although understandable, are there any unintended consequences of protecting yourself by not expressing your emotions?

A common difficulty for many people when it comes to managing, expressing or using emotions, is that we can get caught up with *emotions about emotions*. As we discussed on p. 76 (Chapter 5) and p. 267 (Chapter 16a), we may feel anxious about our anger or sadness, or anger about (a perceived sense) of being weak for experiencing or expressing anxiety or sadness. And shame can be a common experience about all of our other emotions, in the sense that we can feel there is something wrong or flawed with us for feeling this way. We will return to exploring the concept of emotions about emotion in Chapter 16d, and look at the powerful role shame has on emotion regulation problems in Chapter 16e.

So, once we have a better understanding of the struggles we have with expressing certain emotions, we can then think about how we can turn back to the skills we've been developing throughout this book to learn how to practise doing this. Let's look at this together.

Exercise: Managing fears about expressing emotions

One of the key difficulties in expressing emotions is containing and regulating our concerns about doing so. It can be helpful to bring your compassionate mind to help with this struggle.

Take a moment to connect with your soothing rhythm breathing. When you feel ready, bring to mind the qualities of your compassionate self or your ideal compassionate other (Chapter 10) – try your best to connect with a sense of caring-commitment, wisdom and strength.

When you feel ready, from the compassionate part of you, look back on the reasons (above exercise) around your struggle to express an emotion. Consider the following questions:

- What do you, as your compassionate self, recognise about this? What would you want to say about this fear or concern?

- Can you, as your compassionate self, see that it is understandable in some way? How might you validate the fear?

- Given this struggle, how might your compassionate self help you to tolerate any difficulties? What can your compassionate self do to help you to take steps towards expressing this emotion, when appropriate?

If it's helpful, make some notes in response to these questions on a piece of paper.

Once we are able to bring compassion to the things that make it difficult for us to express emotions, it tends to be a bit easier to consider why expressing emotions might be useful. A comparison here might be that if you feel ashamed about something – let's say your sexual urges or fantasies – it might make it quite difficult for you to engage in something natural and pleasurable like sex. However, if you're able to work with the blocks around this (shame) and bring compassion to this block, then things are likely to be a little easier for you. It's similar if we have internal conflicts with our emotions. We will look more at this in Section Six (and you can also access online chapters about too much and too little emotion online at https://overcoming.co.uk/715/resources-to-download).

Three steps to emotion expression

We're now ready to move towards our goal – to help you find ways of expressing difficult emotions to others in a way that is not overly constricted by shame, self-criticism or fear. But we're not going to jump straight into expressing. We will take this in three steps.

As you can guess, it's often engaging with the skills of the compassionate self that facilitates healthy emotional expression. For example, it takes the wisdom to know that, although understandable and unintended, the non-expression, or mindless acting out, of emotions can cause distress to ourselves and others. It takes a commitment to face the difficulties we have in expressing emotion, and a caring motivation to ourselves for why it is important to become more skilled in their area. And it is connecting with compassionate courage and strength that empowers us to tolerate and express our emotions in a helpful way, as well as confront our fears about them. Let's look at this through a number of steps:

Step 1. Preparation for expressing emotions – starting in the shallow end of the pool

If you're learning to play the guitar, it's probably easier to start in your own bedroom, rather than on stage in front of people. The same is the case for learning to express emotions. Take some time to do some preparation for how you are going to express an emotion(s) that you find difficult. To start with, bring to mind an emotion that you struggle to express, or a situation you would usually find it tricky to express that emotion in. For example, it might be that anxiety is an emotion you struggle to express, and the context is when speaking to a colleague about your insecurity in going for a job promotion. Or it could be that sadness is a tricky emotion for you to express, and the context might be in talking to your friends about a recent relationship break-up. Make a few notes, or write a mini script of what you're going to say, and how you are going to do this. For example, Alexis, a client I saw who was struggling to express anger about the way he was being treated by his flatmate (Jamie), wrote out a few ideas about what he could say to express his anger in a helpful way. Here's what he jotted down:

> *Can I speak to you about a few things, please?*
>
> *I wanted to let you know that when you bring your friends home late at night, it makes it very difficult for me to sleep.*
>
> *I get irritated when you play your music late at night, as I have to wake up at 5.30am to go to work.*
>
> *I would like you to think more about the impact on me when you come home late at night.*

It can be helpful to observe other people you know who you rate as good at expressing difficult emotions and feelings – what do you notice about what they do? What emotion(s) do they express? How do they express this? What is their voice tone, facial expression, or body posture as they do so?

It can also be helpful (although of course a little strange at first) to try practising expressing your emotions out loud or in front of a mirror. For some people, it can be useful to role-play expressing difficult emotions with someone who they trust and feel safe with, but who is not the object of the emotion that they want to express. Ask for feedback after this, and any tips or coaching they can give that may help. Some people find it useful to imagine expressing difficult emotions first, before actually doing it. For example, in our sessions Alexis closed his eyes and imagined approaching Jamie, and expressing his angry feelings, but doing this in a way that both expressed his feelings, but also made it likely that he was successful in his goal (to get Jamie to be more thoughtful about how much noise he was making). Finally, although it's not always possible to plan for how and when you can express your emotions (sometimes you'll find yourself in a situation that provides the opportunity), try to bring to mind a situation, person or opportunity in the coming week or two to express an emotion to someone that you would typically shy away from. Try not to pick the most difficult time to do this (e.g. in front of lots of other people, or about a situation in which your emotions are too strong), but if possible, a situation that feels manageable to start with. For example, you may choose to tell your colleague about anxiety you experience around a task at work, or your partner about something they do that frustrates you.

Step 2. Expressing emotion

When it comes to expressing emotions that you find difficult, we're going to do this with the support of your compassionate self. If it helps, take a few minutes before talking to the person you intend to express your feelings to, getting into the wisdom, strength and commitment of your compassionate self which will support you during this exercise. Think about who you're going to choose to express your emotions too. It might initially be clear to you who this is, but you may find your compassionate self holds wisdom that it's more helpful to start voicing your feelings to someone else who is easier to start the process with (e.g. it might be easier to practise this with a friend at first before moving on to someone who may find it harder to listen to you).

Once you have someone in mind, focus on your intention – what is it that you want to get across to the other person? For example, if you're angry with them about something, it's not just 'showing' your anger, but putting a 'wise' and helpful voice to what the angry part of you needs to say, and expressing that in a way that may be heard and appreciated. If it's sadness, it's not just showing sadness (e.g. through tears), but how you can express what has made you sad, and what that sad part needs or would find useful from the other person.

Here are some general things to consider when expressing emotions:

1. *Words take us only part of the way.* Keep in mind that a lot of emotional communication is through our non-verbal behaviours, not just the verbal content, so when you are thinking about expressing emotion consider these two different dimensions of how you are appearing and sounding as well as what you're actually saying or doing

2. *Take the receiver position.* For example, if you were the person experiencing somebody else expressing the same emotion to you, how would this leave you feeling? This can help you to start mentalizing the impact you may have on others in the way you express the emotion. For example, if it's anger you're thinking about expressing, consider what it would be like to see the facial expression or hear a voice tone that goes with this emotion. What impact would this have? Is that what you want? When we take the recipient position, we can begin to think about the effect our emotions have on other people, and then consider the impact we want to have.

3. *Maintaining intention.* Is the way you are intending to express your emotions in tune with your compassionate motivation? Remember, our intention is not to carelessly or purposely cause harm, but rather, use wisdom and a commitment to ourselves to do what we can to convey our feelings in a way that might be more helpful for ourselves and others.

4. *Be sensitive to the flow and interaction.* This means being clear about what your emotion is about, rather than just expressing the emotion itself. So, if it's anger that you're expressing, consider what it is that has made you angry, and how you don't lose this 'reason' by only focusing on telling the person how angry you are!

It's also important to listen and pay attention to feedback that you get as you're expressing your emotions. For example, sometimes we can become so caught up with expressing an emotion that we are no longer aware that the other person has responded appropriately, so we carry on regardless. The classic example here is in expressing anger; the other person recognises they've upset you and starts apologising, but rather than you being able to shift gears and respond to the apology, you're not listening and just want to carry on attacking them. Sometimes this can play out so much that the other person goes from being apologetic to getting angry themselves at you!

Step 3. Working with setbacks

Over time, and with ongoing practice, it's likely you'll find expressing your emotions a little easier. Of course, as with many things, it takes time and practice to develop emotional expression skills, and there will be setbacks, times when you find it harder to express your feelings, and particular emotions might remain tricky to communicate, especially with certain people. Your compassionate self can help you learn from and manage these difficulties, in a way that will help you to continue expressing your feelings.

You may also notice that some of the problems in expressing emotion are less to do with your way of communicating, and more to do with the recipient of your emotional expression. Sometimes the person you express your emotion to may be unprepared for this change (i.e. you becoming more assertive and emotionally expressive) and, for a variety of reasons, may not like and may resist this change. Being compassionate here would involve recognising that, if others have not experienced us expressing emotion before, they may feel confused or threatened, and it may take a while for them to adjust. If this is the case, use your compassionate self to bring validation and understanding to the other person's reaction – how it makes sense that this change might be difficult for them. You may even be able to bring this to their attention. It's important, although understandable, not to be discouraged by this initial response, and to remember that those people who care about us eventually adjust to such changes, and our relationships often deepen as a result of these.

Emotional expression – learning to be assertive

In some ways, the skills that we've been practising here can be seen as a type of assertiveness training – learning how to voice our emotions and feelings more confidently. But we can extend this further. It's fair to say that most of us have had a moment when we've really wanted to ask for something or express an opinion, or stand up to someone, but rather than doing this we've kept silent with our mouth firmly shut! For other people, the problem is saying 'yes' too often, and having to do things that they're not interested in or bothered about (or that actually cause quite a lot of stress). When we're assertive, we find ways to put words to our needs and feelings that may not be being met, and find our way to express ourselves in a manner that could be beneficial to us, and if possible, the person we're communicating with.

While this all sounds great, understandably, many of us find assertiveness difficult. For some people, rather than expressing their views, needs and wishes assertively, they respond in a passive or submissive way. Here, anxiety or shame grip so strongly that their needs or values are squashed. Some struggle with the other extreme of expression, and communicate aggressively, making angry demands, blaming, and even threatening other people. You may have heard of the phrase *passive aggression*, and this describes when you feel angry with someone, but are unable to tell them, and so 'show' this (maybe unintentionally) through your words, voice tone, facial expression or actions.

In each of these situations, it can be difficult to put a direct voice to your feelings, emotions, beliefs or needs in a way that can be heard by the other person. There can be a number of steps that can help you to practice being assertive:

a) Identifying situations where you struggle to be assertive

Take some time to consider the things you find difficult to be assertive about. Maybe this is linked to sharing your feelings with someone, expressing your preferences or needs, or asking for what you want. Perhaps you find it difficult to ask other people to do things for you (e.g. a 'favour'), or to stick up for your perspective or opinion (e.g. with a boss, colleague or friend). Make a few notes on a piece of paper about this.

b) Hold in mind what might be blocking assertiveness

If you find assertiveness difficult, it can be useful to think about why this might be the case. Take a few minutes to reflect on this – what stops you being more assertive than you are at the moment? Maybe there's a fear about what might happen if you start behaving more assertively? Perhaps there is a concern about how others may respond to you (i.e. angrily or critically) if you start being more assertive?

c) Compassion for our struggles with being assertive

Take a moment to get back in the shoes of your compassionate self (or connect with your compassionate other), and the sense of wisdom, strength and commitment. From this part of you, how might you bring compassion to the struggle to be assertive? Are there emotions – such as anxiety or shame – that are making this tough? How could your compassionate self validate, have empathy for, or be supportive towards this difficulty you're having?

d) Developing the language of assertiveness

Before we 'be' more assertive, it can be helpful to plan what we might say, just like an actor practising lines before going on stage. There are different ways to do this, but as ever, it's helpful to do this from your compassionate self. So, take a minute or two to connect with your wisdom, strength and commitment and when you're ready, consider what this part of you would like to say to the other person assertively. It can be useful to follow the below prompts:

- What do you need (what needs or feelings would you like to express)? Try starting this with 'I would like . . .', 'I need . . .', 'I feel . . .', or 'I think . . .'

- Why is this important for you? ('This is important for me because . . .')

- What would you like the person to do (e.g. actions you would like them to take; how they could behave in a different way to you)? This might start with 'I would like you to . . .'

e) Being assertive – using the compassionate self

It's useful now to put this assertive version of you into action. It might be helpful to play this through in mental imagery – imagining how you would approach the person, how you would stand and speak, what your voice tone and pace of speaking would be like in this assertive version. After that, it's useful to start planning for when you're going to engage in this conversation in 'real life'. To do this, take some time to consider when you'll next get a good opportunity to be this more assertive version of yourself. If there isn't a natural opportunity coming up, then it can be useful to manufacture one yourself.

Throughout this process – and more generally using the compassionate self to help explore and engage in difficult emotions – it's sometimes helpful to hold an image or metaphor in mind. For example, some people find it useful to see the compassionate self as similar to elastic – it can allow movement into difficult, scary emotions like anger, but provide a 'home' (a connection and link) to something grounded and solid so that we don't become untethered.

Key reflections

Step 5 of the emotion regulation model focuses on *coping with and expressing emotions*. In this subchapter, we have developed insights and skills linked to how:

- There can be many reasons why expressing emotions can be difficult, and it can be helpful to bring empathy and compassion to these blocks

- Emotions – and their expression – have evolved to serve important functions, and can communicate useful information to other people about how you are, and what you need

- We can learn to express emotions with the help of our compassionate mind

- It can take time for other people to get used to our expressing emotions, so learning to deal with setbacks and difficulties is important

- We can practise being assertive, and use this as a way of getting our feelings, emotions, needs and wants heard

To continue developing your emotion regulation skills, it's important to explore the complexity of how emotions show up in our lives. Take the following situation as an example: you're in a meeting with your boss, someone who you find to be unpredictable and, at times, very critical and denigrating. Also at the meeting are two more senior colleagues, as well as a range of more junior members of staff, including three people who you directly manage. During the meeting, your boss draws attention to a project that you're leading on at the moment. You and the other people working on it have felt that he has been making unreasonable time demands, and, personally, you feel that he has also made unprofessional comments about your management of the project in front of colleagues. As your boss starts to talk about the project and asks you to give feedback on its progress you respond quite angrily, telling him, in no uncertain terms, how hard everyone has been working on the project, and that his demanding approach is not helping any of you. As you finish speaking, still feeling angry, you notice the somewhat shocked facial expressions of some colleagues who are not part of your project. Quickly you shift into an anxious feeling, followed by a gnawing sense of shame and self-criticism, berating yourself for having spoken in the way you did. Your boss then gets very angry, telling you to 'Stop making excuses and do the job you're paid to do,' and as the meeting ends, you walk out of the room feeling anxious, low in mood and ashamed. You go back to your desk and check your emails when a junior colleague approaches and tells you they thought you had been mistreated and should have stood up for yourself and the project more. Upon hearing this, you're then triggered back into anger at your boss for the way he spoke to you, but also anger towards your junior colleague for 'telling' you what you should have done. You take yourself to the toilet, shut yourself in a cubicle, and find yourself feeling low, tearful and like you're 'not up to it'.

Having read over the above scenario, how do you feel? Can you imagine going through this emotional roller coaster? Maybe you've had experiences like this one before (I certainly have), and can recognise the shifting sands of our emotional worlds, and how these can create a lot of distress, confusion and difficulties for us. Some key compassionate insights emerge from this example:

- We can experience multiple emotions within a very short period (or even at the same time)

- Our minds can naturally shift between emotions, but this can be a confusing (and distressing) experience for us

- One emotion can sometimes make it more likely to experience another emotion

- One emotion can block out another emotion, or move us towards a different direction (behaviour), leading to an experience of internal conflict

What might help?

As we have done all the way through this book, the starting point in answering this question is a type of 'not your fault' insight – that is, an appreciation of how and why something happens, without self-blame and self-berating. We call this the psychology of *'no shame and no blame'*. But of course, this is just the starting point. It's also important to learn how to manage such multiple, and often conflicting, emotions, and 'see the wood for the trees'. To help to do this, of course, we turn to our compassionate mind for support.

One way that we can do this is to view our minds as many rather than one, as multi rather than singular. What I mean by this is that, while we often have a sense that we have one 'core' or 'central' self that reacts consistently to situations in the world, it may be more accurate to say we have many different selves, or parts of us, that have quite different ways of see-ing and responding to the same situation. Now, these parts can operate at many levels. For example, they could be on the level of motives (e.g. the caregiving part of you; the care-receiving part of you; the competitive part of you) or behaviours (e.g. the part of you that wants to fight, run away or submit). But for the purposes of this chapter, we are going to look at how different emotional parts may react differently to the same situation.

One of the challenges that many of us face is being able to experience the different parts of us in a flexible, comfortable and helpful way. Often, given a situation that is tricky in some way, different parts of us can be present and respond at the same time. While some people may be aware of, and able to experience and express their different emotional parts as they happen, some of us can become stuck in just one 'self' (e.g. angry or anxious). Moreover, as the different selves often have conflicting urges and needs in response to a situation, the experience of them all being present at once can be rather unsettling. Think about the mixed feelings we can have when criticised in front of other people. A part of us might feel very angry at the person who is doing this, and want to hit out (verbally or phys-ically); another part might feel anxious and want to run away or avoid being 'seen'; while another part might feel sad and hurt, and want to cry. All of these experiences and responses can ripple through us very quickly, and potentially leave us feeling confused, out of control or overwhelmed.

In this chapter, we are going to help you explore three different 'selves', linked to three of our key emotions: anger, anxiety and sadness. We will do this through an exercise called 'multiple selves', in which we will explore these ideas experientially, helping you to learn more about the different parts of you. For this exercise, we are going to use the example of an argument. After trying this, you might want to use a differ-ent example, such as something you feel you've failed at, a setback in life, or a situation in a relationship that you're struggling with. I will guide you through the exercise and illustrate with an example using Simon's experience. Here is a bit of background about Simon.

> *Simon is a thirty-eight-year-old man who came to therapy for*
> *help with managing his anger. He described always having had*

difficulties with anger, and recently he had a falling out with his friend Tony. What started off as a debate about who had the most stressful job, soon turned into an argument about who had achieved more in their career. Simon described getting so 'mad' at Tony that the manager in the restaurant had come over to ask them to leave, as they were disturbing other diners.

As a child, Simon described how he struggled to live up to the expectations of his parents and keep up with the grades that his friends achieved at school. Simon also described periods of being bullied as a teenager and feeling that he wasn't good enough.

Exercise: Multiple selves

To start this exercise, bring to mind an argument or disagreement you had with someone that you care about. Spend a minute or so doing this, remembering what the argument was about, where you were, and who you were arguing with. When you have brought this experience to mind, see if you can move on to the next steps.

Step 1: Listening to the angry part of you

See if you can bring to mind the part of you that feels angry about this argument. Allow yourself time to feel this part of yourself, letting go of any other emotions or feelings you might have about what happened. When you feel connected to your angry part, go through the following steps, making a quick note at each step (e.g. by using Worksheet 2, p. 305).

Thoughts: What thoughts does your angry part have about the argument? What words or phrases come to mind? If it could speak, what would your angry part say about what happened, or what the other person did?

Simon's answer – 'How dare he even start on this? Who does he think he is? He needs to be quiet and be more respectful.'

Body: Try to notice where in your body you can feel your angry part. And if this feeling were to grow and get stronger, where would it move to in your body?

Simon's answer – 'I notice tightness in my stomach, jaw and arms. If the feeling gets stronger, I think my head would explode.'

Behaviour: If this angry part was in complete control, what would it want to do, given this situation? (For example, shout, complain, hit or smash something.)

Simon's answer – 'I would want to grab him by the throat and shake him until he shuts up.'

Memories: Holding in mind your angry part, what memories come to mind?

Simon's answer – 'I remember feeling angry like this when the guys in my class used to laugh at my answers back at school.'

Outcome/needs: What would help your angry part to settle? What does it need? What would it see as a good outcome to the argument?

Simon's answer – 'It needs an apology from Tom for what he said. It needs him to admit that I'm right.'

Once you've got 'into the skin' of your angry part, and completed the above, see if you can gently let it go, slowly allowing this part of you to ease away. Sometimes people find it helpful to validate it for showing up, by saying: 'Thank you, angry self, for explaining your point of view

– that was helpful.' Take a few slow breaths, feeling your way back into a grounded, calm position. Stand up, stretch or move about, if this helps to 'shake off' your angry self.

Step 2: Listening to the anxious part of you

Now we are going to tune in to your anxious self, the part of you that felt (or feels) anxious about the argument or about the potential consequences of the argument. Allow yourself enough time to feel this part of yourself. When you feel connected to your anxious part, take some time to think about the following questions, making a few notes at each step.

Thoughts: What thoughts does your anxious part have about the argument? What words or phrases come to mind? If it could speak, what would your anxious part say about what happened, or its concerns about the consequences of the argument?

Simon's answer – 'He's never going to forgive me for shouting at him – our friendship will never be the same.'

Body: Try to notice where in your body you can feel your anxious part (what physical sensations you experience). If this anxious feeling were to grow and get stronger, where would it move to in the body?

Simon's answer – 'Tension in my stomach and increased heart rate . . . The feeling would move into my legs if it got stronger.'

Behaviour: If your anxious part was in complete control, what would it want to do in response to the situation? (For example, run away, avoid the person, disappear or hide.)

Simon's answer – 'My anxious part wants to run away and not have to deal with this. It wishes it could go back in time and never have talked about it in the first place.'

Memories: Holding in mind your anxious part, what memories come to mind?

Simon's answer – 'I remember being asked to stand up and read out an answer to a question. I was terrified and froze.'

Outcome/needs: What would help your anxious part settle? What would it need? What would it see as a good outcome from this argument?

Simon's answer – 'For this situation to be over and done with – for things to be back to the way they were before.'

Once you completed the above, see if you can gently come out of the 'skin' of your anxious part, and let this part of you ease away. Sometimes people find it helpful to validate it for showing up, by saying: 'Thank you, anxious self, for explaining your point of view – that was helpful.' Take a few slow breaths, allowing your body to slow down. Stand up and move around if that's helpful. When you feel ready, move on to step 3.

Step 3: Listening to the sad part of you

Take a moment to bring to mind the part of you that felt (or feels) sad about this argument or the potential consequences of the argument. Allow yourself time to step into the shoes of this part of yourself. When you feel connected to your sad part, go through the following questions, making a quick note after each one.

Thoughts: What thoughts does your sad part have about the argument? What words or phrases come to mind? If it could speak, what would your sad part say? What concerns does it have about the potential consequences of the argument?

Simon's answer – 'Tony's the only friend who's always been there – he won't want to be friends anymore.'

Body: Try to notice where in your body you can feel your sad part. If this feeling were to grow and get stronger, where would it move to in the body?

> Simon's answer – 'I feel a heaviness in my stomach, chest and throat. If it grew, it would just get heavier.'

Behaviour: If your sad part was in control, what would it want to do in response to the situation?

> Simon's answer – 'For someone to comfort me, for me to feel like I wouldn't be on my own.'

Memories: Holding in mind your sad part, what memories come to mind?

> Simon's answer – 'I just have a picture of me as a young boy, sat on my bed feeling upset and crying after disappointing my parents – I felt completely alone.'

Outcome/needs: What would help your sad part settle? What does it need? What would it see as a good outcome to this argument?

> Simon's answer – 'To stop feeling so alone – to feel connected and liked by Tony.'

Once you have completed this, see if you can gently come out of the 'skin' of your sad part, and let that ease away. Sometimes people find it helpful to validate it for showing up, by saying: 'Thank you, sad self, for explaining your point of view – that was helpful.' Take a few slow breaths, allowing your body to slow down.

Threat emotions – reflections:

- It can be helpful to reflect on what you've learned so far about the different parts of you. What did you learn about the different parts of you in response to the same situation (the argument)? Can you see they often have quite different perspectives on the same situation?

- Did you find one 'part' easier to get into, or think about than another? What do you make of that? Is that something you recognise in other aspects of your life?

- Was there an emotional part that was more difficult to connect with? What do you make of that? Is that something you recognise in other areas of your life?

A common response is to recognise that these three different parts (anger, anxiety, sadness) have very different ways of looking at, thinking and feeling about the same situation, and differ with regards to what they want, and need. They also tend to connect to separate memories. Moreover, the ways the different parts feel, and respond (and what they want) can conflict with one another, and drive you in opposite directions (e.g. to lash out angrily and run away anxiously, at the same time). This is an important reflection, as it can help us appreciate what our minds are up against, and the distress this can cause. And while this is not our fault, having this insight can motivate us to learn how to 'be' with all these different selves, and respond in ways that are helpful. We will return to this later in the chapter.

In my experience (both personally, and as a therapist), it's also common that people find one of these emotional parts easier to connect with and think from, and find (at least) one that is more difficult to connect with. If this was the case for you, this is an important insight in itself; it may help you to understand why you tend to struggle to cope in certain situations, which emotions you might get pulled into more readily, and which you might be blocked with. This can also give us a clue as to what you might need your compassionate self to help you with. For example, your compassionate self might help you to moderate, or keep in balance, the part of you that you readily get drawn into. It may also give space for, or allow, support and strengthen the parts of you that you find difficult to connect with, embody or express in a healthy way.

Tips for multiple self work

- Allow yourself time to move into each 'part' – it sometimes takes a little while to find our way 'in' to each of these emotions, and this can be difficult if we feel rushed

- Keep an eye on 'leakage'. This is when we are with one part of us (e.g. anxious self) and another part of us (e.g. angry self) 'spills in', making us feel and think differently. For example, while describing what the anxious self would like to do in an argument, you notice you have written: 'Punch the idiot in the face'. It's unlikely that an anxious part of us would respond in this aggressive and violent way, and more indicative that we are connected with our angry self instead. If this is the case, spend some time slowing down your breathing rhythm, and then a little longer to connect with the anxious part of you. This leakage is understandable if some emotional selves are easier to connect with than others, as we suggested above

- Try not to worry if you find one, or more, of these parts difficult to connect with. Most people find at least one part more difficult than others to connect with or express. If this happens, take a little longer to try to shift into that self. Try to imagine, if that part (angry, anxious, sad) was present, what it would say, and how it would react in the argument

- Try not to get caught up in whether you did or didn't feel that emotion during the argument. This exercise is about exploring 'as if' scenarios, helping you to learn about your emotions (what each one thinks, wants to do and so forth), and recognising how these different parts of you can get caught up in conflicts that add to your struggles

- Don't feel restricted to just these parts. You may want to do this exercise, but have other parts present, such as shame, guilt, jealousy, competitiveness, pride or caring.

WORKSHEET 2: MULTIPLE EMOTIONAL SELVES

Angry self	Sad self
Thoughts Body Behaviour Memory Outcome	Thoughts Body Behaviour Memory Outcome
Anxious self	**Compassionate self**
Thoughts Body Behaviour Memory Outcome	Thoughts Body Behaviour Memory Outcome

Step 4: How do the different parts relate to each other? Emotions about emotions

As we have discussed throughout the book, sometimes we can struggle with certain emotions because we have other emotions about them. *Emotions about emotions* is a common block to helpful emotion regulation. To help you to look at this, and to deepen your understanding of our different 'selves', the next step in this exercise involves reflecting on how each of the three emotional 'selves' thinks and feels about the others. This step might feel a little strange, but in our experience, it adds to a deeper understanding of why we can struggle in, or feel blocked to, experiencing and expressing certain emotions.

Take a look back on what you've written for your angry, anxious and sad part (Worksheet 2, p. 305). Familiarise yourself again with how each part sees and feels about the argument, and their general outlook. Then see if you can answer the following questions:

- How does the angry part think and feel about the anxious part?

- How does the anxious part think and feel about the angry part?

- How does the angry part think and feel about the sad part?

- How does the sad part think and feel about the angry part?

- How does the anxious part think and feel about the sad part?

- How does the sad part think and feel about the anxious part?

So, what was that like? What have you learned about the interrelations between these different parts of you? One common reflection is that these parts of us don't always get on very well, or sit alongside each other comfortably. This is in part because they have *different patterns to them* – they evolved to orientate our minds and bodies (e.g. the way we think, act and so on) to do different things. In fact, sometimes their patterns seem to compete or conflict with each other. For example, while anger often wants us to challenge or approach someone, anxiety is urging us to move away or avoid them. While this is understandable, it might become tricky for us if one particular part is more easily triggered, or more experienced than another, and keeps wanting to run the show! We can also consider why or how some emotional reactions (or selves) are blocked, inhibited or absent. For example, as discussed in Chapter 4, we may have learned (consciously or non-consciously) that it is safer to be angry than sad. Or notice that we feel anxious about expressing anger, which in turn blocks us from healthy access to assertiveness and getting our needs met. But what can we do when we notice we are struggling with our emotions in this way? Well, it might be helpful to connect with a part of us that can allow, listen to and help all the different selves, and mediate between them. This, of course, would be *our compassionate self.*

Step 5: Bringing compassion to the party

It is important at this stage to try to engage with our compassionate self to bring a different, more helpful perspective to this situation. In these next sections, we are going to see how your compassionate self may bring a perspective to the situation as a whole, but also in working with the different 'parts' (anger, anxiety, sadness) that we looked at earlier.

As we have seen, depending on which part of us is viewing a situation, we are likely to think, feel and want to behave in quite different ways. Knowing this, if we engage our compassionate self, we are likely to approach the same situation with qualities of caring-commitment, wisdom, and strength, and a more balanced perspective, and respond to this in a way that is kinder, wiser and more courageous. To help you see this, have a go at the following exercise.

Exercise: Bringing compassion to the situation

For a minute or two, bring back to mind the argument that you've been using in this chapter. Now, take a few moments to engage in the five steps of practice preparation (p. 115). Engage in your soothing rhythm breathing and friendly facial expression. Allow your breathing to slow, and gently rest your attention in the flow of breathing in, and breathing out. Bring to mind the qualities of your compassionate self – wisdom, strength and caring-commitment. When you feel ready, go through the following steps, answering from the perspective of your compassionate self.

Thoughts/understanding: What thoughts does my compassionate self have about the argument? What understanding or wisdom does it have about what happened, and why it happened?

Body: Where in my body do I feel the strength, caring-commitment and wisdom of my compassionate self?

Behaviour: If my compassionate self was in control, what would it want to do in this situation (e.g. find a way to discuss the issue, rather than argue; help repair any damage caused; find a way to be assertive)?

Memories: Holding in mind your compassionate self, what memories come to mind (e.g. times when you may have acted with or experienced the qualities of compassion in a difficult situation or conflict – or times when you've seen other people act in a compassionate way)?

Outcome: As your compassionate self, what would you see as a good outcome for this argument?

What was it like seeing the argument from the compassionate self's perspective? Did you notice any differences in comparison to the other parts (angry, anxious, sad)? It's often at this step that people get quite a different view of the argument. It's your compassionate self that is able to pull together various aspects of the healthy emotion regulation (the right-hand side of the model in Figure 10, p. 176) in this difficult situation. It is able to have ideas about what led to the argument, can notice different emotions as they turn up inside you, put words to describe those feelings, and validate and understand them. But it can also find a way of regulating them in a way that may be helpful for you and other people.

But we can also take the emotion regulation process further here by looking at how your compassionate mind can help with each of the other 'parts' that we've explored in this chapter.

Compassion for the angry part of me

In Chapter 3 we saw that anger can be a protective feeling, but sometimes can mask feelings of sadness, vulnerability or loneliness. We all experience moments of anger, and it can be helpful if we can find a way to understand and guide this part of us.

Exercise: Compassion for your angry self

For a minute or two, bring back to mind the argument that you've been using in this chapter. Find a comfortable, upright and confident posture in your chair, and spend some time connecting with the soothing rhythm of your breathing. When you feel ready, bring to mind some of the qualities of your compassionate self (caring-commitment, strength, wisdom). When you feel connected with this part of you, bring to mind the angry part of you in the argument above:

- What does your compassionate self understand about your angry part's reaction?

- Given this understanding, what does your compassionate self want to say to the angry part of you? How can it show the angry part validation or empathy?

- What would your compassionate self suggest as helpful for the angry part, given the argument?

- Is there something that it (the compassionate self) would like to do to help the angry self?

Simon's answer: 'It's understandable that you were angry about the argument. It felt like Tony was belittling and dismissing you, and you wanted to stick up for yourself. This unfairness reminds you of the experiences you had at school, and your desire never to feel vulnerable like that again. However, looking back on what he said, he was being a bit "tongue in cheek", and he does like to wind you up. Yes, he ended up saying a few harsh things, but you'd both had a bit to drink by that stage. How about we try to come up with a few ideas of how we could respond to this in a way that is assertive, letting him know why what he said was unfair, but doing this in a way that is grounded and strong, rather than shouting and swearing?'

Compassion for the anxious part of me

In this next exercise, we want to turn the focus of your compassionate mind to the anxious self in the argument. Just as with anger, in Chapter 3 we learned that anxiety evolved to help us pay attention to potential threats, and motivate us to move away or flee as a way of keeping us safe. Let's see if you can use your compassionate self to understand and guide your anxious self in this situation.

Exercise: Compassion for your anxious self

For a minute or two, bring back to mind the argument that you've been using in this chapter. Find a comfortable, upright and confident posture

in your chair. Engage in your soothing rhythm breathing, and slowly connect with the qualities of your compassionate self – caring-commitment, wisdom and strength. When you feel connected to this part of you, read through the questions, making a few notes as you go.

- What does your compassionate self understand about the reactions of the anxious part in response to the argument?

- Given this understanding, what does your compassionate self want to say to the anxious part of you? How could it validate or empathise with it?

- Given its wisdom and caring-commitment, what would the compassionate self want to do for your anxious part?

- How would it like to help or support your anxious part?

Simon's answer – 'I can see why you feel like this; Tony's been your closest friend for twenty years, and it's scary to think that this argument might have a lasting negative effect on your friendship. I also know that anxiety is a tricky emotion for you as it reminds you of all those times at school when you were being bullied. Although it's a scary feeling, I'm here to help out with this; together we can tolerate this feeling and fear – I'll support you through it so we can find a way to patch things up with Tony.'

Compassion for the sad part of me

Sadness can play an important role in signalling distress, often related to the experience of loss, and the need for connection and support.

However, for some of us, sadness may not have been met with care or support from others, and feeling sad can be very difficult. Let's see what your compassionate self can do to understand and support your sad part.

Exercise: Compassion for your sad self

For a minute or two, bring back to mind the argument that you've been using in this chapter. Find a comfortable, upright and confident posture in your chair. Engage in your soothing rhythm breathing, and begin to connect with the attributes of your ideal compassionate self – caring-commitment, wisdom and strength. When you feel ready, from the perspective of your compassionate self, consider the following questions:

- What does your compassionate self understand about the reactions of the sad part in response to the argument?

- Given this understanding, what does your compassionate self want to say to the sad part of you? How would it validate or empathise with it?

- Given its wisdom and caring-commitment, what would the compassionate self want to do for your sad part?

- How would it like to help or support your sad part?

Simon's answer – 'It's really understandable that you're concerned about how this might change your friendship with Tony – you've been great mates for a long time now, almost half your life. It's OK to feel sad about this. I know this isn't an emotion you find easy, and was definitely one that you had to keep hidden when you were growing up, and especially at school. Try to remember that you and Tony have been through a lot together – successes and failures, relationship break-ups, laughter, and tears. It's OK to feel sad about the argument – it shows that it, and your friendship, are important and meaningful to you. I'm here to support you with this.'

See if you can continue to practise this exercise in your day-to-day life. You may choose to use arguments as examples to explore your different emotional parts, but our different selves show up rather commonly in many situations in life, such as:

- Making difficult decisions, when one part of us can feel one thing, and another part another

- An important event, e.g. going to an interview

- A difficult encounter with someone, towards whom we feel ambivalent due to previous experiences

- Disappointments, for example, in relationships, after a setback or failure, or losing something (or someone) that's important to us

Remember when we are learning a new skill, we need to build ourselves up gradually as it can take a while to approach our life in this way. As we have said before, we would not learn to swim in the deep end of the pool, or have our first driving lesson on the busiest motorway.

Key reflections

- We often have multiple emotional reactions to the same situation

- Our emotional selves or parts often turn up with different patterns – they see and react to the same thing with different ideas, thoughts, and urges of how to respond

- We may experience certain emotions as more dominant, and others as difficult to tolerate or experience

- Our compassionate self can help to bring a different, broader and wiser perspective to our life

- Our compassionate self can help to moderate our various emotions, supporting them to have a voice but not run the show

One of the difficulties that many of us face when coping with emotions, is when other emotions turn up about these emotions. The experience of 'emotions about emotions' – sometimes referred to as primary (the initial emotion) and secondary (an emotional reaction about or towards the primary emotion) – can prevent us from effectively regulating our experiences. In fact, we just explored some of these common patterns in Chapter 16d (e.g. anger about anxiety; anxiety about anger), and also go into more detail about them in the online material that you can find at https://overcoming.co.uk/715/resources-to-download, which focuses specifically on emotions that we experience too 'much' or 'little' of. However, in this final section of Chapter 16, we're going to focus on how shame and self-criticism can have a potent, negative impact upon other emotions that we find difficult to manage, and how our compassionate minds can help us to navigate this.

We've all experienced shame at some time in life. Feeling bad about things that we've done in the past, concerns about other people's criticism and judgement of us, feeling that we're a failure or inadequate in some way, or that there's something about us (e.g. a personality trait or something about our physical appearance) that is flawed, lacking or defective. Although it's part of the human condition, for many of us, shame is a deeply unpleasant experience.

Shame is definitely an experience that I'm familiar with – at various times of life shame has felt like one of those personal rain clouds you see someone being followed by in a cartoon! I've experienced shame about my actions, lack of actions, my personality, my appearance, my body . . . well, as you can see, lots of things! As part of these experiences, a common companion of shame has been self-criticism. And like a vine, when self-criticism wraps itself around shame, this tightens the experience in such a way that we can feel constricted and overwhelmed.

So, in this chapter, we're going to look at how shame and self-criticism can have a powerful, negative influence on our capacity to regulate our emotions, and how they can cause and maintain emotional difficulties. We'll then look at how the compassion-based emotion regulation skills you've been acquiring throughout this book, will help you to work with these experiences in a wise and helpful way.

What is shame?

Shame is best described as a multifaceted, social or self-conscious experience. The etymology (or origin) of the word 'shame' is thought to be related to a much older word that meant 'to cover'. This makes intrinsic sense, as it described a common urge many of us have when we feel ashamed. Take a moment to think about this. When you've felt ashamed about something, what was the urge in your body? What did you want to do? A common response is to hide, become smaller, or want to disappear or 'cover up', and conceal the very thing we feel ashamed about.

But it's important here to consider 'what' it is that shame is trying to make us cover up, what it's trying to make us hide. Shame is linked to a type of *social threat*, with a sense that others (real or imagined) will reject, criticise, devalue or see us as inferior or worthless in some way. The thing that we feel they will do this for – that is, something we've done, something about us (e.g. our personality, appearance), or our desires or urges – can vary hugely, but it's the fear of the self as being damaged and held negatively in the mind by others that is crucial in shame.

Sometimes we experience shame in the context of disappointments and feeling not good enough. So, this is not so much that we haven't lived up to our standards, but that we've become an *undesired* or *undesirable self*, both in the eyes of others, but also in how we feel about ourselves. In fact, one research study found when describing shame, research participants linked it to who they didn't want to be – like an *anti-ideal*. They described feeling 'I'm fat and ugly', rather than 'I failed to be thin and pretty' (Lindsay-Hartz et al., 1995). At other times, shame is linked to the disappointment gap, when we feel that our actual self is in close proximity to or similar to our undesired self (hence the sense of shame), but distant – a big 'gap' – to our ideal sense of self.

Why do we experience shame?

While higher levels are associated with emotion regulation problems and mental health distress, in itself, shame isn't 'bad' and may serve important protective functions (Gilbert, 1998, 2010; Jacquet, 2016). We can look at this by initially considering what life would be like if we had *no* shame. Take a moment to think about a *shameless person*; someone with a complete inability to experience shame. Would you like to be close friends with this person? How might this person relate to other people? How might they treat people? What would they be willing to do – or not do for that matter?

Although they might be fun at a party or a night out in a bar or club, the idea of being emotionally close to a shameless person isn't very attractive for most people. Many people get a sense that this type of person could do pretty much anything – be rude, hurt people, take advantage of others – without *caring*. So as far as we know, shame evolved to signal our threat system, urging it to pay attention to important social cues, particularly those related to *social exclusion* (e.g. rejection, ostracism, discrimination), and concerns that we have created negative emotions, thoughts and intentions in other people's minds towards us. It helps us to track how we are living in the minds of other people and may arise when we are approaching or have crossed a line representing social rules, norms or behaviours. It's thought that there is a good evolutionary reason for this. Many thousands of years ago, our ancestors lived in harsh environments where food was scarce, the elements were harsh, and survival was linked directly to living within a group. Being part of the group meant that you looked after and protected others, but were also looked after and protected yourself; you shared food, shelter and responsibility.

However, imagine that within this context you did something that broke the rules or damaged the group in some way – maybe you ate all the food one night after having a few too many drinks (or whatever intoxicant they had access to), stole resources from or badly hurt another group member. Let's imagine that you were caught doing this, and given the severity of your behaviour, you were ejected from the group, having to fend for yourself. Unfortunately, it's unlikely you would have survived for long.

Given this, it seems that shame helps to facilitate group living, to help us monitor our actions and their impact on others, and is tied intrinsically to helping us to avoid rejection, segregation, and ultimately death. If you think about a time you've felt ashamed, and then consider what other people would have thought or felt about you given the thing you felt ashamed about, it's likely you have a sense that their minds were full of judgements, criticism or a desire to want not to be close to you. If shame is experienced over a relatively short time period, and as a passing 'state' (i.e. appropriately in response to circumstances/the environment), and arises at a level that isn't too strong, it may have a useful impact on shaping pro-social behaviour and repairing the 'damaged' sense of self (de Hooge et al., 2013). Unfortunately, when it is more 'trait' like, and is frequently activated, long-lasting and intense, shame can be a terror for the human mind – creating 'loops in the mind' (Chapter 3) and come with a sense of feeling inferior, 'bad', flawed or defective, and alongside this, a sense of being separate, isolated and alone.

The shape of shame

When looking at the experience of shame, it's often helpful to hold in mind the different patterns or shapes that it can come in. As a multifaceted experience, shame includes:

- *An externally focused component, often described as external shame –* here we have a sense of living in the mind of others *negatively,* that they will be judging us, holding negative feelings towards us (e.g. anger, disgust, disappointment), and we have concerns that they will treat us in certain ways (e.g. rejection, criticism)

- *An internally focused component, known as internal shame,* which gives rise to a sense that we're flawed, inadequate, inferior, bad or a failure – that we've become an anti-ideal

- *An emotional component* – here, shame can recruit different threat emotions (e.g. anger, anxiety, contempt, disgust) towards ourselves or others. In this sense, it's difficult to describe shame as an emotion in itself, as it can recruit different threat emotions to its cause. For example, sometimes shame emerges loaded heavily with anxiety, whereas at other times it brings a form of internalised anger, hostility or even disgust. And at other times again, rather than internalising and becoming self-critical, shame comes instead with externalisation, linked closely to anger outwards. As we will see later, internal shame has important overlaps with self-criticism

- *A behavioural or action component* – often this takes the form of wanting to hide, conceal, not be seen (withdraw) or respond submissively or in a placatory way to others. The phrase 'hang your head in shame' gives an indication of how this can affect your body posture. We may also try to strive harder in life, trying to achieve and move away from these feelings of shame and inferiority (Gilbert et al., 2007). However, some forms of shame (referred to in CFT as humiliation; Gilbert, 1997) lead to a desire to get back at, retaliate or punish those that are shaming us

- *A physiological component* – shame triggers the threat system and has been associated with stress hormones and immunological reaction (Dickerson et al., 2004), and changes in the balance between the sympathetic and parasympathetic nervous systems

What impact does shame have on other emotions?

Shame is often described as one of the most painful emotions, and higher levels of shame have been associated with depression (Kim et al., 2011), anxiety (Diana-Mirela & Aurora, 2018), PTSD (e.g. Cunningham et al., 2018), eating disorders (e.g. Duarte et al., 2016) and psychosis (Wood & Irons, 2016). Various research studies have found that shame is associated with emotion regulation problems, such as difficulties with emotional clarity and impulsivity, non-acceptance of emotion and poor access to emotion regulation strategies (Gupta et al., 2008; Zarei et al., 2018), experiential avoidance (Carvalho et al., 2015), emotion suppression (Velotti et al., 2017) and rumination (Cheung et al., 2004; Orth et al., 2006).

It's also helpful to hold in mind that we can experience shame about other emotions. Growing up, although I felt comfortable with sadness, I used to experience shame about expressing fear and anger. It can be helpful at this stage to consider if you feel ashamed about any of your emotions. This might be emotions like anger, anxiety or sadness, but also positive emotions like excitement, joy or contentment. Is there an emotion that you feel most ashamed about? Given the ideas we discussed in Chapter 4, you might have some understanding about why this is, and what events led to you feeling this way.

While it's not our fault that we can experience this, given the nature of shame and how it can often make us want to conceal and hide, you might begin to see that experiencing shame about other emotions and feelings is likely to cause us difficulties in experiencing and expressing those other emotions in a helpful way.

Shame can disconnect us

One way that shame contributes to emotional difficulties is through how it blocks our access to care and social safeness. As shame is linked to fears of being undesirable or damaged in the minds of others, and therefore, to rejection and social exclusion, it can have a potent impact on not only triggering our threat systems, but also blocking us from the soothing and distress-regulating care of other people (or, from a CFT point of view, care from ourselves). If you bring to mind something about yourself that you feel ashamed about (e.g. part of your body, something about your character or maybe a previous behaviour or thing you've done), you might notice that rather than being able to hold friends and family members as potential sources of safeness, care and soothing, they instead become objects of the threat system. Moreover, if you tune in to your own inner voice with this shameful thing in mind, it's likely you'll get a similar response from inside your mind – little compassion, empathy or care, and instead, self-criticism and blame.

There has been lots of research looking at the psychological impact of perceptions (real or imagined) of rejection and exclusion. We know that people who are rejected (compared to those who are accepted) feel worse, which seems to be a combination of reduced positive emotions and increased negative feelings (Blackhart et al., 2009). Some scientists have found the pain of rejection is so unpleasant for humans partly because it runs off the same physiological structures as actual physical pain (Eisenberger et al., 2006). We know that our minds are highly sensitive to signals of rejection. This remains the case even when we're told that rejection was staged, when it was programmed to happen (e.g. in a computer simulation of being rejected in a game; e.g. Zadro et al., 2004), or when the rejection occurred from people who belong to an outgroup that we despise (e.g. a racist, far-right political party; Fayant et al., 2014).

As we learned in Chapter 4, we are all shaped by our experiences in life, and so it might not be surprising to learn that early life experiences that include high levels of rejection are associated with greater shame sensitivity as adults (e.g. Gilbert et al., 2003). We also know that generally, increased shame scores in adulthood are associated with a variety of threat-based early parental experiences (e.g. overprotection, feeling threatened and subordinated; Gilbert et al., 2003), as well as a lack of memories of our parents responding to us in a warm, caring way associated with the soothing system (Matos et al., 2013; Ferreira et al., 2018).

Some of the people I work with as a psychologist have experienced rejection and criticism when they've expressed their emotions as children. Given that the threat system evolved to protect us and keep us safe, it's understandable that we may become more sensitive to our emotions – and emotional expression – as adults. As we have done throughout this book and will come on to below, it's useful to hold these insights gently in our minds; that is, if we are struggling with shame today, we may recognise that this has been shaped by our experiences in life, and that it's 'not our fault'.

Compassion – an antidote for shame?

Given that shame is linked to the threat system, and commonly blocks our connection to others and our self (the soothing system), it's likely that compassion can play a helpful role in down-regulating this experience. In fact, there's a growing research base showing exactly this – that developing greater self-compassion is associated with reductions in shame and self-criticism (Kirby, 2017). There are a number of steps we'll explore in this chapter, and we'll use the example of Tina to help with this.

When Tina first came to therapy, she sat in the chair in a way that seemed like she occupied the least space possible, and when she spoke, I had to strain to hear what she was saying. It took a few sessions for her to begin to feel more at ease, but as she did, she started to put words to deep feelings of shame. Shame about her appearance, shame about her lack of children, for her lack of a partner. She voiced feelings that she was boring and inadequate, and that her friends merely tolerated her as they were 'nice' people. Moreover, if they really knew how flawed she was, they wouldn't want to know her.

Step 1: Emotion regulation model

It's useful to check in first with the emotion regulation model that we introduced in Section Four, and is reprinted overleaf. Holding your difficulties with shame in mind, which step of the emotion regulation model might you be struggling with when it comes to managing and regulating shame?

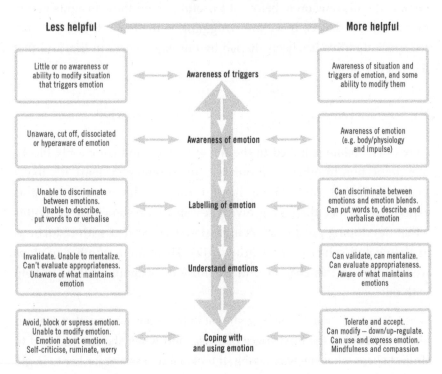

Emotion Regulation Model (ERM)

Less helpful ← → **More helpful**

Less helpful		More helpful
Little or no awareness or ability to modify situation that triggers emotion	**Awareness of triggers**	Awareness of situation and triggers of emotion, and some ability to modify them
Unaware, cut off, dissociated or hyperaware of emotion	**Awareness of emotion**	Awareness of emotion (e.g. body/physiology and impulse)
Unable to discriminate between emotions. Unable to describe, put words to or verbalise	**Labelling of emotion**	Can discriminate between emotions and emotion blends. Can put words to, describe and verbalise emotion
Invalidate. Unable to mentalize. Can't evaluate appropriateness. Unaware of what maintains emotion	**Understand emotions**	Can validate, can mentalize. Can evaluate appropriateness. Aware of what maintains emotions
Avoid, block or supress emotion. Unable to modify emotion. Emotion about emotion. Self-criticise, ruminate, worry	**Coping with and using emotion**	Tolerate and accept. Can modify – down/up-regulate. Can use and express emotion. Mindfulness and compassion

When Tina looked at this model, she recognised that her difficulties in regulating shame loaded mostly on to the bottom two steps of the emotion regulation model. She described finding it very difficult to understand and bring empathy to herself, and instead described a typically invalidating approach to her feelings of shame. Alongside this, she felt unable to cope with feelings of shame when they arose inside her and instead invested time and energy in trying to suppress, avoid, and stay away from shame. Moreover, Tina also realised that she was terrified of her shame, and that self-criticism and rumination tended to fuel this difficult feeling.

Holding shame in mind, once you've identified which step(s) of the emotion regulation model you find most difficult, turn to the relevant chapter(s) in Section Four that link to that step of the model. Take some time to read through the appropriate chapter(s), holding shame in mind as the emotion you'll be working on. Don't rush this; take your time building your skills and ability to regulate specific aspects of shame.

Alongside this, it can be helpful to turn towards shame in a particular way. Let's look at this together in the following steps.

Step 2: Turning towards shame – learning its shape and texture

As we move further into working with shame, it's helpful for us to work with a particular shame experience. It might be helpful to start with one that's less powerful or distressing to you, and over time, work with those that are more distressing. Let's have a look at how to do this.

Bring to mind something that you feel ashamed about. This could be something about yourself – for example, your personality, your appearance or body. It could be something that's happened to you in the past (e.g. a sense of having failed at something), or maybe something that you're struggling with now, such as your performance at work. Spend a few moments allowing this to enter your mind.

With this situation or example in mind, notice what thoughts arise with this thing you feel ashamed about? If shame had a voice, what words would it be saying to you? What emotions is this feeling directing to you? What does your shame part want you to do?

Make a few notes on what you discovered in this exercise. What did you learn about shame? What role is it playing in your life? With this shame-based example in mind, it's useful to consider how compassion can help you to approach and work with this differently.

Step 3: Bringing compassion to shame

Let's try an exercise in which you can use your compassionate minds to help with your shame experience.

Exercise: Bringing compassion to shame

Spend a few minutes to connect with your compassionate self. See if you can find the posture, breathing rhythm, and facial expression that facilitates this, and connect with the qualities of wisdom, strength and commitment. When you feel ready, see if you can use your compassionate mind to turn towards the shame event, experience or sensation.

To begin with, focus on what it is like to use the strength and commitment of your compassionate self with the intention of tolerating the feeling of shame. Draw upon the image of your grounded, upright and stable body posture, soothing rhythm breathing and commitment to face things that can cause distress. Spend a minute or two doing this, holding in mind the shame feeling but doing this as the compassionate self.

When you feel ready, turn to the wisdom of your compassionate self – your understanding of how tricky our minds can be and how we have difficult and painful emotions that were designed for us, not by us. Given what we've discussed in this chapter about the nature, origin and function of shame, see if you can hold this understanding in mind. That shame evolved to help us navigate social groups, to track how we're living in other people's minds, but that like any emotion, it can operate in a way that is too easily triggered and powerful in its response. See if you can recognise how shame is a powerful feeling that human beings experience, and one that has evolved for our survival, and how it arrives with certain fears (for example, rejection and feeling alone). If it helps, hold a phrase or words in your mind about shame: 'This is a powerful feeling that can leave us feeling disconnected, inadequate and alone, and 'Although painful, I understand what this emotion is,

---

why I'm experiencing it and what it's trying to do for me.' Connected to your wisdom, see if you can see 'behind' shame. What is motivating this part to respond like this?

Notice the different thoughts and feelings in your body that come with this sense of shame. Turn towards them with curiosity, and even if they feel unpleasant, intense or are unwanted, remember that as your compassionate self, with your wisdom, strength and commitment, you can tolerate, understand and bring care and compassion to this experience of distress. If you feel they are getting too strong, imagine yourself pulling back, tuning back into your soothing rhythm breathing and when you feel ready, back into the grounded posture of your compassionate self: 'This is a moment of difficulty. I can be with this, it's already here.'

Holding the shame experience in mind and body, consider the following prompts:

- It's understandable that this is a difficult experience because . . .

- What can your compassionate self do to support this part of you?

- What does your compassionate self understand about where this feeling/concern originated?

- What would the compassionate part of you do to help manage any concerns you have about what other people think about you?

- What can your compassionate self do to help you tolerate any negative judgements you're having about yourself?

- Is there something that your compassionate self can learn from where this feeling arose? Is there something that it would be helpful to take responsibility for?

- Can your compassionate self help your shame part to feel connected and welcome?

Take your time reflecting on each of the questions. If it helps, make a few notes on each, and continue to add ideas over a number of days or weeks when you return to it.

It can be useful to consider what else would be helpful here. For example, maybe you could write a compassionate letter about this shame-related difficulty (see Chapter 19 for a guide), or complete a compassionate thought form about this (Chapter 20). Take your time with this and give your compassionate self enough space to provide help and support.

As we begin to turn compassion towards shame, you may notice that it loses a bit of its ferocity and stickiness. For example, Tina initially found this exercise very difficult, but with some practice, noticed that her shame feelings reduced. On reflection, she noted that each of the individual qualities of her compassionate self were important here. It was through the strength of her compassionate self that she could learn to trust that she could tolerate these feelings, and develop confidence that they didn't have to overwhelm her. The wisdom of her compassionate mind helped her appreciate that it wasn't her fault that she was feeling this way, and that there was a difference between what shame was telling her about herself (e.g. no one likes you; you're pathetic and weak) and what she felt when she wasn't feeling such high levels of shame. She was also able to bring wisdom that shame was trying to protect her from being hurt by others (something that she'd experienced growing up), but that the way it kicked in was like an oversensitive car alarm, going off at the drop of a leaf, rather than a car thief. Finally, she recognised that the commitment and care of her compassionate self were important to remind her of her initial intention for coming to therapy – to find a way to become more caring of herself and to find a way to alleviate distress and low mood.

As with anything, take your time with this process. It might be that you start with one thing that you feel ashamed about – maybe something that feels a bit more manageable – and then over time, move towards other things that you experience shame about. Continue to return to this process, using your compassionate mind as an anchor from which to engage in shame feelings.

Self-criticism – shame's best friend

If shame were a character in a film, its partner in crime would likely be self-criticism. Shame-based self-criticism is closely linked to internal shame (p. 318), and commonly has a potent role in either triggering difficult emotions or maintaining them once they're activated. Many studies have found that self-criticism is associated with higher levels of anger, anxiety and shame, and is associated with problematic emotion regulation strategies such as experiential avoidance and low acceptance of emotion (Cunha & Paiva, 2012), rumination and self-harm (O'Conner & Noyce, 2008), and self-harm (Khanipour et al., 2016). This is partly because self-criticism creates loops between our new and old brain (see Chapter 2), but also because self-criticism can affect your brain and your threat physiology / feelings.

When thinking about the impact self-criticism has on emotions that you find difficult to manage, it's important to consider what shape this takes for you. For example, self-criticism often influences what we pay attention to, the content of our thoughts, what we do and so on, as outlined in Figure 18.

Figure 18: Self–criticism shapes multiple aspects of mind

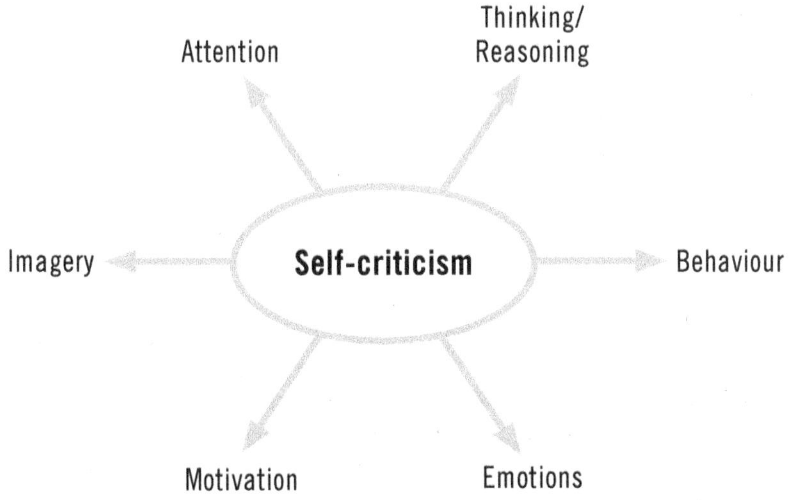

Attention

Thinking/
Reasoning

Imagery

Self-criticism

Behaviour

Motivation

Emotions

Let's take a look at this in more detail, but with a particular focus on how this relates to emotions that you might be struggling with.

Attention: Self-criticism can focus on, or be directed to, a broad range of things in life, but when it comes to emotions, it often turns up in particular ways. Some of us are critical of our appearance, personality, or our abilities, such as our intelligence. Sometimes self-criticism is directed to our mistakes (either current or past), or even to anticipated future mistakes. Often self-criticism involves a comparison with others, in a way that we feel inferior and worse off.

Thinking (content of thoughts): It's useful to become aware of the actual words that we use when being critical with ourselves. For example, there's a big difference between a relatively 'light' type of self-criticism (e.g. 'that was a bit daft'), which often isn't associated with much distress, and self-criticism that is laden with lots of hostility and harshness (e.g. 'you're such a *stupid, useless* piece of shit' or 'you're *pathetic* for showing anxiety'), and far more distressing to experience.

Behaviour: We can act in very different ways as a response to self-criticism. Sometimes we can urge ourselves to work harder, do more or try to achieve, whereas some responses to self-criticism shut us down, making us want to avoid difficult situations and retreat from life. Sometimes self-criticism comes with a desire to punish or hurt ourselves (e.g. through overeating, risk-taking or self-harm), but sometimes it comes with an urge to blame others and externalise.

Motivation: Another way of learning about your self-critic is thinking about the function that it has, or plays, for you – what it's trying to do for you. One way to explore this is to use functional analysis. This is a method of looking at, or discovering, what a particular thought, behaviour, response or emotion serves, what its purpose (or function) is. One way in which we can discover the function of our self-critic is to ask ourselves: what would my fear be if, somehow, I could never be self-critical again? If magically, just reading this book could remove your self-critic, what would your concern be? What would you be concerned about the consequences of how your life would be?

While we can experience an initial relief at the thought of not being self-critical again, soon afterwards there can be a variety of fears that emerge. Here are a few common ones:

- Maybe I'd be really lazy and not get anything done

- I'd make mistakes without realising it

- I'd become arrogant and self-centred

- I'd hurt other people and not care

- I'd become angry and aggressive

So, one thing we can begin to notice here is that self-criticism is often trying to protect us from something unpleasant – it's trying to stop something bad from happening to us or to others (or both). Often under-pinning these types of worries are broader concerns, such as rejection, exclusion, being alone, unlovable or flawed. You might see that these have overlaps with much of what we were discussing earlier in the chapter concerning shame. And in this sense, self-criticism is often tied to our self-identity, which is why it can seem scary to let go of it. We're going to hold on to this wisdom about the self-critic and use it when we use your compassionate mind to work with self-criticism later in the chapter.

Image and emotion: Although the type of words we say to our self is important, self-criticism also comes *with* emotions, and can trigger strong emotional reactions in us. One helpful way of exploring this is through the use of imagery. There's a short but quite powerful exercise to bring this to life. Close your eyes, and spend a few moments bringing to mind the types of things you criticise yourself for, and the way that you criti-cise yourself in these situations. After a minute or so, try to imagine what your self-critic would look like if you could see it in front of you. Take a minute or two to do this. When an image has formed, notice its qualities – its facial expression, voice tone, whether it's bigger or smaller than you, static, moving or making gestures at you. What emotion is it directing to you? What emotions or feelings do you have in the presence of the image of your self-critic, particularly given the emotion it is directing to you? Does it want to see you do well in life? Does it want to see or help you flourish?

I've taken thousands of people through this exercise, and it can be quite interesting to see what image emerges. It can also be quite a surprise just how powerful this exercise is, particularly that many of us live with our self-critics on a daily basis. Of particular interest here for us are the different emotions that the self-critic can send towards us. Commonly, this can be one or more of: anger, rage, disgust, shame, disappointment, fear, anxiety. And upon receiving this, many people are left feeling small, afraid, vulnerable, distressed or defeated – although sometimes it can trigger a different reaction (e.g. anger, aggression). And while some people feel that their self-critic wants the best for them, rarely is there a sense that it wants us to flourish or be happy in life.

Given what you've just looked at, and what you've learned about the emotions that come with and emerge as a consequence of self-criticism, is there anything you can take from this that ties back into your understanding about the difficulties you have with emotions, and more generally, regulating your emotions?

To help become more familiar with your own self-critic, it can be useful to make a few notes with each of these domains.

Why do we become self-critical?

There are lots of ways of looking at this. One is linked to the evolution of our minds; that is, we are self-critical because we have a mind that evolved in a certain way (which we had no influence or control over) that can become self-critical. As far as we know (although we might be wrong), it's unlikely that other animals criticise themselves for overeating or being overweight, or for not being attractive enough or for not being interesting enough when meeting new friends. So, we have a brain that can self-monitor – track how we are living in the mind of others, and then turn in on itself in a way that we can personalise, self-blame and criticise ourselves, stimulating old brain emotions, behaviours and motives (Chapter 3). These loops in the mind can be very painful.

But this underlying capacity to be able to experience self-criticism can get textured by our experiences in life, and often these are linked to interactions with our parents, our peer group, or more broadly, our culture. For Tina, she recalled that her mum could be lovely and supportive at times, but then could suddenly 'switch' in an unpredictable, scary way, shouting and screaming things at her like, 'Why do you always mess things up, you constantly make my life hard,' or 'I don't know why I ever thought you were a good girl.' Tina found that she had internalised some of this 'voice', and would sometimes say similar things to herself. Marta recalled that her father used to be very shaming and critical. Whatever grade she got at school, he would always focus on what she got wrong and would make negative comments about her appearance, behaviour and choice in friends. Marta recognised that she tended to monitor her own performance as an adult, particularly at work and in social scenarios, and be harsh with herself when she perceived she'd messed up on something. The research supports this; in a study that I was involved in many years ago, we found that higher levels of self-criticism today were associated with memories of being treated with rejection and overprotection by parents when growing up (Irons et al., 2006).

Experiences with our peer group can also shape the way we relate to our self, and research studies have shown that remembering being victimised (e.g. hit, left out or coerced to do something you didn't want to) in early adolescence is associated with higher levels of self-criticism as an adult (Kopala-Sibley et al., 2016).

Self-criticism and feared emotions

Earlier in the chapter, we learned that it can be quite scary to imagine not being able to be critical with ourselves. These fears included a concern that we might become selfish, arrogant, lazy, or uncaring. But it's not just these concerns that self-criticism turns up to protect us from – it can also operate to keep emotions that we're fearful of in check. Let's look at a couple of examples:

Self-criticism and the fear of anger toward others

The German philosopher Nietzsche suggested that no one blames themselves without a secret desire for revenge, an idea that Freud developed in his work looking at inverted anger in depression. One concern of letting go of self-criticism for some people is 'if I'm not busy blaming myself for what goes on in my life, I may end up blaming someone else'. It turns out that blaming others can be very difficult – and even scary – for human beings (Gilbert, 2009). Consider an example; imagine a young child being shouted at and blamed for something by their angry, aggressive father: 'It's your fucking fault that we're late, what's wrong with you? Why does it always take you so long to get ready, are you stupid or something?' In the face of angry attacks like this, where do you think it's safe for the child to locate blame? At their father who, after all, hadn't said what time they were due to go out, and who had been watching the football that had finished late? Or could you imagine that this could be quite dangerous, quite scary? That it might trigger further angry attacks: 'How dare you blame me, when we get home I'll show you how naughty children learn to be more respectful.' Or could you see that, in the face of this type of threat, angry feelings of unfairness get turned inwards – 'It must be my fault that this happened and that I upset Dad.' Under these conditions, it's understandable that we can blame ourselves as it's safer to do so, and if self-criticism is operating like this, then it may be that people have learned to be quite afraid of their own anger or externalising and blaming others.

Self-criticism and the fear of sadness

Some people I work with have a concern that if they give up their self-criticism, they might feel very sad, vulnerable and distressed. This can take different forms: sadness about how many years in life they have lost through self-criticism; sadness and grief for the losses of life, or the pain of difficult experiences in early life (e.g. abuse or the death of a parent). So, in these cases self-criticism turns up to stop sadness, to prevent us from feeling vulnerable and exposed to other people's criticism or aggression. Sometimes our concern is that if sadness were to turn up, it would never stop or we would become depressed.

Self-criticism and the fear of aloneness

Some people have been self-critical for many, many years – in fact, one person told me recently that they couldn't remember ever being without their self-critic. Although recognising that it causes distress, the idea of giving this 'voice' up can be associated with a sense of aloneness. There may be different ways that this has developed, but when some children are criticised by their parents, not only does this cause distress (e.g. feeling afraid, angry, sad or ashamed), they can also be left on their own with this experience (the typical 'go to your room and think about what a bad person you've been'). Here, in the activation of threat system emotions and feelings, self-criticism may be the only thing that helps to reduce some of our sense of aloneness. Over many years, our self-critic can become a type of companion, an ever-present acquaintance which, for some people, there can be positive associations and an affiliation with (Tierney & Fox, 2010).

Bringing your compassionate mind to help your self-critic

While understanding how self-criticism impacts your emotions can be helpful in itself, it's also important for us to see if we can bring a different approach to this. Given that self-blame is associated with emotion regulation problems (Garnefski et al., 2001), it's useful to see if we can approach our self-critic with our compassionate mind skills. We'll run through a number of steps to this; take your time with each one.

Step 1: Motivation to work with self-criticism

At first, it might feel like being compassionate to your self-critic – given how unpleasant and aggressive it can be – isn't high up on a list of things you want to do. However, it's useful here to remind yourself about what you discovered earlier in the chapter (p. 327), that self-criticism often serves the function of trying to protect us in some way, particularly from fears of rejection, being criticised or a sense of internal shame/not being good enough. So being compassionate to our self-critic is not about giving it free rein to bully and harass us, and it doesn't mean that we have to do what it's telling us to do, or crucially, believe in what it's telling us. Instead, compassion for self-criticism is learning how to become aware of self-criticism, learning to tolerate and understand that it's often trying to signal a concern or unmet need that we have. Compassion is also about being able to take a different approach, and to practise responding to the relevant concerns and needs differently.

To help with our compassionate motivation towards self-criticism, it's useful here to consider what our motivation would be for other people who are struggling with something, as a mirror for us to consider what would be beneficial for ourselves.

Example: Two teachers

Imagine that a child you care about (e.g. your child, a niece or nephew, a friend's child) is struggling with maths at school – they don't understand some of the concepts and terms being used and feel like everyone else is way ahead of them in class. Given this situation, how would you feel if the image of your self-critic – the one you identified in the exercise on p. 329 – was the teacher of this child who was struggling? How would critical teaching like this leave the child feeling? Would this critical teacher be helpful for the child to deal with their difficulty with maths?

When taking people through this exercise, most people aren't happy with the idea of the image of their self-critic being the teacher of a child who is struggling in this way. That they wouldn't want someone else they care for to experience criticism in this way. But it's interesting that while we wouldn't want our self-critic to be given free rein to take things out on others, it sits inside our heads, chipping away at us at regular intervals.

We can take the above example a step further. Spend a few moments to consider what *sort* of teacher you would like this child to have? Often people come up with qualities like patience, encouragement, kindness, support, warmth and persistence – qualities which are often closely aligned with those of the compassionate self or compassionate other.

But there is also something else important here. Consider for a moment that the critical teacher and compassionate teacher would both be concerned about the child's struggles with maths – they'd both be bothered about this, but it's just that the way they go about focusing on and dealing with this difficulty is vastly different. Why is this important? Well, it can be useful for you – and your self-critic – to know that the compassionate part of you is also concerned about the things that it is. Moreover, instead of trying to get rid of the self-critic, the compassionate self will also keep an eye out for our fears, but try to do this in a way that is helpful, and not harmful to ourselves and others.

Step 2: Awareness of self-criticism and its link to feared emotions

If we're going to work with self-criticism effectively, we first need to become aware of when it's turning up in our life. As we explored in

Chapter 8, awareness is an important skill when it comes to emotion regulation, as it is with becoming more familiar with the frequency and impact that self-criticism has upon our emotions. Sometimes our self-critic is just running in the background, regularly commenting about us, our actions, and the people around us. At other times, it can be triggered by specific situations, or things that we're experiencing. So, it helps to start noticing when self-criticism shows itself, and how this relates to emotions that we struggle to regulate. For example, Kathy was looking forward to meeting her friend Gill for lunch, and so was upset when Gill cancelled at the last minute. Being upset like this – particularly sad and distressed – then triggered a secondary, self-critical response, in which Kathy started to beat herself up: 'Pathetic – someone cancels lunch and look at the state of you; no one else would react as dramatically as this.' As a result, this self-attack left her feeling ashamed and beaten down as if there was something wrong with her.

It can be helpful to use Worksheet 3 opposite to track the frequency of your self-criticism, and how it links to difficulties you have with emotions. In particular, column 4 helps to focus our minds on what impact self-criticism has upon our emotions, which can build a clearer picture of the consequences of self-criticism on our emotional landscape. The final column (column 5) helps us to consider whether self-criticism was serving as a protective or safety strategy in the situation, stopping us from feeling or expressing a certain emotion. This can be helpful to track, as it can give a better sense of what we may need to bring our compassionate mind skills for.

WORKSHEET 3: SELF-CRITICISM LOG – TINA

Date	What was I doing? What triggered my self-criticism. What was I feeling?	What did I say to myself? What was the focus of my self-criticism?	Why was I critical? What was my criticism trying to do?	How did self-criticism impact on my emotion(s)?	If the self-critic wasn't there, what emotion might I have felt/been able to express instead?
21/7/2018	Lunch with friends – one couple have just got engaged, one shared that they were expecting a baby. I felt upset.	I told myself there was something wrong with me for being single and compared myself negatively to them.	I was critical because I fear that otherwise, I'll ignore that I'm single, and not push myself to meet someone.	I felt ashamed and inferior.	Sadness and loneliness.
23/7/2018	Trying on outfits for my birthday party. I felt unattractive and ashamed.	I started focusing on all the parts of my body that I don't like, and telling myself 'you're ugly'.	Being self-critical tries to make me focus on losing weight and looking more attractive so I won't be alone.	Anger (at myself), ashamed, and low in energy/motivation that I can change.	Sadness.
27/8/2018	Checking Facebook and Instagram – seeing friends on holiday together having fun. I felt left out.	Comparing my life with other people – I had a sense that I was inadequate and boring.	Prepare me in case other people criticise me for being boring and dull.	Anxious and sad.	Anger (that I'd not been invited). Loneliness.

WORKSHEET 3: SELF-CRITICISM LOG

Date	What was I doing? What triggered my self-criticism. What was I feeling?	What did I say to myself? What was the focus of my self-criticism?	Why was I critical? What was my criticism trying to do?	How did self-criticism impact on my emotion(s)?	If the self-critic wasn't there, what emotion might I have felt/been able to express instead?

Step 3: Compassionate engagement of the self-critic

As we learned earlier in this chapter, self-criticism is associated with the threat system. In fact, research has found that when we're self-critical, and when we're self-reassuring, caring and supportive of ourselves, these are associated with different regions in our brain (Longe et al., 2010). And obviously, from a CFT perspective, self-compassion draws more upon the physiology of the soothing system. This next phase involves using your compassionate mind to engage with your self-critic. We are going to guide you using the skills that you've developed throughout this book, and show how these can be used to help you.

Exercise: Using our compassionate self to work with self-criticism

To start with, find a place to sit in an upright but comfortable position. Take your time to bring awareness to the here and now, connecting with your soothing rhythm breathing and friendly facial expression. After a minute or two, bring to mind the qualities of your compassionate self – wisdom, strength and caring-commitment. Take a few moments to see if you can step into the shoes of your compassionate self and connect with your compassionate facial expression, voice tone and body posture. When you feel connected with this part of you, imagine that you can see the image of your self-critic in front of you – the image that you developed earlier in this chapter. Gently direct the qualities of your compassionate self towards your self-critic. See if you can use the following as a guide:

Strength and confidence – sometimes in the face of our self-critics, we can begin to feel threatened, anxious or overwhelmed. To help with this, focus on the strength and groundedness of your compassionate self. Notice your upright body posture and the ability that this part of you has to tolerate difficulties. If you do feel a bit overwhelmed, you might imagine taking a couple of steps back from the image of your self-critic, tuning back into your soothing rhythm breathing, and reconnecting with the strength of your compassionate self.

Wisdom and understanding – once you feel able to be in the presence of this image, we can now work on bringing wisdom and understanding to it. So, upon looking at your self-critic, what can you understand about it? What is it trying to do for you? Can you see what emotions sit behind the self-critic, or what fears it has about you, or the world around you? Sometimes when we look behind it, we can see that the self-critic is actually feeling quite threatened or afraid of something else. If that's the case, see what it feels like to hold empathy for the thing that the self-critic is worried or concerned about.

Caring-commitment – holding on to your desire to be caring and supportive, how might you communicate this to your self-critic? As your compassionate self, what would you like to say or do for your self-critic? Given your understanding about what sits behind it, try to focus your desire that this could cease – that the self-critic would no longer have to be so concerned about these fears, that it would no longer be distressed and that it could find peace. Is there a way you could help the self-critic with its concerns, but maybe in a more caring and wise way?

As you engage in these steps, there might be an opening to how hard it's been for the self-critic over the years, trying to stop bad things from happening in your life. There might even be a sense of feeling compassion for how hard it's been working, how tired it is. If this is the case, see what it's like to offer your support to it.

If during this exercise you feel you're getting overwhelmed or anxious in the face of the self-critic, or on the other hand, getting angry and wanting to attack it, this is a sign that you've moved out of your compassionate self. If this is the case, try to ground yourself again in your upright body posture, your soothing rhythm breathing and the sense of groundedness of your compassionate self. Try to refocus on your intention to be supportive and helpful, and in particular, remember that the self-critic is doing what it does to protect you, even if the way it does this is unpleasant, painful or full of threat.

When you feel ready, allow the image of your self-critic to fade from your mind. Tune back into your soothing rhythm breathing for a few moments. When you feel ready, bring yourself back into the room.

What did you notice from doing that exercise? What was it like to bring compassion to your self-critic, and in particular, to what sits behind it? Did anything change with the image of your self-critic (e.g. it's size, sense of its power, or the way it was relating to you)? If you started to get caught up in your threat system during this exercise (e.g. you felt scared by the self-critic, or started getting angry or critical towards it), please hold in mind this does happen sometimes, so you're not on your own. If so, it can be useful to consider what your compassionate self would need (for example, what qualities, or skills you could engage in that you learned in Section Three) that would help it to remain in the presence of self-criticism, tolerating any distress and remaining grounded and stable.

It's also useful to keep an eye out for becoming self-critical for your struggles to be compassionate for your self-criticism! This is quite common actually, and sometimes when people notice this is happening, it can bring a smile to their face and recognition again that we have a tricky brain, but that self-criticism is a common response when we find something difficult. Again, your compassionate self gets this, it understands that these are the types of things that can happen when we experience setbacks, and instead, try our best to return to our caring intention to work with our difficulties in a helpful and supportive way.

Step 4: Changing self-criticism to compassionate self-correction

Rather than trying to take away our self-critic (which tends to trigger the threat system, as it is often trying to protect us), compassion for self-criticism is about how we can guide our self-critic differently. This may involve paying attention to the concerns and fears that often sit underneath it, but also helping to shape and guide *how* it voices its concerns and worries to us. We refer to this as *compassionate self-correction*, where our compassionate self helps us turn towards difficult emotions in life, and motivates us to take responsibility to work on them (engage in helpful emotion regulation), in a way that is encouraging, supportive and wise. If you have a look at the table below, we can consider some of the differences between self-criticism and compassionate self-correction when trying to manage difficult emotions.

Shame-based self-criticism	**Compassionate self-criticism**
Here are some common reasons linked to self-criticism. Self-criticism is associated with threat-based emotions (fear, shame and anger) and relates to:	Self-correction involves a desire to do our best, to be open to our limitations and to want to learn and improve skills. It focuses on:
• A wish to punish and condemn • Fear of failure • Blaming and shaming • Feelings of disappointment with oneself, anger and frustration • Avoidance of situations • Social comparisons, where the self is inferior and judged against specific standards	• A desire to improve • Growth and enhancement • Giving support, encouragement and kindness • Acknowledgement of what goes well and considers areas for development • Appreciation and acceptance of the self as a whole, in an unconditional way

Hopefully, you'll be able to see from this table, self-compassion is not about letting ourselves off the hook, or just about being nice or kind to ourselves. Instead, we're focusing on developing a compassionate part of us that can help us to manage difficulties we face in life – like painful emotions – but with wisdom, strength and commitment, and a willingness to correct ourselves in a helpful and supportive way.

So, the next time you notice self-criticism, try and see this as an opportunity. Use the above table to become aware of how much you're tracking the left-hand side of the table, and hold in mind whether this is really the part of you that can help you move forward and learn from what has triggered the self-criticism. Instead, using the skills of your compassionate self, remind yourself that you are going to try to address the problem, but try to do this by focusing on the ideas on the right-hand side of the table. If it helps, write a compassionate letter to yourself (see Chapter 19) for something that you've been self-critical about, but this time trying to use the right-hand side of the table to guide how you focus and reflect upon the situation that triggered your self-criticism. After you finish the letter, read it through in a supportive, caring voice tone, and notice what it's like to focus upon this difficulty differently. Keep this type of practice going, training yourself to switch from a shame or self-critical voice, to a compassionate, supportive one.

Key reflections

- Shame is a powerful emotion and evolved to help us navigate social groups and the risk of making transgressions, mistakes and hurting people

- At high levels, shame can be one of the most debilitating emotions

- Self-criticism often turns up with shame experiences, and can further inhibit helpful emotion regulation

- Self-criticism has different functions and is often trying to protect us from a variety of fears

- Compassion – and in particular, the different qualities of wisdom, strength and commitment – can help us to turn towards, understand and bring light to shame and self-criticism

SECTION FIVE

Deepening your emotion regulation skills

Now that we've started to practise different emotion regulation skills for each of the five steps of the model, we're going to turn to how to help you strengthen and deepen your skills in this area. We'll do this across four separate chapters, each of which draws upon multiple levels of the emotion regulation model that we've been working on in Section Four:

1. The compassion PDA

2. Cultivating positive emotions

3. Compassionate letter writing

4. Compassionate thought balancing

17 'Turning up for yourself' – the compassion PDA (pre, during and after)

When I'm working with my clients and members of the general public on compassionate mind training, many people are keen to have practical tools to help guide and apply their developing skills. A method that I've developed to help them with this is called the compassion PDA (Irons & Beaumont, 2017). PDA stands for 'pre', 'during' and 'after' – three overlapping but separate stages of engaging in something that we find threatening or difficult. We can use this as a way to work with situations that trigger difficult emotions.

I started using this approach when working with sportswomen and men, after learning about their approach to training and competitions. Let's take the example of Serena Williams or Usain Bolt preparing for a big event that brings up nerves, and a sense of anxiety. Using a PDA can be useful for them to consider what would be helpful before the event happens (pre), what they need to hold onto or do during the event itself (during), and finally, what they need to do once the event has finished (after).

For both Serena and Usain, in the 'pre' phase of the event, they might prepare by doing lots of fitness training (running, lifting weights) and eating healthily. It might also be important for them to work with their coach on specific skills (e.g. perfecting the start of the race, or a backhand volley), as well as making tactical plans for the event itself. For the 'during' phase (the day of the event), both would need to warm up properly, eat certain foods and as the event starts, focus on their tactics. In the 'after' phase, there's also a variety of important things to focus on (for example, warming down) to minimise injury and facilitate recovery; discussing their performance with their coach, considering what they did well and what they could do differently in the future, and so on.

I've always thought it's interesting that for emotionally stimulating and difficult 'events', we tend not to take the same approach to warming up and warming down. So, here's a chance to give this a try, and take a similar approach to work with things that cause us difficult emotions. First, let's look at the example of Rhian, and how she used this approach. Rhian came to see me struggling with social anxiety. She described having always been quite a shy and introverted person, but that she used to enjoy spending time with friends and meeting new people. Unfortunately, when she was at university, she'd gone to a party with some people from her course that she didn't know very well. When she got there, no one talked to her, and she found herself standing on her own, feeling awkward and ashamed, before leaving after 20 minutes. We spent some time helping Rhian to understand how her threat system had been shaped by this, and she engaged well with exercises that we've worked on together in Section Three (compassionate mind training skills). Rhian was very motivated to bring change to her life and didn't want to miss out on being with her friends and having fun. After introducing the idea of the compassion PDA to her, we spent some time together looking at how her compassionate self would help her with future parties. With each of the three stages (pre, during and after), we first spent some time thinking about what difficulties and distress she envisioned at each step (threat system activation). We then spent some time helping her to embody her compassionate mind (e.g. by first taking 5 minutes to embody her compassionate self – see the exercise on p. 155), so that she was approaching these difficulties 'warm', and from the part of her that was wise, strong and committed to helping herself. Worksheet 4 outlines what Rhian came up with.

WORKSHEET 4: RHIAN'S COMPASSION PDA

Threat-based situation: Going to a party with friends. Worried that I'll say something stupid, act strangely, make a fool of myself, and have to head home. After, I'll beat myself up relentlessly for being an idiot.

Pre (P)	During (D)	After (A)
Difficulty (threat system focus): Before the party, I'll worry that I'll say something stupid, and nobody will want to speak to me. Focusing on all potential problems.	**Difficulty (threat system focus):** During the party, I'll probably monitor how I'm getting on, criticising myself for having problems and focusing on other people's facial expressions and thinking they think I'm boring.	**Difficulty (threat system focus):** In the hours and days after, I might ruminate over everything that happened, picking over the things I did wrong, and beat myself up for being weak and boring.
Compassionate Mind – what will help? It's helpful to spend time regularly practising mindfulness and soothing breathing, as this helps to calm me and step out of 'loops in the mind' and catastrophising. It's also useful to spend time talking with Rich, as he always helps me to feel supported and encouraged when I'm doubting myself. It's also useful to remember why I want to do this, why it's important to me – that I enjoy people's company, dancing and going to parties.	**Compassionate Mind – what will help?** On the day, I'll do some breathing practice and compassionate self practice (particularly my courage and posture) before leaving home. I'll have a prompt on my phone about my intention to be courageous and strong, and I'll listen to the encouraging voice message from my compassionate self. I'll hold in mind that it's a party for a friend who I really value, so it's important for me to be there. It's worth experiencing anxiety for this.	**Compassionate Mind – what will help?** Afterwards, it's going to be really important not to let my threat mind do all the judging – so mindfulness will be my friend here. I think a compassionate letter to myself would be useful, deliberately embodying my compassionate mind rather than my threat mind. It would be helpful to speak to Rich again as he'll know this might have been tough for me. I'll try to step back from criticising myself and focusing only on the things that seemed to go wrong, and hold in mind what went well, what I enjoyed, and the fact that I managed to face something I find difficult.

Rhian found that by using the compassion PDA, she was more prepared for anxiety and shame linked to going to the party. During the next few parties she went to, she used this approach to plan and prepare how best to 'turn up for herself' – how to embody her inner Serena Williams!

Exercise: Your compassion PDA

So, holding in mind Rhian's PDA, take some time to consider how you could use this as a guide with a struggle you're having with an upcoming situation that triggers difficult emotions for you. To start with, write down in the first column the situation that you're finding difficult at the moment, or that is coming up in the near future. Try to pick something that is associated with an emotion that you find difficult to manage (e.g. anxiety, anger, sadness, shame).

Just as Rhian did, start by thinking about what the threats or difficulties are likely to be pre, during and after this emotionally tricky situation or event. With this in mind, spend some time getting in contact with the part of you that can helpfully direct your PDA – your compassionate self. From this wise, strong and caring part, take your time to think through what might help before, during and after facing this challenge. Here are some tips for each:

Pre: Consider what steps you could take that would help in the lead-up to engaging in this difficult situation. Are there things that could help you prepare for this event (e.g. things you need to find out or learn, or maybe something you can practise)? Maybe there are some important things to mindfully 'keep an eye on', and step back from if you notice them starting up – for example, worrying that it won't work out, or imagining worst-case scenarios about what you will feel. If this happens, remember that you have a variety of skills from Section Three to draw upon (e.g. mindfully noticing these loops, and bringing yourself back into the here and now). It can also be helpful here to hold in mind your motivation – why doing this thing is important to you. In this sense, we can appreciate (with wisdom) that we are likely to feel difficult emotions, but still engage in the action anyway as we know this is more important.

During: As you engage directly with the thing that triggers difficult emotions for you, it can be helpful to hold in mind the following questions:

- What would your compassionate self help you to do right now?

- What qualities of your compassionate self – wisdom, strength, caring-commitment – might help you to manage this difficult thing?

It can also be helpful to consider what would help you to 'do' the thing you find difficult at the time – for example, would it be useful to have some support from a friend? What other skills from Section Three could you bring online to support you in doing this?

After: After you've completed the difficult activity, what would be helpful for you now? Really think about this – and if possible, do this from your wise, understanding compassionate self. If it's gone well, what would be a wise thing to do now? How could you learn from what happened, and allow a sense of appreciation of what you were able to do? If it didn't go well, what would help you tolerate the disappointment, sadness, anger or anxiety that might emerge? What would prevent you from getting caught up in self-criticism or unhelpful rumination? What could you learn from this for the future?

Although it can feel a bit strange to use this structure at first, over time many people (including myself!) have found this a useful way to guide the process of engaging in events that trigger difficult emotions, and in particular, of 'using' the compassionate self for encouragement and support. Sometimes I describe embodying your compassionate self like this as a way of *'turning up for yourself'*. If you can, try it out initially with two or three different scenarios. As you get more confident using the idea, it's likely you'll be able to develop more in-depth, and nuanced PDAs. Try to use the form in Worksheet 5 (next page) to guide you on this, or find further blank versions at https://overcoming.co.uk/715/resources-to-download.

WORKSHEET 5: YOUR COMPASSION PDA

Threat-based situation:

Pre (P)	During (D)	After (A)
Difficulty (threat system focus):	Difficulty (threat system focus):	Difficulty (threat system focus):
Compassionate Mind – what will help?	Compassionate Mind – what will help?	Compassionate Mind – what will help?

You can use this approach with any emotion (and in fact, any situation) that you find threatening or distressing in some way. As with all of these skills, try to practise this approach as often as you can, and take notes on what it was like to bring your compassionate self to difficulties in this way.

Key reflections

In this chapter, we've looked at how:

*   When engaging with difficult emotions and the situations linked to them, there can be three phases at which we encounter emotional difficulties – before it occurs (pre), while it's happening (during), and once it's finished (after)

*   We can draw upon our compassionate self to help with the emotion regulation process at each of these stages

18 Cultivating positive emotions

Over the past ten years, there has been increasing interest in, and evidence for, how positive emotions can play a powerful role in helping to regulate negative emotions. Research has highlighted that cultivating and experiencing positive emotions can balance negative, threat-based emotions like anxiety and anger (e.g. Garland et al., 2010). Some of this work has highlighted the potential for positive emotions to 'broaden and build' psychological processes such as attention, social relationships, resilience, exploration and fulfilment in a way that can be emotionally healthy (Fredrickson, 2013).

It's important here though to reflect on what our relationship is like with positive emotions. As Rick Hanson, the American psychologist, points out (2013), in the brain, 'positives are like Teflon, negatives are like Velcro'. Given the struggle to survive, evolution has built into our nervous system a negativity bias, and various studies have found that we respond more quickly to threats than we do to positives. In this sense, 'bad is stronger than good', and naturally, negative emotions are likely to 'knock offline' positive emotions. There's nothing wrong with this, it's absolutely not our fault – in fact, it makes complete sense; better to experience intense fear or panic as a snake emerges from the grass and disturbs the pleasure and excitement of your scenic picnic with friends, rather than you not reacting and being bitten! But, the power of our threat system means that we can easily get caught in threat-spirals, heating up distress and inhibiting helpful emotion regulation. Moreover, the more this happens, the more we ignore or become blocked to noticing and taking in all the positives that are around us. So, given this, it can be helpful for us to do what we can to level the playing field a little – to allow more space for positive emotions to play the beneficial role that they can do if and when they have the chance to, and crucially, our attention and intention to do so.

From a CFT point of view, it is important to keep in mind different types of positive emotion. In Chapter 3 we outlined the three system model of emotions, which suggests that there are (at least) two different types of positive emotion. One – including emotions like excitement and joy (known as the drive system) – evolved to energise us, taking us towards things that could be beneficial (e.g. resources), and leaving us feeling good (and therefore acting as a reinforcer) when we succeed. This type of positive emotion is likely linked to the neurochemical dopamine and associated with the sympathetic nervous system. The other type of positive emotion – including emotions like contentment, safeness, calmness (known as the soothing system) – may have initially emerged to sit alongside 'rest and digest', and give rise to a sense of peacefulness or calm when we are not threatened, and not striving to achieve anything. It's likely that these emotions are more closely associated with the parasympathetic nervous system, and neuropeptides like oxytocin. Research has found that both of these emotion systems are associated with lower levels of self-criticism, depression, anxiety and stress (Gilbert, 2008).

Given all of this, it seems prudent to consider how we might increase our contact with these different types of positive emotion. We actually spent some time doing this already; in Chapter 9, we explored a number of exercises (e.g. soothing breathing, and safe place imagery) that can give rise to and help us cultivate these emotions of the soothing system, and it may be helpful to spend some more time practising these exercises as a way in to positive emotion cultivation. But in this chapter, we are going to extend some of what we started in Chapter 9, and look at further ways to deliberately cultivate positive emotions. We'll do this by:

- Paying more attention to positive emotions
- Using memory to stimulate positive emotions
- Using gratitude and appreciation to build positive emotion

Pay attention to positive emotions

What we pay attention to tends to get 'bigger' in our minds. Unfortunately, this means that if we are locked into the emotions of our threat system (e.g. anxiety, anger), then it can be difficult to notice and connect with positive emotions. As we learned in Chapter 8, this is where attention training and mindfulness can help us to orientate to the here and now, rather than getting caught in living in the future, the past, or relating to ourselves in critical ways. Mindfulness can also help us notice, identify and connect with positive emotions as they arise; and by doing so, this opens the possibility that we can allow them to 'breathe'. There are a few steps to this:

1. Set yourself an intention – that over the coming 24 hours, you will try to notice when you experience positive emotions. This might be the pleasure of a cup of coffee, or having a warm, relaxing shower. It might be the feeling of talking to a friend or loved one or doing some exercise.

2. When you notice the presence of positive emotion, pay attention to it – not in a 'grabby', tense way, but rather, gently move your awareness towards it.

3. As you pay attention to it, choose to stay mindfully attentive to it, maybe for 10 seconds, or longer if you can. Try to savour this feeling, to hold it lightly like you might a delicate flower.

4. As you hold awareness of this positive emotion, see if you can feel into its shape. What sensations do you notice in your body? Is the feeling low, medium or high intensity? What's the urge in your body, given the presence of this emotion? And what thoughts or images are passing through your mind that are associated with this positive emotion?

5. Like rubbing moisturising cream into dry skin, allow the positive emotion to sink in, absorbing it into your body and mind.

6. Finally, try to hold the intention to notice and savour positive emotions whenever they show up in the future. Sometimes to start with, it can be helpful to put a reminder on your phone which flashes up 'notice the positive' or something similar, a number of times throughout each day. Over time, with practice, it's likely you'll get better at doing this without prompts.

If it helps, make a few notes afterwards about this experience; this can further allow the experience to be maintained, and help us become more familiar and acquainted with these types of emotions.

Recalling positive emotions

In Chapter 9, we learned that if we focus on memories linked to feelings of soothing and contentment, this can re-trigger the same feelings that we experienced at the actual time of the event, thus helping to build the soothing system. It turns out that we can do the same thing for emotions like excitement and joy, which are more closely linked to the drive system. Here's one way that we can begin to connect with this.

Exercise: Connecting with positive memories

Spend a few moments connecting with your soothing rhythm breathing. Allow your body to slow down with the out-breath. When you feel ready, bring to mind a memory of a time when you experienced an intense feeling of joy or happiness. Try to recall within this memory as much detail about this as possible: where you were, who was there, what was happening. Focus if you can on sensory aspects of this memory – what you could see, smell, hear. Try to bring back to mind your emotions of joy or happiness. If you can, notice where this feeling is located in your body. Using your mindfulness skills, gently allow yourself to connect with as much of this memory as you can. Savour the feelings of joy and happiness – allow yourself as much time as you would like, just to be with this memory. When you feel ready, open your eyes.

As with the practices we introduced in the previous chapters, it's useful to create space to practise this memory exercise regularly. To help with this, you might find the following written version of the exercise also helps with the process of connecting with drive system emotions.

Exercise: Memory writing

Taking the above idea of focusing on positive emotion memories, we can also elaborate this type of feeling by spending time focusing on this through writing. If you can, spend 15 to 20 minutes on this exercise (this is the amount of time that researchers suggest when they have investigated this), and try to repeat it over two or three consecutive days.

Spend a few moments connecting with your soothing rhythm breathing. When you feel ready, bring to mind the most 'wonderful' experience in your life – the happiest, most joyful or ecstatic moment or experience that you have had. Spend some time holding this experience in mind. Notice where you were, who was there, what was happening. Really focus on the feelings and emotions that are associated with this memory. When you feel ready, spend time writing about this memory in as much detail as you can. What did you think, feel and experience at the time? Try to write for as long as you can.

Over the coming week(s), put some time aside so that you can practise these exercises. Notice how these leave you feeling, how they sit alongside any different emotions that you're experiencing (e.g. anxiety, anger) and what it's like to create more space for balance between positive and negative emotions.

Gratitude and appreciation

Reconnecting with previous events that gave you positive emotions can help you to familiarise yourself with the usefulness of spending time with pleasant feelings. Similarly, this next exercise focuses on helping us to become more mindful, aware and appreciative of things that we've experienced. Given the dominance of our threat system, it's easy (although not our fault) to be dragged into paying attention to unpleasant and difficult things in life. It's important to remember the phrases 'what we focus on expands' and 'we become what we pay attention to'. In recent years, researchers have found that deliberately focusing on and paying attention to things in life that you're grateful and appreciative for can lead to increased levels of well-being (e.g. Davis et al., 2016). Being aware of the things we appreciate in this way does not mean that we ignore the pain in our lives; rather this noticing can bring a bit more perspective and balance in how we feel. A helpful way to develop this is to practise regularly the following exercise.

Exercise: Three good things

Take a few moments to connect with your grounded, upright body posture, friendly facial expression, and soothing breathing. When you feel ready, look back over your day, and write down three 'good things' that happened. This could be a wide variety of things, such as having had a nice meal with a friend; being treated kindly by a shop assistant; having had a good night's sleep; getting a compliment from someone. It does not matter how big or small these things are, as long as they give you a sense of happiness, joy or excitement.

1. _____

_____

2. _____

_____

3. _____

_____

It's important that we invest time focusing upon positive experiences so that they have an opportunity to 'stick' in our brains. To do this, we are going to spend some time exploring each of the positive experiences you identified above, one at a time.

Good event 1: _____

- What led to this good event happening?

- How did this event leave you feeling? (Spend some time bringing the situation/event back to mind, in as much detail as you can)

- What could you do so that more of these events happen in the future?

Plan: Repeat this step for each of the three good events you noted down for the day. Remember, the key is to try to give this exercise enough time and space so that it can embed in your mind. To help with this, it is important to repeat the 'good things' exercise throughout a week, each day focusing the spotlight of your mind on three positive experiences. As with everything else, the more you practise this way of focusing, the more these positive experiences and the emotions that come with them will take root in your brain!

Key reflections

- Positive emotions can be cultivated and developed

- Positive emotions can help to balance out or regulate negative emotions, like anxiety and anger

- We can use mindfulness, memory, writing and savouring in different ways to build access to positive emotions

19 Compassionate letter writing

For thousands of years, humans have used writing as a powerful and cathartic method of managing experiences, emotions and fears. Whether through storytelling, poetry, literature or diary-keeping, people have used writing as a way of emotional expression and regulation. Over thirty years ago, an American psychologist, Professor James Pennebaker, started investigating the psychological and physical effects of writing about things that we are struggling with. Intriguingly, he found that writing about difficulties in a particular way was associated with positive health and psychological effects over time (Pennebaker & Smyth, 2016), in comparison to people who just wrote about non-relevant, unemotional difficulties.

In the compassionate mind approach, we use insights based on Pennebaker's, but as you can probably guess, with a slight 'compassion' twist. There are many ways to write compassionate letters, but in this chapter, we will explore one that utilises the various steps of the emotion regulation model we covered in the previous section. To help you to start writing compassionate letters, we will walk you through a number of steps. Over time and practice, you'll find your own style and a format that works for you.

Before writing – engage your compassionate mind

A helpful phrase to keep in mind when using the compassionate mind approach is: 'which part of you is doing the work'. So, we could write a letter from an angry part of us, or from an anxious part, and depending on the reason for writing the letter, writing from different 'parts' of you could be useful (using Chapter 16d as a guide). However, to facilitate helpful emotion regulation, it's key to write the letter from the part of you that is wise, strong and caring – your compassionate self. To start this process, bring to mind an emotion, or an emotionally stimulating situation, that you've been struggling with recently – the thing that you're going to spend time focusing your letter on. Once you have this in mind, and before you put pen to paper, find a quiet place to sit, and, with an upright body posture, spend a few moments mindfully connecting with your soothing rhythm breathing. When you feel ready, spend a little time connecting with the qualities of your compassionate self – caring-commitment, wisdom and strength. Take as long as you need to feel connected to these qualities. From this part of you, tune in to your compassionate intention and motivation in writing this letter. Try to focus on your desire to be sensitive to the difficulty and your willingness to find ways to alleviate this suffering. Really focus your compassionate intention on trying your best to do this in the coming letter (spend 30 seconds or so just holding this in the front of your mind).

Exercise: Compassionate letter writing

Step 1: Identifying and labelling a difficult emotion/situation that you are struggling with

So now it's time to start actually putting pen to paper (or if you'd prefer, fingers to keyboard!). We start all of our letters with an address to ourselves – so this could be something like 'Dear Chris', or 'Hello me'. Use the language that feels comfortable and personal to you.

Then begin to put words to the nature of what the struggle is, what you're going to focus the letter on. Try to identify not only the difficulty, but also the distressing emotion(s) it has led to. We're going to use Carly here as an example. Carly came to therapy looking for help with relationship problems. In terms of difficult emotions, she described bouncing between anger at the way her partner had been treating her, and intense anxiety that he may end the relationship.

To start the letter, Carly wrote:

> Dear Carly,
>
> I know that life is really tough at the moment, and you've been feeling upset, anxious and angry. There have been lots of arguments with Pete recently, and it seems like a long time since you've both 'got on'. Part of you wants to shake him out of this, but another part is terrified that the writing is on the wall for the relationship and that he'll leave you.

Step 2: Validation and empathy for the struggle

As we looked at in Chapter 15, when we're struggling and distressed, it can help to try to validate and empathise with this experience. When distressed, many of us have a tendency to invalidate our distress and find it difficult to understand why we are feeling as we are. So, step 2 involves bringing your compassionate mind – its wisdom and caring-commitment – to validate how we're feeling. For example, Carly wrote:

> It's really understandable that you're feeling upset and angry with everything that's been happening, particularly given how disconnected and unresponsive Pete has been these past few weeks.

Following this, we can look further into the situation and your struggles by bringing empathy and understanding to the situation. Here, Carly wrote:

> I can understand that you've been finding this all difficult, because you really thought that your relationship with Pete was getting to a stage where you might get engaged – in fact, everything seemed to be going so well, and I know you've felt confused by how quickly things have changed. It also makes sense that you've been feeling panicky and worried about Pete ending the relationship – this reminds you of how David was before he broke up with you five years ago, and it seems likely that your threat system is reacting to the similarities here. Because of this,

I can understand that your anger comes on quite strong as a way of trying to protect you and not letting you be in a weak or vulnerable position.

Step 3: Understanding of your attempts to manage your emotions – not your fault

As we have explored elsewhere, we can often bring unhealthy approaches to managing and coping with our emotions (the left-hand side of the emotion regulation model). However, as we've also explored through this book, it can be helpful to try to put these in context: that we're all socially shaped, have tricky brains that get caught up in 'loops', and can learn a way of relating to our emotions that can in itself cause further problems. It can be helpful to outline your own attempts to manage your emotions as 'not your fault'. This is what Carly wrote:

I know that you've been trying to manage your anxiety and fear of rejection by being as nice and kind as you can be with Pete, and by checking with him how he's feeling about you. This makes sense as a way of minimising your fears of splitting up and being on your own. This is also likely to be linked to your previous painful experiences with David. I want you to know that this isn't your fault – you're just trying your best to manage a really scary situation.

Step 4: Taking responsibility – coping with the difficult emotion

Although it's understandable that we engage in a variety of protective strategies to manage our difficult emotions, it may not be very compassionate to sit by allowing these – and the unintended consequences they lead to – without trying to bring change. Compassion often involves taking responsibility for the way that we think, feel and behave – and it may be helpful here to do the same. So, step 4 involves considering what might help you to manage some of the tricky and distressing emotions we can experience. For this step, Carly wrote:

While it's not your fault for how you've been feeling and responding to Pete, it's likely that when you keep asking how he's feeling, this is making him more frustrated and adding to your distress. It might be helpful to think about how you can take responsibility for your distressing emotions: a first step, for example, might be to try to become more aware of how your anxious feelings are linked to fears of rejection, and more mindful of your urge to respond in an anxious or angry way. Remember to use your breathing rhythm and your wisdom, strength and caring-commitment to accept and tolerate this feeling, rather than bouncing to anger and aggression as a way of protecting yourself.

Now that we've started to commit to change and take responsibility, it is important to think about how we can bring our compassionate minds to influence how we are thinking and behaving in this situation. So, it's helpful to reflect on new perspectives, intentions and actions that you're intending to take going forward. In a way, this is trying to consider how your compassionate self will try to manage the struggle. So, if your compassionate self was the 'part' of you that was directing the traffic, how would it do this in a way that brings its wisdom, strength and caring-commitment? At this step, Carly wrote the following:

It might be helpful here to try to speak to Pete about how things are at the moment, but to do this in a different way than you have tried in the past. Although this might be scary, letting him know how you've actually been feeling, and why you've been responding to him in the way that you have been. And, rather than after a long day at work, maybe it would be wise to speak sometime this weekend when you're both a little more relaxed.

Step 5: Working with blocks, difficulties and setbacks

Wouldn't it be great if everything that Carly just suggested worked out really well? Of course, we all know that unfortunately, bringing change in these sorts of situations is very difficult, and in fact, we often meet setbacks and failures when we try to change things. These setbacks can, in themselves, lead to us becoming more critical with ourselves and ultimately, feeling even worse than before. So, it can be helpful here to consider what difficulties or setbacks you might experience in your attempts to support yourself and bring change to this situation. Carly wrote:

> Try to keep an eye on when you begin to ask him regularly for reassurance, or notice your urge to attack him. If you can, use these setbacks as opportunities from which to learn and practise new ways to grow, rather than bash yourself. Remember that this is completely understandable, given your previous experiences and how your threat system has been shaped. It could also be helpful to reread this letter, and to remember that it might take a while to work through all of this.

Step 6: Compassionate commitment to bringing change

To finish off the letter, see if you can convey a sense of support and commitment from your compassionate self in the letter. For example, Carly finished her letter with:

> Try to remember that I'll be here for you to help with all of this – you're not on your own. I'll be here whenever you need some support. Although things are hard and may continue to be in the coming days, remember your motivation to engage with this distress and take steps to bring change to this, to work through some of the difficulties with Pete.

After writing – compassionate reading

The final step of the process is to read the letter back to yourself, but before you do, consider which part of you is going to do the reading.

Without intending to, it could be quite easy for your threat system to come online here (e.g. an anxious, angry or self-critical part) and this is likely to bleach the potential helpfulness of the letter. Instead, spend a few minutes connecting back to the qualities of your compassionate self, try to read the letter back to yourself slowly, and gently, allowing the words to connect with your motivation to be helpful and supportive. Also, try to read it through in your own mind in a warm and caring voice tone.

Although everyone develops their own style when writing letters, here are a few reflections to consider as you continue to practise compassionate letter writing:

Helpful tips:

- Try experimenting with using the first person (I) and second person (you). Some people find it harder using the first person (e.g. 'I can see that the difficulty I have with anger is not my fault') rather than the second person (e.g. 'It's not your fault you've struggled with anger'). Try out both ways, and see which is the easiest or most powerful for you

- Don't worry if your letter isn't quite 'right', or perfect. This exercise is about the intention to approach emotions that you're struggling with, with various qualities of compassion (for example, care, empathy and support), rather than the end product

- As you're writing the letter, remain aware of which 'part' of you is doing this – while we can start the letter with a very compassionate voice, if we're not careful, the tone and content can quickly shift to a more cold, critical or demanding one

- The structure outlined above is only one way to approach letter writing. This is not a 'one size fits all' approach, so feel free to experiment, and find your own style over time

- It may be helpful to reread your letters on a weekly or monthly basis, always doing this with a warm, caring inner voice tone

- Remember that letter writing is like any skill – it takes some practice to get into the flow. Try to create space at various times in the coming weeks and months to write letters to yourself when you notice difficult emotions showing themselves

Key reflections

In this chapter, we've looked at how compassionate letter writing can be a powerful way to engage with difficult emotions:

- Letter writing can help to focus the skills of your compassionate self, by bringing wisdom about the struggles you're having, and a commitment to help yourself manage these, in a supportive and caring way

- Letter writing can utilise various steps of the emotion regulation model and help you bring compassion to your difficult emotions

20 Using compassionate thinking to manage your emotions

As we continue our journey, we're now going to work on how bringing a compassionate focus to our thinking can help manage distressing emotions and feelings. As Marcus Aurelius, the famous Roman emperor, said: 'If you are distressed by anything external, the pain is not due to the thing itself but to your estimate of it, and this you have the power to revoke at any moment.' In a similar vein, the Greek philosopher Epictetus suggested: 'People are not disturbed by things, but by the views they take of them.'

Many of us realise that our thinking can have a massive impact on the way we feel. Let's look at an example of this. Let's say you're lying on the sofa, and begin to notice that your chest is a bit tight, with a slight pain on the left-hand side. If you start thinking: 'Jeez, I'm having a heart attack. I'm going to die,' it's fair to expect an increase (possibly significant) in I'm-having-a-heart-attack-related anxiety, in contrast to if your thoughts are, 'I knew I shouldn't have eaten that curry so quickly – I always get bad heartburn when I eat spicy food quickly.'

Many therapies have recognised the powerful impact our thoughts can have on our feelings. For example, a type of therapy called cognitive behavioural therapy (CBT) – which CFT has a number of overlaps with – suggests that much of our mental distress is related to the way we think about things, and in particular, to the content of our interpretations and reflections of events and situations. As an approach, it focuses on how we can become aware of 'negative' or 'distorted' thoughts or interpretations, and find a more balanced and accurate way of thinking about things. In more recent years, other talking therapies have emerged, such as acceptance and commitment therapy (ACT) and mindfulness-based approaches. Rather than focusing on the content of our thoughts being key in leading to distress (and as a consequence, trying to change the content of thoughts), these approaches suggest it is the process – for example, the way we relate to our thoughts – that has a greater impact on our emotions and feelings. So, from these perspectives, change in distress comes from learning to notice the way we are thinking, and, rather than trying to get rid of, challenge, or change the content of our thoughts, accept them as 'mental experiences', rather than see them as 'facts'.

In this chapter, we will explore how in CFT, we hold *both* of these perspectives as important. So, we will explore how, by bringing a more compassionate stance to the content of our thoughts, as well as to our relationship with them, we can reduce distressing feelings.

Understanding the way we think

We could spend a long time getting technical about this, but at this stage, it may be helpful to remind ourselves of a few points that we touched on in Section One of the book.

1.   *Evolutionary backdrop*

     The origins to the way we think lay with our evolution and biology. Through hundreds of millions of years, and particularly in the last one or two million years, we experienced a rapid expansion of certain parts of our brains, such as the cortex, and in particular, the frontal cortex. This in turn gave rise to the biological structures that underpin thinking, capacity to imagine, worry, ruminate and self-monitor. These abilities were *designed for us, not by us*.

2.   *Our thinking was designed around a 'better safe than sorry' principle*

     As increasingly complex, new brain abilities evolved, our capacity for reflection, planning and imagination had the potential for not only great benefits to us but also some problems. As we explored in Chapter 3, in a threat context (such as a lion running towards us, or someone with a balaclava holding a large knife in their hand), thinking in too much detail about what is happening is likely to slow down old brain survival responses such as fight or flight.

From a CFT perspective, we would suggest that our thinking operates on a 'better safe than sorry' principle whereby, under high-threat scenarios, it either shuts down or becomes narrowly focused on the threat, shifting from complexity and reflection to:

- *Jumping to conclusions* in which ideas about danger come to mind quickly and we hold firm beliefs even in the absence of evidence for such

- *Overgeneralising* whereby we globally apply a bad experience to others (e.g. experiencing rejection in one relationship, we conclude that this will happen in all our other relationships)

- *Dichotomous thinking*, so that experiences in life are viewed in 'black or white' ways, often with a negative bias to them

It can be helpful here to recognise that when you're thinking becomes threat-focused like this, this is not your fault; it's just what tends to happen to our thinking under threat circumstances. In this sense, these represent 'glitches in the system' in which our new brain is powerfully influenced by old brain motives and emotions. This is often OK in the short term but becomes 'tricky' if elaborated over time and, as we learned in Chapter 3, can drive a lot of distress and difficulties with emotions. Compassionate thinking often starts with this de-shaming understanding of the reality of our evolved thinking patterns, rather than clinging onto expectations of how they ought to be, or how we would like them to be.

3. *Genes can influence thoughts*

The genes we inherit from our parents – which we have no control over – can have a significant effect on the pattern of our thinking. For example, Beevers et al. (2009) found that a group of healthy adults who had a particular variation in a gene linked to brain-derived neurotrophic factor (BDNF; related to growth of brain cells) had significantly higher levels of rumination (the tendency to focus repetitively on unpleasant events, thoughts and emotions) than adults who didn't share the same variation of gene. This is important as we have many, many studies showing that higher levels of rumination are associated with a variety of mental health problems, including depression. While these types of gene variant studies are quite new, and often contain small numbers of participants, they point towards how, just like with our eye colour and weight, our genes can have an impact upon the way our mind works.

4.   *We are socially shaped*

Our thinking can also be influenced by our personal experiences in life. For example, a large body of research has found that certain types of experiences in life, for example, being criticised, rejected or abused (e.g. Irons et al., 2006; Manfredi et al., 2011), are associated with higher levels of rumination, worry and self-criticism. While we may have the evolutionary and genetic predisposition to ruminate or self-criticise, these are not fully formed from birth, and, instead, become evident following certain interpersonal experiences. In other words, like many other things, we tend to internalise or mirror how others have talked to and treated us.

Taking perspective – not your fault

Given our exploration of some of the reasons why we think in the way we do, an important concept emerges that we also explored earlier in the book. You did not choose to have a brain that evolved to have the capacity to think in certain ways, nor to have genes that make you more (or less) likely to think in certain ways, nor to have experiences that shape your thinking. In this sense, it can be useful to hold in mind that the patterns of thoughts you experience are *not your fault*.

Consider this idea for a moment. Can you remember the day you woke up and decided: 'Right, that's it, from today on I'm going to really focus on ruminating on the past, and all the things I've messed up in my life,' or

'I've had enough of the way I think, my new year's resolution is to dedicate myself to worrying about things in the future as much as humanly possible'? My guess is that the answer is probably 'no'. For most of us, we just find ourselves with a mind that tends to get caught up with certain types of thinking, such as worry, rumination or self-criticism; in many ways, we are the reader of the book, rather than the author.

The relationship between threat emotions and thinking patterns

If you remember, our thinking is naturally biased by threat system activation, but our thinking is also influenced by the type of threat emotion we are experiencing (e.g. anger, anxiety or shame). Let's take a look at a few examples:

Emotion	Style of thinking	Content of thinking
Anxiety	Worry	'I've got to give a talk on Monday, I'll make mistakes and mess it all up'
		'The pain in my stomach is terrible – I think there's something seriously wrong with me, maybe it's cancer'
		'I'm going to have a heart attack'
	Rumination	'Maybe if I'd spent more time revising then it would have worked out better'
		'Was it something that I said in the meeting that led her to respond like that? Or maybe it was when I forgot to text her on her birthday?'

Anger	Rumination	'How dare she say that to me in the meeting – who does she think she is? Why didn't I tell her what I thought of her?'
	Self-criticism	'I'm such an ugly, useless, fat piece of shit'
	Other-criticism	'He's the one who messed this up, he should apologise to me and realise that!'
Sadness	Hopelessness/feeling trapped	'This will never change; I will always feel depressed' 'I'll always be on my own – it's always been like that and always will be'
Shame	Self-criticism	'I'm no good – I always screw things up' 'It's my fault this has happened – I'm such an idiot'

Thought monitoring

Given the association between patterns of thinking and threat emotions, it can be useful to purposefully pay attention to the type of thoughts you're having, and how they're linked to emotions. There are lots of different ways to do this but one way many find useful is to use the 'thought-emotion monitoring form' (opposite page) to track this. The purpose of this form is to help you track the type of thoughts linked to different threat system emotions, and how you attempt to deal with these. We'll use the example of Claire, a woman in her early twenties who came to therapy for help with persistent anxiety.

Thought-emotion monitoring form

Time of day	Type of thought e.g. worry, criticism, blame, rumination	Content of thought e.g. thoughts about work, family, health, the future	What threat emotion was this associated with?	How did you deal with the thought? E.g. ignored thought, acted on the thought
Morning	Worry	I'm not going to be able to cope with the meeting later	Anxiety, shame	Tried to push it out of my mind – told myself I was daft for thinking and feeling like that
Afternoon	Worry	Why has my section of the meeting been put to the end? It must be because it's not as interesting as other people's contributions	Anxiety, shame	I went for a cigarette to distract myself
Evening	Rumination and self-criticism	Why did I mess that up at work – I always make mistakes I'm such a loser	Shame, anger (at myself)	I drank three large glasses of wine, smoked a lot and ordered pizza. I kept checking Facebook to stop myself thinking

Time of day	Type of thought e.g. worry, criticism, blame, rumination	Content of thought e.g. thoughts about work, family, health, the future	What threat emotion was this associated with?	How did you deal with the thought? E.g. ignored thought, acted on the thought
Morning				
Afternoon				
Evening				

Have a go at completing your own thought-emotion monitoring form (see opposite page).

Reflections: What did you learn about your thoughts from this exercise? Did you notice any patterns?

It might be that this exercise was quite useful in itself, and helped you to become more aware of certain types of thinking patterns that are common to *you*. Remember this step can reflect the first psychology of compassion – enabling you to become more sensitive to that which causes you distress. Beyond noticing the type of thoughts/loops, noticing the way you reacted to your thoughts and emotions (i.e. with invalidation, self-blame or with strategies like distraction or blocking/suppression) is also important. While these ways of coping are understandable, as we explored in Chapters 5 and 15, they are likely to contribute to ongoing difficulties with distress and difficult emotions.

Threat system thinking vs compassionate thinking

So far in this section, we've been focusing on an understanding of our patterns of thinking, and learning to focus our minds on noticing these, and our responses to them, but without trying to change the content of these thought patterns. In this next section, we're going to focus more on this, specifically by looking at ways of bringing your compassionate mind to facilitate a greater balance to the content of your thoughts. In CFT we do this by learning how to create a certain type of emotional tone and content to our thinking that is supportive and compassionate. We refer to this as 'compassionate thought balancing', and we will explore this on the next page.

To help with this process, it can be useful to contrast threat system-based thinking with compassionate-based thinking.

	Threat system thinking	Compassionate thinking
Focus	Narrowly tied to the cause or trigger of the threat	Open and reflective – able to see the 'wood for the trees'
Form	Repetitive, ruminative and lacking flexibility	Flexible and balanced – able to notice but not over-identify, or fuse with thought(s)
Content	Non-rational, negative content – 'better safe than sorry'	Underpinned by care, support, warmth and compassion
Intent	To deal with or avoid threat. The intent is guided by the nature of threat and related emotions. For example: • Linked to anger, the intent is focused on revenge, punishing or dominating • Linked to anxiety, the intent is focused on appeasement, avoidance or submission	To validate and empathise To learn, grown, move forward To offer support and grow

Developing compassionate, balanced thinking

To develop compassionate thinking, first, it might be helpful to consider what compassionate thinking is not. Compassionate thinking is not just positive thinking, although of course, it might include positive thoughts or perspectives on a situation at times. Rather, in contrast to threat system-based thinking, compassionate thinking has a more balanced, empathetic and supportive focus, form, content and intent. So, this isn't just about being 'nice' or thinking 'positive', but about how we can bring wisdom and perspective-taking to our struggles. It's also not just about rationality though; as well as a more rational content in our thoughts, compassionate thinking involves bringing a particular type of emotional tone that is linked to a genuine desire to be more caring, supportive and warm.

We will work on how we can do this using the following steps and exercises.

Exercise: Thought-emotion form

To help you begin to bring a different perspective to your thinking, we're going to use a common tool that is often used in other thera- peutic approaches, such as cognitive behavioural therapy (CBT), but with a bit of a twist. The thought form provides a way to outline the type and content of thoughts that may be related to your dis- tress, and then helps you to develop a more balanced way of dealing with this situation. It's important to emphasise here that this is not about thinking 'positively'; instead, it's how we can bring wisdom, understanding, supportiveness and ultimately, greater balance and flexibility of thinking and reflection about distressing emotions and their triggers.

In this exercise, we will look at how we can use our compassion- ate minds – and in particular, compassionate thinking – to support us at times of emotional struggles. We're going to explore this by using Marta's example of falling out with her best friend. We will then provide you with the opportunity to apply this to your own emotional difficulty. Marta's responses are listed in Worksheet 6 on p. 384, and there is a separate blank worksheet (Worksheet 7) for you to complete on p. 386.

Marta's story

Marta is a thirty-five-year-old single woman. She works long hours in a busy law firm, and outside work spends most of her time with a group of friends from university. On a night out last week, Marta got very drunk and, for a joke, brought up a few of Jennifer's (her best friend's) recent embarrassing dating experiences. The next day, Jennifer sent a long text message saying how hurt she was about what Marta had said and, since then, had refused to respond to Marta's calls or messages. This left Marta with a mix of feelings – anxiety that Jennifer may end their friendship, shame about her drunken behaviour, and guilt about the hurt she had caused. During the past week, Marta had struggled to sleep at night and called in sick from work because she was feeling so distressed at what had happened.

Step 1:

There are two steps to working with this form. The first step involves completing columns one to three on the thought form (p. 386), in which you bring to mind a recent situation that you found difficult, and consider the types of threat-based thoughts you had and how these left you feeling. Take a look at what Marta identified as key thoughts and emotions linked to this difficult situation. Once you've read this, take some time to think about a recent situation you experienced that triggered a distressing emotion. Using the blank form or a separate piece of paper with the same headings/columns, make some notes for columns one, two and three.

Step 2:

The second step involves bringing a more balanced way of thinking to the situation (column four in the form on p. 386). Before trying this, it's important that you take some time connecting with the part of you that can look at this situation in a more balanced, sensitive and helpful way. Spend 2 or 3 minutes engaging your compassionate mind, initially connecting with your soothing breathing, and then linking in with the qualities of your compassionate self – caring-commitment, wisdom and strength. You will also notice that there are different subheadings (empathy and validation for your distress, compassionate attention, compassionate thinking and compassion-ate behaviour) in column four. Let's have a look at the subheadings (taking one at a time), again using Marta's answers as an example (p. 384).

Empathy and validation for your distress

As we discussed earlier in the book, a common struggle for many people is to invalidate their emotional experiences, indicating that something is wrong with them. So, an important step when we're doing this work is to start with where we are – to validate our feelings and to under-stand empathetically how it makes sense that we feel the way we do. Here, Marta responded:

> It's understandable that you're feeling very distressed about what happened. Jen has been your best friend for so many years, and it's scary and really upsetting to imagine that what hap-pened might end your friendship.

Compassionate attention

When our threat emotions are triggered, our attention and thinking often get dragged along in tow, further fuelling distressing feelings. So, it's important to notice where your attention is being pulled to, and instead, try to direct this in a more helpful way. This might be noticing and stepping back from negative, catastrophic 'loops in the mind', or trying to focus on something that provides a broader and more helpful context (e.g. by paying attention to occasions when things have been different/when things went well). Marta responded:

Try to step back from worst-case scenario thoughts where you can. Remember that you and Jen have fallen out many times over the years, but always find a way to patch things up again.

Compassionate thinking

Rather than beating ourselves up (self-criticism), replaying the event over and over searching for why we did something (rumination), or getting caught up with catastrophic predictions of how things might end up in the future (worry), it's important to step out of threat-system thinking, and find a more balanced, helpful alternative in a way that has the intention to be supportive and caring. As we discussed earlier, compassionate thinking isn't so much about being nice, but about the intention to be helpful and supportive, rather than react out of fear, anger or shame. As a prompt, it can be useful to consider what you might say to a friend who was going through a similar struggle, or trying to take a different perspective. Marta responded:

I made a bad mistake, but I never intended to hurt Jen. I feel really sad for hurting Jen, and for how she must be feeling let down by my actions. I will do my best to make this up to her – I can and will be a better friend to her in the future.

The following 'tips and hints' box lists some generic examples of compassionate thoughts. Over time and practice, you'll find your own statements that are helpful for the particular situation you're struggling with.

Tips and hints: Examples of compassionate thoughts/

statements

- It is understandable that I feel like this

- Life is hard and other people experience situations like this

- I have had difficult times in the past and have worked through them (perhaps actively think of examples demonstrating this is true)

- My automatic 'better safe than sorry', threat-detection system has been activated, so I'm likely to think in a biased way. This is understandable and not my fault

- This moment of pain/sorrow/suffering is a natural part of life and will pass

- This is a moment of distress and suffering – everyone has moments like this in life

- Like all emotions, this will stay for a while but at some stage fade away

- The thoughts are just events in my mind, rather than reflections about me

- Just because this is hard, it doesn't mean that things will always be hard

- Although unpleasant, my compassionate self can help me to tolerate this

- Perhaps I can look at the bigger picture – is there anything I'm missing, or minimising because my mind is only focusing on negative experiences?

- If a good friend were experiencing a similar situation, I'd say to them . . .

WORKSHEET 6: MARTA'S COMPASSIONATE THOUGHT RECORD

Column 1 Triggering events	Column 2 Unhelpful or upsetting thoughts and images	Column 3 Feelings and emotions	Column 4 Compassion-focused alternatives – 'helpful' or 'balanced' thoughts	Column 5 Understanding and change in feelings
What actually happened? What was the trigger?	*What am I thinking about others and their thoughts about me? What am I thinking about myself?*	*What are my main feelings and emotions?*	*What would I say to a friend? What compassionate alternatives might there be?*	*Write down any change in your feelings*
'I got drunk on a night out with friends and said some horrible things about my best friend. Since then she's not been speaking to me.'	'Jen's never going to forgive me – she won't be my friend anymore.' 'The other girls will be on her side.' 'I can't believe I said what I did – I messed up massively. I'm such an idiot.'	'I feel anxious, ashamed and alone.'	**Empathy for my distress** 'It's understandable that you're feeling very distressed about what happened. Jen has been your best friend for so many years, and it's scary and really upsetting to imagine that this might end your friendship.' **Compassionate attention** 'Try to step back from worst-case-scenario thoughts where	'I still feel bad for what I did, but less ashamed than previously.' 'I want to be a better person and make it up to her.'

you can. Remember that you and Jen have fallen out many times, but always find a way to patch things up again.'

Compassionate thinking

'I made a bad mistake, but I never intended to hurt Jen. I realise we all mess up sometimes. I feel really sad for hurting Jen, and for how she must be feeling let down by my actions. I will do my best to make this up to her – I can and will be a better friend to her in the future.'

Compassionate behaviour

'Although it is hard, I am going to tolerate my fear about the relationship ending and keep on trying to make contact. When I get a chance, I'm going to apologise and work on a way to not repeat this type of behaviour in the future. I'm going to speak to the other girls that were out that night, and find a way through this.'

WORKSHEET 7: COMPASSIONATE THOUGHT RECORD

Column 1 Triggering events	Column 2 Unhelpful or upset-ting thoughts and images	Column 3 Feelings and emotions	Column 4 Compassion-focused alternatives – 'helpful' or 'balanced' thoughts	Column 5 Understanding and change in feelings
What actually happened? What was the trigger?	What am I thinking about others and their thoughts about me? What am I thinking about myself?	What are my main feelings and emotions?	What would I say to a friend? What compassionate alternatives might there be?	Write down any change in your feelings
			Empathy for my distress	
			Compassionate attention	

Compassionate thinking	**Compassionate behaviour**

Compassionate behaviour

Along with bringing a different way of thinking about the distressing situation, we also want to employ your compassionate self to engage in wise action. For example, if you are avoiding a situation or finding something difficult to do, how can your compassionate self help you? What can you do that might bring about positive change? Can you ask for support from a family member or a friend, so that you can move in a direction that will help you to alleviate some of your difficulties?

> *Marta's answer – 'Although it is hard, I am going to tolerate my fear about the relationship ending and keep on trying to make contact. When I get a chance, I'm going to apologise and work on a way to not repeat this type of behaviour in the future. I'm going to speak to the other girls that were out that night, and find a way through this.'*

Once you have completed your responses in column four, engage your soothing breathing and compassionate self and spend some time reading over what you've put down in this column, with a warm, caring inner voice tone. Then write down how you feel now in column five.

> *Marta's answer – 'I still feel bad about what I did, but I'm more connected to feeling sad and guilty for hurting Jen than worrying about the type of person I am, or whether I'll be left alone. I really want to make this up to her.'*

Top tips – using thought forms

- Try using this thought form across different occasions when you experienced emotional difficulties

- Before you try to engage in column four, spend some time getting connected to your compassionate mind. See if you can connect to your soothing breathing and the caring-commitment, wisdom and

> strength of your compassionate self. When you feel connected, use this part of you to bring a new, compassionate perspective in the final column
>
> - Try not to feel like there is a 'right' way of doing these forms – just use the example given on p. 384, but mostly, allow yourself to be guided by your compassionate self

Compassionate flash cards/notes on your smartphone

In my clinical work, I often find that compassionate thought forms can make a significant difference in helping people better manage their emotions – in fact, I also find that they're very helpful personally, when I'm dealing with emotional difficulties. However, it's not always possible to carry spare forms around in your pocket or bag so that they're available to use when you need them! One way to navigate this is to use flash cards, or even your smartphone to record your thoughts.

There are different ways to do this. You could write down some supportive, helpful statements on the flash card (or smartphone), and then access these when you need to. Again, the key thing here is to read them from a compassionate part of you, with a warm and caring voice tone. You might also find it helpful to have something else that prompts you to engage with yourself with greater compassion; for example, a picture or a phrase that is meaningful to you. The motivation here is to try to use this to stimulate a more caring, supportive way of thinking about, and coping with, the difficulty that you're experiencing.

Key reflections

- In this chapter, we've looked at how bringing a compassionate approach to thinking about distressing situations and emotions can help to create a more balanced perspective, and regulate the emotional experience

- Thought forms can be a helpful way to work through an emotional difficulty in a step-by-step way

SECTION SIX

Compassionate futures – sustaining your compassionate mind

As we come to the end of this book, and your journey working with emotional difficulties, it may become clear that this is a stage of the journey, rather than the destination itself. We've covered an awful lot in this book. Ideas about what emotions are, why they can cause us difficulties, and explored the concept of emotion regulation. We've discussed evolutionary ideas, loops in the mind and the three systems emotion regulation model. We've spent time developing various 'compassionate mind' skills, such as mindfulness, breathing and imagery. And we've also spent some time thinking about and seeing how we can use a compassion-focused emotional regulation approach to working with our difficult feelings and emotions. I hope that through all of this, you've been able to learn a lot more about yourself and your emotions, and how developing compassion may help you to deal with them.

21 Sustaining healthy emotion regulation

As with many things in life, setbacks are often the rule, not the exception! So, opening our minds to be aware of this reality, and finding ways for us to work in a supportive and understanding way with this is a great example of embodying compassion. In this chapter, we will explore healthy ways to deal with setbacks, but before we do this, it can be helpful to hold in our minds what we've learned and accomplished while working through this book. To do this, it can be useful to make a few notes on some paper, your computer or phone in answer to the following questions:

- What have I learned during the book?

- What has changed? How do I manage my emotions differently now?

- What challenges have I faced while doing this?

- What skills have I developed in working with difficult emotions?

- What challenges do I face in continuing to develop my emotion regulation skills in the future?

Try to reflect on these questions through the lens of your compassionate mind – the part of you that will help give an accurate reflection of how you're getting on, and what might be needed going forward.

Continue to work out!

We've been using comparisons to physical health throughout this book, and another one might be helpful here too. For a moment, consider how this book has been like doing an eight-week introductory training schedule at your local gym . . . hard at first, but over time you begin to notice some changes! But just like the gym, if you stop engaging in the practices and skills that you've learned throughout this book, it's likely some of the progress you made will dissipate. So, it's important to continue to pick the book up from time to time, rereading sections again, and as time progresses, recognise that the nature of our emotions and difficulties we have with them can evolve.

With this in mind, it might be helpful for you to connect one last time in this book to your compassionate self. Take a few moments tapping into your breathing rhythm and then qualities of your compassionate self. When you feel ready, what would your compassionate self see as some of the difficulties you might face with your emotions in the weeks and months ahead? Given this awareness, what wise intention could you hold, or action could you take, that will help you work with these difficulties?

Deepening emotion regulation skills – online chapters

As with learning a new language, musical instrument or sport, we develop and deepen our abilities as we spend more time practising and applying what we know already. It's similar to your emotion regulation skills. With this in mind, and appreciation for the wisdom, strength and commitment that you've already shown in turning towards difficult emotions throughout this book, I wanted to provide some further bonus material online that you might find beneficial. The focus of these extra chapters is on specific emotions that we may experience particular difficulties with, and broadly, the concepts of:

1. *Too much emotion:* This is when we struggle with an emotion that turns up too often, too powerfully, or for too long, and which we feel unable to down-regulate in a helpful way.

2. *Too little emotion:* When we struggle with an emotion because it turns up too infrequently, or too quietly when triggered, or over which we have little ability to experience or express (or more generally,

'up-regulate') in a way that would be helpful to us or others if we could.

This online material looks at specific emotions that we can have 'too much' or 'too little' of – anger, anxiety and sadness. They build upon the material that you've been working through in this book, and upon the skills you've developed in using your compassionate mind to approach emotional difficulties. They can be accessed for free here: https://overcoming.co.uk/715/resources-to-download

I hope you find them helpful!

Conclusion

I'd like to take this opportunity to thank you for reading this book, and for having the courage to try to work with whichever emotions you find difficult in life. Please do have a look through the resources section at the end of the book, and check out www.balancedminds.com for some audio guides similar to the ones that we've gone through in the text here. You might also find it helpful to look at www.balancedminds.com for local or online compassionate mind training (CMT) courses that can support the development of your compassionate mind skills.

At the end of our journey together, I would like to wish you all the best with your ongoing travel. Know that I will also continue to use the insights and skills outlined here when working with my emotions too! So, for all of you:

May you continue to have the commitment, wisdom and strength to approach your difficult emotions with compassion, and the dedication to work to alleviate these in wise and skillful ways.

Compassionate wishes,

Chris

References

Aldao, A., Nolen-Hoeksema, S., & Schweizer, S. (2010). Emotion-regulation strategies across psychopathology: A meta-analytic review. *Clinical psychology review, 30*(2), 217–237.

Arch, J. J., & Craske, M. G. (2006). Mechanisms of mindfulness: Emotion regulation following a focused breathing induction. *Behaviour Research and Therapy, 44*(12), 1849–1858.

Baer, R. A., Lykins, E. L., & Peters, J. R. (2012). Mindfulness and self-compassion as predictors of psychological wellbeing in long-term meditators and matched non meditators. *The Journal of Positive Psychology, 7*(3), 230–238.

Beevers, C. G., Wells, T. T., & McGeary, J. E. (2009). The BDNF Val66Met polymorphism is associated with rumination in healthy adults. *Emotion, 9*(4), 579.

Blackhart, G. C., Nelson, B. C., Knowles, M. L., & Baumeister, R. F. (2009). Rejection elicits emotional reactions but neither causes immediate distress nor lowers self-esteem: A meta-analytic review of 192 studies on social exclusion. *Personality and Social Psychology Review, 13*(4), 269–309.

Bowlby, J. (1988). The role of attachment in personality development. *A secure base: Parent-child attachment and healthy human development,* 119–136.

Brach, T. (2013). *True refuge: Finding peace and freedom in your own awakened heart.* Bantam.

Caldwell, Y. T., & Steffen, P. R. (2018). Adding HRV biofeedback to psychotherapy increases heart rate variability and improves the treatment of major depressive disorder. *International Journal of Psychophysiology, 131,* 96–101.

Carney, D., Cuddy, A. & Yap, A. (2010). Power posing brief nonverbal displays affect neuroendocrine levels and risk tolerance. *Psychological Science, 21*, 1363–1368.

Carter, C. S. (2017). Oxytocin and Human Evolution. In R. Hurlemann & V. Grinevich (eds), *Behavioral Pharmacology of Neuropeptides: Oxytocin. Current Topics in Behavioral Neurosciences, 35*.

Carvalho, S., Dinis, A., Pinto-Gouveia, J., & Estanqueiro, C. (2015). Memories of shame experiences with others and depression symptoms: The mediating role of experiential avoidance. *Clinical Psychology & Psychotherapy, 22*(1), 32–44.

Chalmers, J. A., Quintana, D. S., Maree, J., Abbott, A., & Kemp, A. H. (2014). Anxiety disorders are associated with reduced heart rate variability: a meta-analysis. *Frontiers in Psychiatry, 5*, 80.

Cheung, M. P., Gilbert, P., & Irons, C. (2004). An exploration of shame, social rank and rumination in relation to depression. *Personality and Individual Differences, 36*(5), 1143–1153.

Coan, J. A., Schaefer, H. S., & Davidson, R. J. (2006). Lending a hand: Social regulation of the neural response to threat. *Psychological Science, 17*(12), 1032–1039.

Condon, P., Desbordes, G., Miller, W. B., & DeSteno, D. (2013). Meditation increases compassionate responses to suffering. *Psychological Science, 24*(10), 2125–2127.

Cunha, M., & Paiva, M. J. (2012). Text anxiety in adolescents: The role of self-criticism and acceptance and mindfulness skills. *The Spanish Journal of Psychology, 15*(2), 533–543.

Cunningham, K. C., Davis, J. L., Wilson, S. M., & Resick, P. A. (2018). A relative weights comparison of trauma-related shame and guilt as predictors of DSM-5 posttraumatic stress disorder symptom severity among US veterans and military members. *British Journal of Clinical Psychology, 57*(2), 163–176.

Darwin, C. (1872). *The Expression of the Emotions in Man and Animals.* London: Fontana Press.

Davis, D. E., Choe, E., Meyers, J., Wade, N., Varjas, K., Gifford, A., . . . & Worthington Jr, E. L. (2016). Thankful for the little things: A meta-analysis of gratitude interventions. *Journal of Counseling Psychology, 63*(1), 20.

Depue, R. A., & Morrone-Strupinsky, J. V. (2005) A neurobehavioral model of affiliative bonding. *Behavioral and Brain Sciences;* 28: 313–395.

Cândea, D. M., & Szentagotai-Tăta, A. (2018). Shame-proneness, guilt-proneness and anxiety symptoms: A meta-analysis. *Journal of Anxiety Disorders, 58,* 78.

Dickerson, S. S., Gruenewald, T. L., & Kemeny, M. E. (2004). When the social self is threatened: Shame, physiology, and health. *Journal of Personality, 72*(6), 1191–1216.

Diedrich, A., Hofmann, S. G., Cuijpers, P., & Berking, M. (2016). Self-compassion enhances the efficacy of explicit cognitive reappraisal as an emotion regulation strategy in individuals with major depressive disorder. *Behaviour Research and Therapy, 82,* 1–10.

Duarte, C., Ferreira, C., & Pinto-Gouveia, J. (2016). At the core of eating disorders: Overvaluation, social rank, self-criticism and shame in anorexia, bulimia and binge eating disorder. *Comprehensive Psychiatry, 66,* 123–131.

Eisenberger, N. I., Jarcho, J. M., Lieberman, M. D., & Naliboff, B. D. (2006). An experimental study of shared sensitivity to physical pain and social rejection. *Pain, 126*(1–3), 132–138.

Fayant, M. P., Muller, D., Hubertus Joseph Hartgerink, C., & Lantian, A. (2014). Is ostracism by a despised outgroup really hurtful? A replication and extension of Gonsalkorale and Williams (2007). *Social Psychology, 45*(6), 489.

Finlay-Jones, A. L., Rees, C. S., & Kane, R. T. (2015). Self-compassion, emotion regulation and stress among Australian psychologists: Testing an emotion regulation model of self-compassion using structural equation modeling. *PloS one, 10*(7), e0133481.

Fonagy, P., Gergely, G., & Target, M. (2007). The parent-infant dyad and the construction of the subjective self. *Journal of Child Psychology and Psychiatry, 48*, 288–328.

Fehr, B., & Russell, A. (1984). Concept of emotion viewed from a proto-type perspective. *Journal of Experimental Psychology: General, 113*(3), 464–486.

Ferreira, C., Mendes, A. L., & Trindade, I. A. (2018). Do shame and perfectionistic self-presentation explain the link between early affiliative memories and eating psychopathology? *Psychology, Health & Medicine, 23*(5), 628–634.

Fraley, R. C. (2002). Attachment stability from infancy to adulthood: Meta-analysis and dynamic modeling of developmental mechanisms. *Personality and Social Psychology Review, 6*, 123–151.

Fredrickson, B. L. (2013). Positive emotions broaden and build. In *Advances in Experimental Social Psychology* (Vol. 47, pp. 1–53). Academic Press.

Frijda, N. H. (1986). *The Emotions*. Cambridge: Cambridge University Press.

Garnefski, N., Kraaij, V., & Spinhoven, P. (2001). Negative life events, cognitive emotion regulation and emotional problems. *Personality and Individual Differences, 30*(8), 1311–1327.

Garland, E. L., Fredrickson, B., Kring, A. M., Johnson, D. P., Meyer, P. S., & Penn, D. L. (2010). Upward spirals of positive emotions counter downward spirals of negativity: Insights from the broaden-and-build theory and affective neuroscience on the treatment of emotion dysfunctions and deficits in psychopathology. *Clinical Psychology Review, 30*(7), 849–864.

Gilbert, P. (1997). The evolution of social attractiveness and its role in shame, humiliation, guilt and therapy. *British Journal of Medical Psychology, 70*(2), 113–147.

Gilbert, P. (1998). What is shame? Some core issues and controversies.

In P. Gilbert & B. Andrews (eds), *Series in affective science. Shame: Interpersonal behaviour, psychopathology, and culture* (pp. 3–38). New York, NY: Oxford University Press.

Gilbert, P. (2009). Introducing compassion-focused therapy. *Advances in Psychiatric Treatment, 15*(3), 199–208.

Gilbert, P. (2010). *The Compassionate Mind: A New Approach to Life's Challenges.* New Harbinger Publications.

Gilbert, P. (2015). An evolutionary approach to emotion in mental health with a focus on affiliative emotions. *Emotion Review, 7*(3), 230–237.

Gilbert, P., Broomhead, C., Irons, C., McEwan, K., Bellew, R., Mills, A., Gale, C. & Knibb, R. (2007). Development of a striving to avoid inferiority scale. *British Journal of Social Psychology, 46*(3), 633–648.

Gilbert, P., Cheung, M. S. P., Grandfield, T., Campey, F., & Irons, C. (2003). Recall of threat and submissiveness in childhood: Development of a new scale and its relationship with depression, social comparison and shame. *Clinical Psychology & Psychotherapy: An International Journal of Theory & Practice, 10*(2), 108–115.

Gilbert, P., & Choden (2013) *Mindful Compassion.* London: Constable and Robinson.

Gilbert, P., McEwan, K., Catarino, F., & Baião, R. (2014). Fears of negative emotions in relation to fears of happiness, compassion, alexithymia and psychopathology in a depressed population: A preliminary study. *Journal of Depression and Anxiety,* S2 (01).

Goldberg, S. B., Tucker, R. P., Greene, P. A., Davidson, R. J., Wampold, B. E., Kearney, D. J., & Simpson, T. L. (2018). Mindfulness-based interventions for psychiatric disorders: A systematic review and meta-analysis. *Clinical Psychology Review, 59,* 52–60.

Graser, J., & Stangier, U. (2018). Compassion and Loving-Kindness Meditation: An Overview and Prospects for the Application in Clinical Samples. *Harvard Review of Psychiatry, 26*(4), 201–215.

Gross, J. J. (2015). Emotion regulation: Current status and future prospects. *Psychological Inquiry, 26*(1), 1–26.

Gupta, S., Zachary Rosenthal, M., Mancini, A. D., Cheavens, J. S., & Lynch, T. R. (2008). Emotion regulation skills mediate the effects of shame on eating disorder symptoms in women. *Eating Disorders, 16*(5), 405–417.

Hanson, R. (2013). *Hardwiring Happiness: The Practical Science of Reshaping Your Brain and Your Life.* Random House.

Hayes, S. C., Wilson, K. G., Gifford, E. V., Follette, V. M., & Strosahl, K. (1996). Experiential avoidance and behavioral disorders: A functional dimensional approach to diagnosis and treatment. *Journal of Consulting and Clinical Psychology, 64*(6), 1152–1168.

Hebb, D. O. (1949). *The Organization of Behavior.* New York: Wiley & Sons.

Heinrichs, M., Baumgartner, T., Kirschbaum, C., & Ehlert, U. (2003). Social support and oxytocin interact to suppress cortisol and subjective responses to psychosocial stress. *Biological Psychiatry, 54*(12), 1389–1398.

Hoffman, S. (2016). *Emotion in Therapy: From Science to Practice.* London: Guildford Press.

Irons, C., Gilbert, P., Baldwin, M. W., Baccus, J. R., & Palmer, M. (2006). Parental recall, attachment relating and self-attacking/self-reassurance: Their relationship with depression. *British Journal of Clinical Psychology, 45*(3), 297–308.

Jacquet, J. (2016). *Is shame necessary?: New uses for an old tool.* Vintage.

Jazaieri, H., McGonigal, K., Jinpa, T., Doty, J. R., Gross, J. J., & Goldin, P. R. (2014). A randomized controlled trial of compassion cultivation training: Effects on mindfulness, affect, and emotion regulation. *Motivation and Emotion, 38*(1), 23–35.

Johnson, E. A., & O'Brien, K. A. (2013). Self-compassion soothes the savage ego-threat system: Effects on negative affect, shame, rumination, and depressive symptoms. *Journal of Social and Clinical Psychology*, 32(9), 939–963.

Kabat-Zinn, J. (2003). Mindfulness-based interventions in context: Past, present, and future. *Clinical Psychology: Science and Practice, 10*, 144–156.

Kashdan, T. B., Ferssizidis, P., Collins, R. L., & Muraven, M. (2010). Emotion differentiation as resilience against excessive alcohol use: An ecological momentary assessment in underage social drinkers. *Psychological Science, 21*(9), 1341–1347.

Khanipour, H., Hakim Shooshtari, M., & Bidaki, R. (2016). Suicide probability in adolescents with a history of childhood maltreatment: the role of non-suicidal self-injury, emotion regulation difficulties, and forms of self-criticism. *International Journal of High Risk Behaviors and Addiction, 5*(2), e23675–e23675.

Kopala-Sibley, D. C., Zuroff, D. C., Leybman, M. J., & Hope, N. (2013). Recalled peer relationship experiences and current levels of self-criticism and self-reassurance. *Psychology and Psychotherapy: Theory, Research and Practice, 86*(1), 33–51.

Kim, S., Thibodeau, R., & Jorgensen, R. S. (2011). Shame, guilt, and depressive symptoms: A meta-analytic review. *Psychological Bulletin, 137*(1), 68.

Kirby, J. N. (2017). Compassion interventions: the programmes, the evidence, and implications for research and practice. *Psychology and Psychotherapy: Theory, Research and Practice, 90*(3), 432–455.

Kircanski, K., Lieberman, M. D., & Craske, M. G. (2012). Feelings into words: contributions of language to exposure therapy. *Psychological Science, 23*(10), 1086–1091.

Kraft, T. L., & Pressman, S. D. (2012). Grin and bear it: The influence of manipulated facial expression on the stress response. *Psychological Science, 23*(11), 1372–1378.

Kuyken, W., Watkins, E., Holden, E., White, K., Taylor, R. S., Byford, S.,

. . . & Dalgleish, T. (2010). How does mindfulness-based cognitive therapy work?. *Behaviour Research and Therapy, 48*(11), 1105.

Lin, I. M., Tai, L. Y., & Fan, S. Y. (2014). Breathing at a rate of 5.5 breaths per minute with equal inhalation-to-exhalation ratio increases heart rate variability. *International Journal of Psychophysiology, 91*(3), 206–211.

Lindsay-Hartz, J., de Rivera, J., & Mascolo, M. F. (1995). Differentiating guilt and shame and their effects on motivation. In J. P. Tangney & K. W. Fischer (eds), *Self-conscious emotions: The psychology of shame, guilt, embarrassment, and pride* (pp. 274–300). New York, NY, US: Guilford Press.

Longe, O., Maratos, F. A., Gilbert, P., Evans, G., Volker, F., Rockliff, H., & Rippon, G. (2010). Having a word with yourself: Neural correlates of self-criticism and self-reassurance. *NeuroImage, 49*(2), 1849–1856.

Matos, M., Duarte, C., Duarte, J., Pinto-Gouveia, J., Petrocchi, N., Basran, J., & Gilbert, P. (2017). Psychological and physiological effects of compassionate mind training: a pilot randomized controlled study. *Mindfulness, 8*(6), 1699–1712.

Matos, M., Pinto-Gouveia, J., & Duarte, C. (2013). Internalizing early memories of shame and lack of safeness and warmth: The mediating role of shame on depression. *Behavioural and Cognitive Psychotherapy, 41*(4), 479–493.

Manfredi, C., Caselli, G., Rovetto, F., Rebecchi, D., Ruggiero, G. M., Sassaroli, S., & Spada, M. M. (2011). Temperament and parental styles as predictors of ruminative brooding and worry. *Personality and Individual Differences, 50*(2), 186–191.

Orth, U., Berking, M., & Burkhardt, S. (2006). Self-conscious emotions and depression: Rumination explains why shame but not guilt is maladaptive. *Personality and Social Psychology Bulletin, 32*(12), 1608–1619.

Kemp, A. H., Quintana, D. S., Gray, M. A., Felmingham, K. L., Brown, K., & Gatt, J. M. (2010). Impact of depression and antidepressant treatment on heart rate variability: a review and meta-analysis. *Biological Psychiatry, 67*(11), 1067–1074.

Kokkonen, P., Karvonen, J. T., Veijola, J., Läksy, K., Jokelainen, J., Järvelin, M. R., & Joukamaa, M. (2001). Prevalence and sociodemographic correlates of alexithymia in a population sample of young adults. *Comprehensive Psychiatry, 42*(6), 471–476.

Nummenmaa, L., Glerean, E., Hari, R., & Hietanen, J. K. (2014). Bodily maps of emotions. *Proceedings of the National Academy of Sciences, 111*(2), 646–651.

Opialla, S., Lutz, J., Scherpiet, S., Hittmeyer, A., Jäncke, L., Rufer, M., . . . & Brühl, A. B. (2015). Neural circuits of emotion regulation: A comparison of mindfulness-based and cognitive reappraisal strategies. *European Archives of Psychiatry and Clinical Neuroscience, 265*(1), 45–55.

Oxford Dictionary (2018). Oxford University Press, Oxford, viewed 14 July 2018, https://en.oxforddictionaries.com

Pandey, R., Saxena, P., & Dubey, A. (2011). Emotion regulation difficulties in alexithymia and mental health. *Europe's Journal of Psychology, 7*(4), 604–623.

Panksepp, J. (1998) *Affective Neuroscience*. Oxford University Press.

Pascuzzo, K., Moss, E., & Cyr, C. (2015). Attachment and emotion regulation strategies in predicting adult psychopathology. *SAGE Open, 5*(3), 2158244015604695.

Pennebaker, J. W., Smyth, J. (2016). *Opening up by writing it down: The healing power of expressive writing* (3rd ed.). New York, NY: Guilford

Pond Jr, R. S., Kashdan, T. B., DeWall, C. N., Savostyanova, A., Lambert, N. M., & Fincham, F. D. (2012). Emotion differentiation moderates aggressive tendencies in angry people: A daily diary analysis. *Emotion, 12*(2), 326.

Priel, B., & Shahar, G. (2000). Dependency, self-criticism, social context and distress: Comparing moderating and mediating models. *Personality and Individual Differences, 28*(3), 515–525.

Richards, H. J., Benson, V., Donnelly, N., & Hadwin, J. A. (2014). Exploring the function of selective attention and hypervigilance for threat in anxiety. *Clinical Psychology Review*, 34(1), 1–13.

Roemer, L., Williston, S. K., & Rollins, L. G. (2015). Mindfulness and emotion regulation. *Current Opinion in Psychology*, 3, 52–57.

Sapolsky, R. M. (2004). *Why zebras don't get ulcers*. London, UK: St Martin's Press.

Sifneos, P. E. (1973). The prevalence of 'alexithymic'characteristics in psychosomatic patients. *Psychotherapy and Psychosomatics*, 22(2–6), 255–262.

Scoglio, A. A., Rudat, D. A., Garvert, D., Jarmolowski, M., Jackson, C., & Herman, J. L. (2018). Self-compassion and responses to trauma: The role of emotion regulation. *Journal of Interpersonal Violence*, 33(13), 2016–2036.

Small, D., Lerner, J., & Fischhoff, B. (2006). Emotion Priming and Attributions for Terrorism: Americans' Reactions in a National Field Experiment. *Political Psychology*, 27(2), 289–298.

Spinkins, P. (2017). Prehistoric origins: The compassion of far distant strangers. In P. Gilbert (ed.), *Compassion*. Taylor and Francis.

Stracke, F., Martin, L. L., & Stepper, S. (1988). Inhibiting and facilitating conditions of the human smile: A nonobtrusive test of the facial feedback hypothesis. *Journal of Personality and Social Psychology*, 54(5), 768.

Tierney, S., & Fox, J. R. (2010). Living with the anorexic voice: A thematic analysis. *Psychology and Psychotherapy: Theory, Research and Practice*, 83(3), 243–254.

Tomkins, S. S. (1970). Affect as the primary motivational system. In M. B. Arnold (ed.), *Feelings and emotions: The Loyola symposium* (pp. 101–110). New York: Academic Press.

Trompetter, H. R., de Kleine, E., & Bohlmeijer, E. T. (2017). Why does positive mental health buffer against psychopathology? An exploratory study on self-compassion as a resilience mechanism and adaptive emotion regulation strategy. *Cognitive Therapy and Research, 41*(3), 459–468.

Tsai, J. L., Knutson, B., & Fung, H. H. (2006). Cultural variation in affect valuation. *Journal of Personality and Social Psychology, 90*(2), 288.

Velotti, P., Garofalo, C., Bottazzi, F., & Caretti, V. (2017). Faces of shame: implications for self-esteem, emotion regulation, aggression, and well-being. *The Journal of Psychology, 151*(2), 171–184.

Williams, D. P., Cash, C., Rankin, C., Bernardi, A., Koenig, J., & Thayer, J. F. (2015). Resting heart rate variability predicts self-reported difficulties in emotion regulation: A focus on different facets of emotion regulation. *Frontiers in Psychology, 6*, 261.

Wood, L., & Irons, C. (2016). Exploring the associations between social rank and external shame with experiences of psychosis. *Behavioural and Cognitive Psychotherapy, 44*(5), 527–538.

Zadro, L., Williams, K. D., & Richardson, R. (2004). How low can you go? Ostracism by a computer is sufficient to lower self-reported levels of belonging, control, self-esteem, and meaningful existence. *Journal of Experimental Social Psychology, 40*(4), 560–567.

Zarei, M., Momeni, F., & Mohammadkhani, P. (2018). The Mediating Role of Cognitive Flexibility, Shame and Emotion Dysregulation Between Neuroticism and Depression. *Iranian Rehabilitation Journal, 16*(1), 61–68.

Zhou, T., & Bishop, G. D. (2012). Culture moderates the cardiovascular consequences of anger regulation strategy. *International Journal of Psychophysiology, 86*(3), 291–298.

Index

'5-4-3-2-1 grounding' 273

A

acceptance and commitment
    therapy (ACT) 369–70
accepting emotions 263–5, 277
acting techniques 154–9
action tendencies 14
adaptive advantages 25
affect regulation system *30*
affection 11, 57
'after' phase (PDA) 347–8, *349*, 351
alexithymia 72–3, 214
alleviating distress 90–3
anchor for the mind *see* mindfulness
anger 27
    cardiovascular responses 53
    and compassion 96
    and emotion dysregulation 67
    emotions about emotions 76–8,
        306–7
    emotions 'family tree' *221*
    listening to 298–300
    'multiple selves' 297
    style of thinking 374
    wisdom of emotions *246*
    at work 295–6
anti-ideal 315–16
anticipating future situations
    196–7
anxieties 27
    avoiding 253

emotions about emotions 76–8,
    306–7
emotions 'family tree' *221*
fears of compassion 171
listening to 300–3
'multiple selves' 297
style of thinking 373
wisdom of emotions *246*
arousal 15, *143*, 144, 183
assertiveness 291–3
attachment 57, 58–61
attachment theory 60–1
attention 15, 106–9, 205
    defining 106
    mind awareness 107
    mindful body scan 118–20
    mindfulness 111
    power of 108–9
    and self-criticism 328
    soothing rhythm breathing 133
    top tips 123–4
    training and awareness 111
    triggers of difficult emotions
        183–91
avoidance, blocking and
    suppression 75
awareness of emotions 177, 205–10
    ERM 69, 71–2, *202*
    locating on body 206–7
    worksheet *81*
awareness of self-criticism
    335–6

awareness of triggers 181–200
  of difficult emotions 183–91
  emotion regulation 177
  ERM *69, 181*
  external triggers 187–9
  internal triggers 189–91
  managing emotions 70–1
  worksheet *81*

B

'bad' emotions 21
basic emotions 219–20
Bateman, Anthony 240
behaviour
  and impulses 204
  old brain competencies 40
  and self-criticism 328
'being and non-wanting' 56
blaming others 332
blocked, thwarted or disappointed
  situations 186
blocking assertiveness 292
blocking compassion 168
body language 154 *see also* posture
Bolt, Usain 347
bonding 57
Bowlby, John 58–9, 60
brains 102–3
breathing
  affecting mind and body 131–2
  and CFT 132–4
  and posture 129
  slowing down 133, 134–6
breathing rhythms 132
bringing compassion to shame
  exercises 324–6
bringing compassion to the situation
  exercises 308

Buddha 109
bullying 144

C

calm-place imagery 147–8
calmness 27, 56, *221*
care and affection signals 59
caring 33–4, 58–61, 86–7 *see also*
  motivation
caring-commitment 152, 157, 164–5,
  340
children punished for anger 52
cognitive behavioural therapy (CBT)
  369
commitment 234, 262, 266
compassion
  alleviating distress 90–3
  care for well-being 86–7
  definitions 85–6, 149
  and emotional difficulties 4–5
  empathy 89
  fears 168, 171
  fears, blocks and resistances
    (FBR) 168–9
  and friends and family 145
  many faces of 94–6
  misunderstandings 169–71
  and motivation 100
  non-judgement 90
  sensitivity to distress 87, 95
  shadow and difficult emotions
    96–7
  and shame 321–6
  skills *94*
  sympathy 87–8
  three flows of 98–9
  tolerating excesses of drive
    system 56

compassion-focused emotion
  regulation skills (CERS)
    awareness of emotion triggers
      181–200
    awareness of emotions 201–13
    coping with and using emotions
      251–69
    expressing emotions and
      assertiveness 282–94
    intensity of emotions 270–81
    labelling emotions 214–29
    managing shame and self-
      criticism 314–43
    multiple emotional selves 295–
      313
    understanding emotions 230–50
Compassion Focused Therapy (CFT)
  xxiii, 4, 5, 62–4, 128
compassion for others 98
compassion for the angry part of me
  309–10
compassion for the anxious part of
  me 310–11
compassion for the sad part of me
  311–13
compassion from others 98
compassion PDA (pre, during and
  after) 347–53
compassionate acceptance 265–7
compassionate attention 91
compassionate behaviour 92, 388–9
compassionate circles 94
compassionate commitment to
  bringing change 366
compassionate feelings 93
compassionate flash cards 389
compassionate image 275
compassionate imagery 91

compassionate intention 261–3
compassionate ladder 171–3
compassionate letter writing 361–8
    compassionate reading 366–7
    exercises 362–6
    helpful tips 367–8
    managing emotions 364
    setbacks 365–6
    taking responsibility 364–5
    validation and empathy for the
      struggle 363–4
compassionate memory exercises
  153–4
compassionate mind
    benefits 97
    creating 149–50
    developing 93–4
    modifying trigger situations 193–5
    self-criticism 333–43
    and writing 361–2
compassionate mind training
  ('CMT') 5, 55–6, 96–7, 103–5, 173
    see also attention; compassionate
    self; mindfulness; soothing system
compassionate motivation 101–2
compassionate other 161–7
compassionate people 95–6
compassionate reason and thinking
  91–2
compassionate self 149–67
    acting techniques 154–5
    assertiveness 293
    core qualities 150–3
    cultivating 153–4
    distress tolerance 261–3
    embodying 159–61
    exercises 155–8, 159–61, 262–3,
      339–41

memory 153–4

multiple selves 307–9

validating emotions 234–6

compassionate self-correction 341–3

compassionate self-criticism 342

compassionate sensory focusing 92

compassionate thinking 369–90

   developing 378–83

   supporting emotional struggles 379

   thought record *384–7*

   and threat system thinking 377–8

competitive cultures 55

conflicts in threat system emotions 31–2

contentment 27, 56

contentment, soothing and affiliative-focused system *see* soothing system

coping with and using emotions

   CERS 251–4

   ERM 69, 74–5, *252*

   worksheet *81*

coping with emotions 178, 251

'core'/'central' self 296–7

creating a calm place exercise 146–7

creating ideal passionate other exercise 164–6

criticism 144

D

Darwin, Charles 283, 284

depression 171

describing ourselves 48

dichotomous thinking 371

difficult emotions 2–3, 5

   accepting 263–5

author's story 3–4

compassion 4–5, 96–7

recognition of 247–9

shaping 50

discriminating between emotions 225–6

disgust 27, *221*, *246*

distress regulation 58–61

distress to physical pain 25

distress tolerance 88–9, 256, 260–1

drive-excitement system 32–3

drive system 29, 33, 53–6, 62

duration 18

'during' phase (PDA) 347, *349*, 351

E

embarrassment 28

emotion awareness chart 207–9

emotion brain triggers *143*

emotion daily review exercises 218–19

emotion dysregulation 66–7, 70

emotion expression 286–91

emotion patterns 203–5

emotion regulation

   and compassion 97

   compassionate mind 175–9

   defining 65–6

   and self-reflection 80

   and shame 319

   worksheet *81*

emotion regulation model (ERM) 68–75

   awareness of emotions *202*

   awareness of triggers *181*

   coping with and using emotions *252*

difficult emotions *176*
labelling emotions *215*
shame 321–3
understanding emotions *231*, 240–1
emotion regulation skills 257, 345, 394–5
emotion regulation strategies 68
emotion regulation systems *30*
emotional communication 289
emotional experience 219–22
emotional intensity 277–9
emotions xxi–xxv, 11–21
    adaptive advantages 25
    changing with new situations 13
    definitions 11–12
    discriminating between 225–6
    evolution 24–5, 29, 36, 39
    'family tree' *221*, 223
    and feelings 19–20
    functions 26–8
    'good or bad'/'healthy or
        unhealthy' 21
    importance 1–2
    lacking control 78–9, 270
    life without emotion experiment
        23–4
    and moods 20
    and motives 26
    old brain competencies 40
    regulating xxii
    relevance radar 16–17
    shaping *50*
    as a story 17–19, 270
    'threat processing' xxi–xxii
    wisdom of emotions 243–7
emotions about emotions 76–9,
    267–8, 284, 306–7, 314

émouvoir 11
empathy, compassion 89
envy 28
Epictetus (Greek philosopher) 369
evolution xxi, 24–5, 36, 39, 58, 370
evolved function 27–8, 29
experiences 48–9, 51–2, 54–5, *372*
expressing emotions 282–94
    exploring difficulties exercises
        284
    learning to be assertive 291–3
    managing fears exercises 285
    three steps to 286–91
expression *14*, 16, 18
external maintainers of emotion *248*,
    249
external shame 317–18
external triggers *143*, 187–9

F
facial expressions 137–8, 154, 165
falling in love 107
fear of anger toward others 332
feared emotions 332, 335–6
fears *see also* anxieties *246*
fears of compassion 168, 171
feedback 290
feelings *14*, 16, 19–20, 227, 369
'felt-sense' imagery 145
Ferster, Charles 52
first psychology of compassion
    86–90, 93, *94*, 149
focused attention 113–14, 182–3
Fonagy, Peter 240
frequency 18
friends and family 145

G

genes 371–2
Gilbert, Paul 4, 29, 265
'good' emotions 21
gratitude and appreciation 358–60
Greek philosophers 243
Gross, James 65
grounding techniques 272–4
guilt 27, *246*

H

Hanson, Rick 354
happiness 27, *246*
harm avoidance 26
'healthy' emotions 21
heart rate variability (HRV) 131–2
Hoffman, S. 12
holding hands 63
Hong Kong 56

I

ideal compassionate other 161–7
imagery 142–8, 205
images
  compassionate other 165
  and emotion 329–30
  'felt-sense' 145
  and motivations 110
  notes 147
imagination 40, 278
infants' emotional distress 59–60
inner talk 138–40
insecure attachment styles 60
intensity of emotions 18, 255–6
  decreasing 272–7
  increasing 277–80
  modifying 271–2

online materials 280–1
internal maintainers of emotion
  248–9
internal shame 318
internal triggers *143*, 189–91
internalising emotions 53
invalidating emotions 233, 236
Irons, Chris 3–4

J

jealousy 28
joy 27, 53–4, 221, *246*
jumping to conclusions 371

K

Kabat-Zinn, J. 111
key attributes (first psychology) 93,
  94
Kraft, T. L. 137

L

labelling emotions 177, 214–29
  ERM 69, 72–3, *215*
  exercises 224–5, 227
  mixed emotions 226–8
  present moment labelling 217–18
  worksheet *81*
lacking control 78–9, 270
language of assertiveness 292–3
learning from the past exercises
  184–5
letting people of the hook 169
life without emotion thought
  experiment 23–4
listening to emotions 28, 74–5, 243–7
listening to the wisdom of emotions
  exercises 244–5

loops in the mind 41–7, 189
low-arousal positive emotions 56

M

maintaining intention 289
managing emotions 3–4, 364, 369–89
   compassionate balanced thinking
     378–82
   patterns of thoughts 372–4
   thought monitoring 374–7
   threat emotions 373–4
   threat system 377–8
   understanding the way we think
     370–2
'map of emotions in the body' *206*
Marcus Aurelius 369
memories
   compassionate self 153–4
   and emotion labelling 224–5
   and imagery 142–8
   multiple selves exercises 299, 301,
     302
   soothing memory exercise 141–2
   and working models 59
memory writing exercise 358
mentalizing 73–4, 240–3
mind awareness 106–8, 111–12
mind-mindedness 107
mind wandering 110
mindful body scan exercises 118–20
mindful eating exercises 125
mindful walking exercises 124–5
mindfulness
   compassionate mind 106–8
   cycles of *114*
   of daily life 124–6
   definitions 111–12

difficult emotions 257
   difficulties with 122–3
   external focus 116–18
   intensity of emotions 274
   internal anchor 118–22
   managing emotions 112–13
   paying attention 227
   practicing 113–22
   therapies 369–70
   top tips 123–4
mindfulness of breathing exercises
   120–2
mindfulness of emotions
   distress tolerance exercises 257–9
   shape and pattern exercises
     210–13
mindfulness of sound exercises
   116–17
mindfulness practice log 126, *127*
mixed feelings 226–8, 297
modifying situations 193
modifying the intensity of emotions
   271–2
modifying triggers 191–6
moods 20
motivation *14, 15 see also* caring
   and compassion 100
   features of emotions 205
   and self-criticism 328–9, 334–5
motives
   and emotions 26, 28
   old brain competencies 40
'*motivus*' 26
multiple emotional selves 149,
   295–313
   compassion 307–9
   compassion for angry self 309–10

compassion for anxious self
310–11
compassion for sad part 311–12
different selves 296–7
emotions about emotions 306–7
exercises 297–303
multiple self work 304
worksheets *305*

N

negative emotions 97, 354
neurons 102
new brain competencies 40–1, 43, 44, *45*, 276
niceness 169
Nietzsche, Friedrich 332
'no shame and no blame' psychology 296
non-judgement 90
non-verbal behaviours 289
'not doing' 56
'not your fault' insight 296
noticing internal triggers to difficult emotions exercises 190–1

O

old brain competencies 40, 43, 44, *45*
'old brain–new brain' loops 41–7, 107, 110, 170
older adults 197
online materials 394–5
open-awareness mindfulness practice 114
overgeneralising 371
Oxford Dictionary of English 12, 106
oxytocin 57

P

pain 25, 63
painful feelings 251
parasympathetic nervous system 34
'passions' 11
passive aggression 291
patterns of emotions 203–5, 210
patterns of 'mind' 102–3
patterns of thinking 276
patterns (shaping) 317–18
paying attention 109
peacefulness 56
Pennebaker, James 361
physical activities 275–6
physiological responses to threats 29
physiology 14, 204
planning 41
'plays the body' 107–8
positive emotions 354–60
  compassionate mind 97
  different types 355
  and drive system 33
  fearful of expressing 283
  gratitude and appreciation 358–60
  paying attention to 355–7
  recalling 357–8
  regulating negative emotions 354
positive memories exercises 357
posture 128–30, 129–30, 272–3
power of attention 108–9
'pre' phase (PDA) 347, *349*, 350
present-moment awareness 187
present moment labelling 217–18
Pressman, S. D. 137
pride 28
primary emotions 219–20, 314

problematic emotion regulation 68
process of emotions 17–18
proximity seeking 59
psychologies of compassion 86–94,
  149

R
range of emotional experiences
  219–22
recalling positive emotions 357–8
receiver positions 289
recuperation 56
reflections and threat emotions
  302–3
regulating 18
rejection 320–1
relevance radar 16–17
remembering 111
reproduction 53
resistances to compassion 168–9
responses (validation) *see* validating
  emotions
'rest and digest' system 57
restless minds 109–11
ruminating 41, 43, 68, 79

S
sadness 27
  emotions 'family tree' *221*
  listening to 301–2
  'multiple selves' 297
  signalling distress 311–12
  style of thinking 374
  wisdom of emotions *246*
safe emotions *221*
safe haven 59
science of compassion 97

second psychology of compassion
  90–4, 149
secondary emotions 314
secure bases 59
self-awareness 40
self-compassion 98–9, 321
self-criticism 314–43
  compassionate engagement
    339–42
  compassionate mind 333–43
  and compassionate self-correction
    341–3
  and compassionate self exercises
    339–41
  compassionate to 334–5
  evolution 330–1
  fear of aloneness 333
  fear of anger toward others 332
  fear of sadness 333
  and feared emotions 332
  frequency 336
  image and emotion 329–30
  and rumination 79
  self-protection 334
  and shame 315, 321, 327–30
  shaping the mind 327–9
  threat system 339
self-criticism log 336–8
self-monitoring 40
self-protection to dangerous
  situations 51
self-reflection 34–5, 46, 80
sensitive to distress 95
sensory information 142 *see also*
  imagery
setbacks 290–1, 365–6
settling 18

shadows 96–7
shame 27, 76–8, 314–43
  behavioural/action component
    318
  and compassion 324–6, 326
  definitions 315–16
  disconnecting 319–21
  emotion about emotion 76–8
  emotional component 318
  emotions about emotions 284–5
  ERM 321–3
  experiencing 316–17
  externally focused component
    317–18
  facilitating group living 317
  impact on other emotions 319
  internally focused component 318
  physiological component 318
  and self-criticism 315, 327–30, 342
  shape 317–18
  social threat 315
  style of thinking 374
  wisdom of emotions *246*
  without self-criticism 329
shameless people 316
shaping (patterns) 317–18
'situation selection' 196–8
skills of compassion (second
  psychology) 93, *94*
skills-training *94*
slowing down 56, 133, 134–6
smartphones 136–7, 389
social exclusion 316, 320
social shaping 372 *see also*
  experiences
social threats 315
soothing affiliative system 56–8

soothing breathing exercises 260–1
soothing memory exercises 141–2
soothing rhythm breathing (SRB)
  130–4
  exercises 133
  friendly facial expression
    exercises 138
  inner speech exercises 139
  intensity of emotions 274
  slowing down 134–6
  tips and hints 134
soothing system 33–5
  accessing 63
  emotions 56
  evolutionary function 57
  experience-dependent 57–8
  experience shaping 62
  imagery exercises 146–7
  regulating threat system 63
  and sympathetic nervous system
    34
sportswomen and men 347–8
stability of mind and body 260–1
stable body posture exercises 129–30
stimulating feelings 144
'story' of emotions 17–19
strength
  compassionate self exercises 157,
    262, 339–41
  and courage 152–3
  difficult emotions exercise 266
  ideal passionate other exercises
    164
  self-criticism exercises 339–41
  validating emotions exercise 234
stress 171
suppressed emotions 3–4, 68

survival 53
survival threats 51
sustaining healthy emotion
  regulation 393–5
sympathetic nervous system 34, 131,
  355
sympathy 87–8

T

taking responsibility 364–5
talking with friends 276
technology 136–7
thinking
  features of emotions 205
  genes influencing 371–2
  and imagery *14*, 15
  impact on feelings 369
  not your fault 372–3
  and self-criticism 328
  socially shaped 372
  understanding 370–2
thinking-feeling loops 43, 46
thinking patterns 373–4
thought-emotion form exercises
  379–82
thought-emotion monitoring form
  375–6
thought experiments 23–4
thought monitoring 374–7
threat emotions 302–3, 373–4
'threat processing' xxi–xxii
threat system emotions 31–2, 50–3
threat system thinking 377–8
threat systems
  abusive parents 52–3
  dominant emotion processing
    system 30

experiences shaping exercises 61
and safety 282–3
self-criticism 339
self-protection system 29–31
'situation selection' 196
and soothing system 34, 63
threat-spirals 354
types 51–2
and wisdom 197
threats
  'better safe than sorry'
    approaches 51
  loops in the mind 41–6
three flows of compassion 98–9
three good things exercise 359–60
three steps to emotion expression
  286–91
three system model (Gilbert) 29,
  34–5, 170
tolerating difficult emotions 255–6,
  261–3
tone of voice 138–40, 157
too little emotion 394
too much emotion 394
touch 57
triggering difficult emotions 183–91,
  196–7
triggering emotions 18
'turning up for yourself' 351
two teachers example 334–5

U

understanding emotions *see also*
  wisdom of emotions
  emotion regulation 177–8
  ERM 69, 73–4, *231*
  mentalizing 240–2

validating 233–7
worksheet *81*
understanding the way we think 370–2
undesired/undesirable self 315
'unhealthy' emotions 21
unpleasant emotions xxii
using compassionate self to validate emotions exercises 234–6
using memory and imagination to validate feelings exercises 238

V

validating emotions 233
   compassionate self 234–6
   difficult emotions 247
   exercises 239–40
   responses 237–40
voice tone 138–40, 157

W

weakness 169
Western cultures 54
Williams, D. P. 132
Williams, Serena 347

wisdom
   compassionate self 151–2
   compassionate self exercises 156, 262
   difficult emotions exercises 266
   ideal passionate other exercises 164
   selecting situations 196–9
   self-criticism exercises 340
   threat system-inducing material 197
   validating emotions exercises 234
wisdom of emotions 243–7 *see also* understanding emotions
working with setbacks 290–1, 365–6
worksheets
   compassion PDA *349, 352*
   emotion regulation *81*
   multiple emotional selves *305*
writing
   compassionate letters 362–6
   intensity of emotions 274–5, 279–80
   psychological and physical effects 361